# ATI NURSENOTES

# Maternal–Newborn
## Core Content At-A-Glance

### Includes "Study and Memory Aids"

*Edited by:*
**Sally Lambert Lagerquist, RN, MS**

*Author:*
**Janice McMillin, RN, EdD**

# NurseNotes
# Maternal–Newborn
## Core Content At-A-Glance

*Edited by:*

**Sally Lambert Lagerquist, RN, MS**

Former Instructor in Undergraduate and Graduate Programs
and Continuing Education in Nursing
University of California, San Francisco, School of Nursing
President, Review for Nurses, Inc., and RN Tapes Company
San Francisco, California

*Author:*

**Janice McMillin, BSN, MSN, EdD**
Instructor of Maternal–Child Nursing at CSU, Sacramento
Clinical Coordinator of Family Birth Center,
Methodist Hospital of Sacramento, California

Assessment
Technologies
Institute™, LLC

Acquisitions Editor: Bob Cole
Assistant Editor: Melissa Wells
Project Editor: Sally Volkoff
Production Manager: Don Walde
Programer: Trevor Gunter
Art Director: Hara Allison
Graphic Design-Illustrator: Allen Croswhite and Eric Osterback
Design Production: Hara Allison
Indexer: Laura Steen and Melissa Wells

Copyright © 2007 by Sally Lambert Lagerquist. All rights reserved.
This book is protected by copyright. No part of it may be reproduced, stored in a retrieval system, or transmitted, in any form or by any means–electronic, mechanical, photocopy, recording, or otherwise–without the prior written permission of Sally Lambert Lagerquist, except for brief quotations embodied in critical articles and reviews. Printed in the United States of America. For information write ATI 12603 Hemlock, Overland Park, KS 66213

**Library of Congress Cataloging in Publications Data**
Lagerquist, Sally
Nurse notes : maternal–newborn/Janice McMillin; edited by Sally Lambert Lagerquist.
p.cm.
Includes bibliographical references and index.
ISBN 0-9760063-4-0
1. Maternity nursing—Outlines, syllabi, etc.  2. Maternity nursing—Examinations, questions, etc.  I. McMillin, Janice. II. Lagerquist, Sally L. III. Title.
[DNLM: 1. Maternal–Child Nursing—examination questions.  2. Neonatal Nursing—outlines.
WY 18.2 B663n 2007]
RG951.B66 1997-2007
610.73'678'076–dc20
DNLM/DLC
for Library of Congress                                                                                        96-9117
                                                                                                                          CIP

Care has been taken to confirm the accuracy of the information presented and to describe generally accepted practices. However, the authors, editors, and publisher are not responsible for errors or omissions or for any consequences from application of the information in this book and make no warranty, express or implied, with respect to the contents of the publication.

The authors, editor and publisher have exerted every effort to ensure that drug selection and dosage set forth in this text are in accordance with current recommendations and practice at the time of publication. However, in view of ongoing research, changes in government regulations, and the constant flow of information relating to drug therapy and drug reactions, the reader is urged to check the package insert for each drug for any change in indications and dosage and for added warnings and precautions. This is particularly important when the recommended agent is a new or infrequently employed drug.

Some drugs and medical devices presented in this publication have Food and Drug Administration (FDA) clearance for limited use in restricted research settings. It is the responsibility of the health care provider to ascertain the FDA status of each drug or device planned for use in their clinical practice.

9  8  7  6  5  4  3  2  1

# Contributing Author to Previous Edition

Irene M. Bobak, RN, PhD, FAAN
Professor Emerita, Women's Health and Maternity Nursing
San Francisco State University
San Francisco, California

# Dedications

"For everything there is a *season*"  (*A, B* ... After all of my 7 new
    books are in print!)

A time (with **Tom**, my mate of 37 years) *to plant* year 'round
    (more wisteria, trumpet vine and morning glory)
...and a time *to pick* (with gratitude, what "gifts" our
    son, **Kalen** planted)

A time *to be born* (our second grandchild)
...and a time *to die* (in memoriam, to my 93-year-old mother)

A time *to break down* (what once was)
... and a time *to build up* (what can soon be — more space
    and a new place for our daughter, **Elana** and her
    family)
... and a time *to laugh* (with our mechutanim, **Jo**, **Carol** and
    **Gail**)
... and a time *to dance* (with 3-year-old **Kaya** — our very special
    first grandchild)

A time *to throw away stones* (that have little purpose)
... and a time *to gather stones* together (with **Kalen** and **Lara**
    and build bridges)

A time *to embrace* ... (**Sally** and **David Volkoff**, who are more
    than cousins — they're our friends, who have cared
    and shared!)

A time *to seek* (new ventures in cyberspace with **Dan**, our
    son-in-law, who can make so many exciting ideas
    happen with his versatile skills)
... and a time *to lose* (the clutter in our life)

A time *to keep* sweet memories (and make new ones
    with some special long-term friends — **Ayaus**,
    **Bobak, Colombraros, Cohens, Gyepes, Nelsons,**
    **Shillings, Stecchis** and **Tenches**)
... and a time *to throw away* (all that is broken)

A time *to love* (all those who have added joy to our life)
... and a time for *peace* ...

Sally

# Dedications

To my husband Mike, my best friend and humorist, who keeps me laughing and makes life fun. Thank you for listening to my endless nursing stories. I am blessed by God with your endless love and devotion.

To Rachel, my daughter. I am so proud of you for your many accomplishments and hard work in nursing school.

To Justin, my son. I am proud of you for becoming a United States Marine.

To my parents, John and LaVerne Mahony, who have always fostered my dreams.

I am truly thankful for great nursing role models, Dr. Mollyn Bohnen and Dr. Louise Timmer. Thank you for your wisdom and encouragement. I can only hope to fill your huge shoes.

This book is for my nursing students, whose enthusiasm and joy in learning inspire me. Each time I see the excitement of a nursing student participating in a birth for the first time, I recognize myself and remember why I became a perinatal nurse. I have never grown tired of my *choice* to be a nurse. Remember to be proud of being a nurse and never forget "where you came from" when you have the responsibility of mentoring the next generation of nurses.

Finally, I thank the Lord for His endless grace and blessings so richly given to me.

Jan McMillin

# Acknowledgements

You are all that which spells your name (and more!)


**D**etermination, with a smile, that this book will surely be
   "delivered"
**O**verall involvement, from conception (of design) to viewing
   results
**N**urturing these ATI book projects all the way, with impressive
   patience, quick-wit humor and a marketing vision


**M**eticulous attention to the "face" (the cosmetic look) and
   "body" (the substance) of this book
**E**xpert coordination of various stages of development
**L**aboring under complex circumstances to deliver the
   finished product
**I**nspirational — your commitment of time and intense
   involvement was amazing!
**S**upportive of my passion for making this book better
   than ever!
**S**olving production conundrums so very skillfully
**A**ccommodating to the need for all the "re-dos"


**H**igh performance in "parenting" this product with me
   and the ATI/Element Media Productions team
**A**ttitude of "can do" and flexibility — even at zero hour!
**R**esponsiveness to sights and sounds that said PLEASE HELP
   to push this 6th book through
**A**rtistic eye for formatting and consistency


   I gratefully acknowledge you — **Don Walde**, **Melissa Wells** and
**Hara Allison**.  You have given "your all" to produce this member
of a new "family of 6!"

   A heart full of thanks also to Molly, Laura, Eric, Trevor, Allen and all the folks at
Element Media Productions who worked all the way with me ...through much, much
laboring before the joyful delivery of this, the 6th product, in the new ATI series.


Sally Lagerquist

# Foreword

It is a pleasure to endorse resources for students and faculty that really work!

Faculty now has an important role in assisting the student in condensing and organizing the essential knowledge that can be translated into competent and safe nursing practice. With the exploding amount of knowledge in nursing and health care, students are often frustrated because they need to know so much. They ask questions from faculty like, "what is on the test?" and "what do I need to know?" The *ATI NurseNotes* are an incredibly easy synthesis of critical material that students need to master. Using the *NurseNotes* series along with the major nursing textbooks enhances students' comprehension of complex concepts and their application to clinical practice. The feedback from students themselves has been very positive. They comment that the *NurseNotes* save them time as they learn and review core content because concepts are graphically presented, chapters are short (yet comprehensive), with summaries and test questions at the end of each chapter to identify their problem areas.

The faculty finds that the *NurseNotes* series helps to organize their own presentations of material to students in a way that helps elevate the students' mastery of core content.

John M. Lantz, RN, PhD
Dean and Professor
School of Nursing
University of San Francisco
2130 Fulton Street
San Francisco, CA 94117

Sally Higgins, RN, PhD, FAAN
Professor and Chair of the Department of
  Family Health
University of San Francisco
2130 Fulton Street
San Francisco, CA 94117

I have found the Maternal-Newborn text to be extremely useful in the undergraduate family health course that I teach. Its concise review of all of the essential content makes it an extremely user-friendly text, particularly for students who struggle as they try to take in a tremendous amount of material during the 14 week semester. Many of my previous students have sworn that they never would have successfully completed all of the course objectives without this volume.

Linda Walsh CNM, MPH, Ph.D.
Faculty
University of San Francisco
2130 Fulton Street
San Francisco, CA 94117

# Preface

### What's New In This Edition

This book was originally written by Dr. Irene Bobak, a national nursing expert and author of best-selling maternity textbooks for over 20 years; and updated for this edition by Dr. Janice McMillin, who, has updated and enhanced the information on contraception, discharge guidelines and labor management to include new developments. Questions have been updated and new format questions have been included to reflect the new format of the NCLEX® examination. It is intended for busy nursing students who need to cover the most important information in the shortest time.

## Purpose

1. To help nursing students learn *faster, easier*, and retain vital information with this guided study written in an easy-to-read format. This will enable students to use their other large textbooks as reference sources.
2. To help graduate nurses update and build on their nursing knowledge as they prepare for certification exams.

## Features That Make This Book Stand-out From All Other Nursing Content Review Books

1. **Time-savers:** Numerous charts (**28**), illustrations (**30**), and extensive pharmacology boxes (**4**) outline a great deal of information in few pages. Save valuable study time with quick-access *index* to instantly locate pages that cover key content such as **36** *diets*, over **75** *diagnostic tests*, **35** maternal-newborn *emergencies*, **18** *positions*, and **58** *hands-on care.*
2. **Visual:** Unique use of icons throughout the content review sections helps important content stand out.

| | | | |
|---|---|---|---|
| ! | Alert | | Lab values |
| | Diagnostic tests | | Meds |
| | Emergency | | Nutrition/diets |
| | Hands-on care | | Standard precautions |
| | Hand-washing | | Steps of nursing process |
| | Hazard | | Study and memory aids |
| | Home health care/teaching | | Warning |
| | Key points | | |

There is also a purposeful use of **bold face** and *italics* within the text to identify content related to *diets, positions*, what to *avoid*, and *drugs*. These visual methods have proven to be particularly beneficial in boosting retention.

3. The most up-to-date, comprehensive (yet succinct!) coverage of a variety of topics, for *beginning* and *advanced* nurses already in practice, as well as for *repeat* test-takers.

4. **Self-assessment**: Questions and answers at the end of each chapter include *fact-packed* rationale for *each* option. Learn more from the most complete explanations!

5. **Free disk**: An integrated exam covers all essential areas in maternity and newborn care.

6. **One-of-a-kind sections** in each chapter: *key points, summary, key words,* and *study and memory aids.*

7. An **extensive appendix** section includes a 32-page (over **1200** terms) *glossary;* **350** need-to-know *acronyms* and *abbreviations; quick guide to* **28** *common clinical signs* (e.g. Chadwick's); an index to quickly locate key content throughout the book, such as *diets* 🍎, *diagnostic tests* 〰, *hands-on nursing care* ☞; index to help locate *test questions* covering each step of the nursing process ◄, client needs and subneeds, and categories of human functions; an index to **13** *memory aids* (mnemonics); list of NANDA-*approved diagnoses;* and a list of *health care agencies* and *resources.*

## How to Benefit from this Book

1. Use the key *words* and key *points* section at the beginning of each chapter to *anticipate* the content that will be covered in the chapter.

2. Use the extensive *glossary* (over 1200 definitions of terms relevant for maternal-newborn care) in the appendix as an *end-of-course review* to ensure that you have retained what you need to know.

3. Use the various *indices* in the appendices to pull out for study and review *separate* key topics such as *diets, diagnostic tests and medical procedures, maternal-newborn emergencies* ⊕, and *nursing skills and procedures* (hands-on care) necessary for beginning nursing students to master, including *positioning* and care of the client with *tubes.*

I wish you much success as you prepare for nursing exams with the aid of *NurseNotes: Maternal–Newborn.*

Sally Lambert Lagerquist, RN, MS
Editor, *ATI's NurseNotes series*

# How to Use the ATI NurseNotes Series

The *ATI NurseNotes* series was written to lower students' stress while increasing mastery of essential subjects (i.e. core content), by presenting concise information in a visual way to enable an at-a-glance approach to increasing understanding and retention.

Students can use this series as a basis for doing care plans (care maps) at the *beginning* of and *throughout* a course, as well as an *end–point* review for the course exam or for *NCLEX-RN® review*. This is the only nursing review series with content and practice questions that *directly relate to the NCLEX-RN® test plan blue print*.

## Step-By-Step Approach To the Most Effective Use of This Book By Students

❖ Quickly glance at the *outline* at the start of each chapter to see what topics/conditions will be covered.

❖ Go over the *key words* that are basic and *need-to-know*.

❖ Carefully read the **summaries** of key points ✐ at the start of each chapter to be aware of what you need to understand and retain as the key points when you read through the chapter.

❖ Look over the outline format that is used, noting that there is a brief *introduction*, followed by concisely worded description of *physiology* and a relevant *risk factors/causes*, and incidence.

❖ Spend significant time going over the *assessment* section, especially the diagnostic tests/procedures and any related lab data. Note that the symbol in the margins ⧖, quickly identifies diagnostic tests.

❖ Briefly glance at the *nursing diagnosis*, which can relate to pathophysiology, with implications for nursing interventions.

❖ Spend the most concentrated time in the section: *nursing plan* (i.e., the general goals)/ *implementation* (i.e., specific interventions). Pay special attention to *diets* 🍎, *positioning, hands-on care aspects* ☞, *medications* ▭, *infection control situations* ▲, hazards ⚡, and *home health care/teaching* 📖.

❖ Next, study all the information in table format, the words and phrases that are in **boldface** (very important) and *italic* type, as well as boxed content and shaded areas. These visual cues are time-savers for the reader because they serve the same purpose as when students spend time doing their own highlighting and underlining for emphasis. These visual cues allow for faster learning!

❖ Look at the end of each chapter for a synthesis of need-to-remember points about the condition(s), diets, drugs and diagnostic tests/procedures.

❖ Now take the *test questions* at the end of *each* chapter. Read the rationale not only for the best answer, but also the rationale for all the other options. Determine your percentage correct; if it was less than 85% correct (this is a higher benchmark than you'd expect to find on the licensure exam), then we suggest that you re-read that chapter.

❖ When you have completed all the chapters in the book for an end-point review, be sure to go through the content-packed **appendices**. The indices there can also lead you to pages where specific content (e.g. diets) and specific questions (e.g. safety and infection control) are located in the book. For example, this means that you can go through the book and only review all the diets; then you can go through the book and do a review of all the tubes or positioning etc.

❖ Follow this approach before you use the 275 questions on the *CD* in this book as your final "test and assess."

## Suggestions for Instructor's Use of the Books in the ATI NurseNotes Series

While these books offer a <u>synthesis</u> of essential content in a condensed format, the instructor can then use lecture time to focus on <u>expansion</u> of content, to illustrate key concepts with <u>clinical scenarios</u> (to use in conjunction with *ATI Nursing Q&A: Critical Thinking Exercises* and the 75 case scenarios).

❖ These books can increase time for the focus of the instructor's lecture to be on a re-emphasis of more <u>complex</u> concepts (e.g. acid-base).

❖ If any clinical experience in the nursing program is reduced in scope, the instructor can select from these books certain chapters for special supplemental coverage to fill in those gaps. In that way, their lectures can be <u>tailored</u> to the particular needs of the nursing program.

❖ Instructors can use these books to point out <u>major</u> nursing care problems, to <u>separate</u> them from secondary ones; and to provide a *hands-on care skills assessment checklist* (see ☞ throughout the chapters), with an opportunity to learn and fill in gaps in the how-to aspects of nursing care.

❖ A focus on sections in these books that cover **assessment** data is another way the instructor can point out patterns, relationships and make appropriate inferences based on assessment data.

❖ The instructor should also call students' attention to the many appendices that provide **multiple ways** that students can use these books for self-assessment in addition to the usual end-of-chapter questions and questions on the *CD*. For example, show students how they can do a focused review of <u>special topics</u> (e.g. use the index in an Appendix to locate throughout the book a review of diets, diagnostic studies/procedures, common tubes, positioning of the client.) They can also review by <u>questions</u> throughout the book which directly relate to the NCLEX-RN® Test Plan (e.g. by client needs/subneeds), by nursing process steps; and by level of complexity of questions (from basic knowledge/comprehension to application and analysis.)

❖ These books can help *new* instructors to zero-in on core content, and can give *experienced* lecturers more time to focus on clinically-based anecdotal illustrations.

# Contents

## Appendixes

# List Of Illustrations

# List of Tables

# List of Pharmacology Boxes (*See* also **Tables 1.2, 4.3**)

# Growth and Development

## Chapter Outline

## 🗝 Key Points

- Knowledge of a woman's reproductive anatomy and physiology is essential to health promotion/maintenance.
- Factors such as immunizations, life-style, environment, and nutrition affect the functioning of the immune defense system.
- Common etiologic factors of impaired fertility include *male* factors (e.g., decreased sperm production, varicocele) and/or *female* factors (e.g., tubal occlusion, short luteal phase, endometriosis).
- Preconception counseling is designed to promote/maintain good health to afford the developing embryo/fetus the best environment for development/growth (one that allows the newborn to achieve the genetic potential).

## Key Words

"ACHES"
BBT (basal body temperature)
Calendar method
Contraception
Dysmenorrhea

Fertile days (of menstrual cycle)
Fibrocystic breast disease
Hot flushes (flashes)
Impaired fertility
Interruption of pregnancy
Living ligature
Mammography
Menstrual cycle
   Menarche
   Menopause
   Menstruation
   Ovulation
Mittelschmerz
"PAINS"
PID (pelvic inflammatory disease)
Preconception care
Premenstrual syndrome (PMS)
Safer sex practices
Spinnbarkeit
STD (sexually transmitted disease)
Sterilization
TSS (Toxic Shock Syndrome)

# Biologic Foundations of Reproduction

**General overview:** This review of the structures, functions, and important assessment characteristics of the reproductive system provides essential components of the database required for accurate nursing judgments. Comparing normal characteristics and established patterns with nursing assessment findings assist in identifying client needs and in planning, implementing, and evaluating appropriate goal-directed nursing interventions.

## Female Reproductive Anatomy

I. **Structure of pelvis (Figure 1.1)**
   A. Two hip bones (right and left innominate: sacrum, coccyx).
   B. *False pelvis*—upper portion above brim; supportive structure for uterus during last half of pregnancy.
   C. *True pelvis*—below brim; pelvic inlet, midcavity (curved passage having a short anterior wall and a much longer concave posterior wall), pelvic outlet comprise this structure. Fetus passes through this during birth.

II. **Pelvic measurements**
   A. Diagonal conjugate—12.5 cm or greater is adequate size; measured by examiner.
   B. Conjugate vera (true conjugate)—11 cm is adequate size; measured by x-ray. (rarely done)
   C. Obstetric conjugate—measured by x-ray. (rarely done)
   D. Tuber-ischial diameter—9-11 cm indicates adequate size; measured by examiner.

III. **External genitalia (vulva, pudendum) (Figure 1.2)**
   A. *Mons veneris* (mons pubis)—fatty subcutaneous tissue covered with pubic hair; protects symphysis.
   B. *Labia majora*—folds of adipose tissue; form internal borders of vulva; cover and protect labia minora.
   C. *Labia minora*—two located within labia majora; lubricate vulva and protect with bacteria-fighting secretion; sensitive to stimuli.
   D. *Clitoris*—small erectile tissue; sensitive to sexual stimulation; analogous to the man's glans penis.
   E. *Vestibule*—between labia minora; contains:
      1. *Urinary meatus*—opening of urethra.
      2. *Skene's glands*—paraurethral glands.
      3. Vaginal opening (*introitus*).
      4. *Hymen*—thin membrane at opening of vagina.
      5. *Bartholin's glands* (paravaginal)—produce alkaline secretions that enhance sperm viability, motility.

IV. **Internal structures (Figure 1.3)**
   A. *Vagina*—outlet for menstrual flow, depository for semen; lower birth canal.
   B. *Cervix*—uterine outlet.
   C. *Uterus*—muscular organ, composed of corpus (body), isthmus (lower uterine segment during pregnancy), and cervix; houses and nourishes embryo and fetus during gestation. See also **Figure 1.3A and B.**
      1. The thick uterine myometrium consists of elastic and connective tissue, blood, and three smooth muscle layers (longitudinal, figure-eight , and circular  fibers).
      2. The primary function of the outer longitudinal fibers is to assist with effacement and dilatation of the cervix and to expel the fetus. These fibers are found mostly in the fundus.
      3. The figure-eight fibers of the middle layer (also known as the "living ligature") provide hemostatic action because the interlaced fibers encircle large blood vessels.
      4. The primary function of the circular muscle fibers of the inner layer is to retain uterine contents during pregnancy and prevent regurgitation of menstrual blood through the fallopian tubes into the abdomen during menstruation.
   D. *Fallopian tubes*—two tubes stretching from cornua of uterus to ovaries; transport ovum; site of fertilization is in the outer two-thirds (in the ampulla of the tubes).

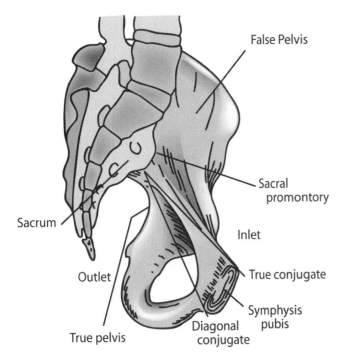

**FIGURE 1.1   THE FEMALE PELVIS.**

(From SL ©Lagerquist {ed}. *Little Brown's NCLEX–RN® Examination Review*. Boston: Little, Brown; out of print)

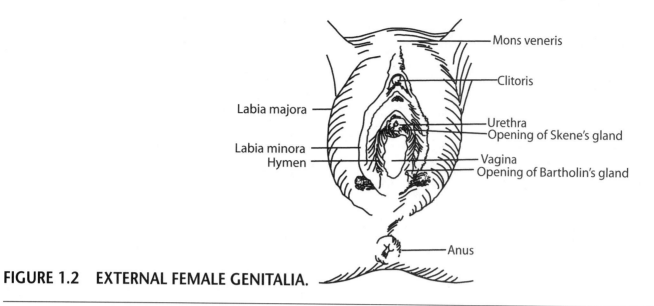

**FIGURE 1.2   EXTERNAL FEMALE GENITALIA.**

**FIGURE 1.3   FEMALE INTERNAL REPRODUCTIVE ORGANS**

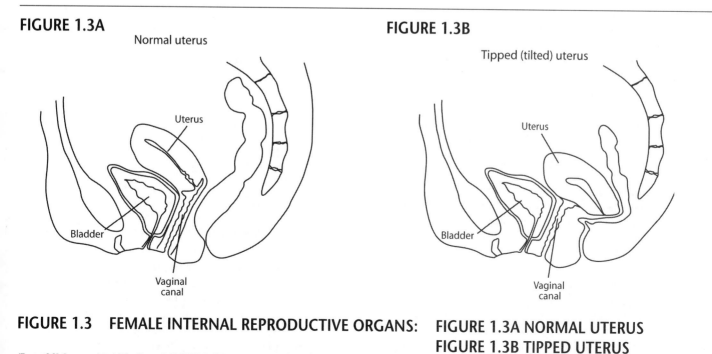

**FIGURE 1.3   FEMALE INTERNAL REPRODUCTIVE ORGANS:**   **FIGURE 1.3A NORMAL UTERUS**
**FIGURE 1.3B TIPPED UTERUS**

(From ©SL Lagerquist. *Little, Brown's NCLEX-RN® Examination Review*. Boston: Little, Brown; out of print)

### TABLE 1.1 MENSTRUAL CYCLE: A FEEDBACK MECHANISM

| Phases/Events | First "Half" Cycle | | | Second "Half" Cycle | |
|---|---|---|---|---|---|
| Length | NOTE: 8 d to several weeks or months | | O | NOTE: Constant: 14 d | |
| Anterior pituitary hormones | Follicle stimulating (FSH): follicular phase | | V | Luteinizing hormone (LH): luteal phase | |
| Ovarian hormones | Estrogen | | U | Progesterone and estrogen until start of ischemic phase 3 d before menstruation | |
| Endometrial response | Bleeding → 5 days (range: 3-6 d) | Proliferative phase → | L A T I O N | Secretory phase → | Ischemic 3 d |
| Cervical mucus response | Dry (no mucus) | • Increasingly viscous, opaque <br> • No ferning | | • Cloudy, sticky; impenetrable to sperm <br> • No ferning | |
| BBT | Individualized; often below 98.6°F (37°C) | | | After slight drop, rises about 0.4° to 0.8°F (0.2-0.4°C) | |

## Female Reproductive Physiology

I. **Reproductive hormones**

   A. *FSH* (follicle stimulating hormone)—secreted during the first half of cycle; stimulates development of graafian follicle; secreted by anterior pituitary.

   B. *ICSH or LH* (interstitial cell stimulating hormone, luteinizing hormone)—stimulates ovulation and development of corpus luteum; secreted by anterior pituitary.

   C. *Estrogen*—assists in ovarian follicle maturation; stimulates endometrial thickening; responsible for development of secondary sex characteristics; maintains endometrium during pregnancy. Secreted by ovaries and adrenal cortex during cycle and by placenta during pregnancy.

   D. *Progesterone*—aids in endometrial thickening; facilitates secretory changes; maintains uterine lining for implantation and early pregnancy; relaxes smooth muscle. Secreted by corpus luteum and placenta.

   E. *Prostaglandins*—substances produced by various body organs that act hormonally on the endometrium to influence the onset and continuation of labor. A medication that may be used to facilitate onset of second trimester abortion; also used to efface the cervix prior to induction of labor in term pregnancies.

II. **Menstrual cycle**

   A. The **menstrual cycle** is a complex interplay of events that occur simultaneously in the hypothalamus and pituitary glands, the uterine endometrium and cervix, and the ovaries. The menstrual cycle—a feedback mechanism—is presented in **Table 1.1**.

   B. Important terms

   1. **Menarche**—onset of menses; occurs at about age 13. Initial cycles are irregular, unpredictable, painless, and anovulatory in the majority of girls. Ovulatory periods tend to be regular, monitored by progesterone;

may be associated with *dysmenorrhea* (painful uterine cramping).

   2. **Menstruation**—vaginal discharge of blood and fragments of the two upper layers (the functional layer) of the endometrium; cyclic; occurs in response to dropping levels of estrogen and progesterone. *Menses* refers to the normal flow during menstruation. Average blood loss: 50 mL (range: 20-80 mL). First day of bleeding is the first day of the cycle.

   3. **Ovulation**—maturation and release of egg from ovary; generally occurs 14 days *before* first day of next cycle (first day of bleeding).

   4. **Ovulation-associated events:**

      a. **BBT** (basal body temperature)—slight drop.

      b. **Cervical mucus**—abundant, thin, clear (egg-white) mucus with **spinnbarkeit** (mucus stretchable from 4 cm, often up to 10 cm); dries in a fern pattern (arborization); facilitates sperm transport; pH rises (becomes more alkaline) from about 7.0 to 7.5 to facilitate sperm viability and mobility.

      c. **Mittelschmerz** (intermenstrual pain) occurs 1.7 days after peak of cervical mucus and 2.5 days before increase in BBT.

      d. **Fertile days:** 3 days before through 1 day (24 hr) after ovulation.

   5. **Fertilization**—impregnation of ovum by sperm.

   6. **Implantation**—fertilized ovum attaches to uterine wall for growth.

III. **Menopause**—normally occurring cessation of menses with gradual decrease in amount of flow and increase in the time between periods at end of fertility cycle; average age, 53. Early menopause rare but may be influenced by hypothyroidism, surgical ovarian removal, overexposure to radiation.

A. Women say that the most distressing symptoms are hot flushes ("flashes") and night sweats. These are due to hormonal stimulation of the sympathetic system resulting in vasomotor instability with changeable vasodilation and vasoconstriction.

B. Treatments during menopause for symptom relief: hormonal replacement therapy (there is controversy surrounding HRT; it has been shown to increase a woman's risk of cardiac disease); *vitamin* E and also antidepressants, such as venlafaxine can be used for *hot flushes*; vaginal lubricants for *dyspareunia* (painful intercourse), and exercise, calcium and Fosamax for *osteoporosis*.

---

## FIGURE 1.4    BREAST SELF-EXAMINATION

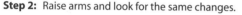

**Step 1:** Look at the breasts in the mirror with shoulders straight and arms on hips. Here's what to look for:
- Breasts that are their usual size, shape, and color.
- Breasts that are evenly shaped without visible distortion of swelling.

Look for following changes
- Dimpling, puckering, or bulging of the skin.
- A nipple that has changed position or an inverted nipple (pushed inward instead of sticking out).
- Redness, soreness, rash, or swelling.

**Step 2:** Raise arms and look for the same changes.

**Step 3:** While at the mirror, gently squeeze each nipple between finger and thumb and check for nipple discharge (this could be a milky or yellow fluid or blood).

**Step 4:** Feel breasts while lying down, using right hand to feel the left breast and then left hand to feel the right breast. Use a firm, smooth touch with the first few fingers of the hand, keeping the fingers flat and together.

Cover the entire breast from the top to the bottom, side to side—from the collarbone to the top of abdomen, and from armpit to cleavage.

Follow a pattern to be sure to cover the whole breast. Begin at the nipple, moving in larger and larger circles to reach the outer edge of the breast. Feel all the breast tissue just beneath the skin with a soft touch. Begin examining each area with a very soft touch and then increase pressure to feel the deeper tissue, down to the ribcage.

**Step 5:** Feel the breasts while standing or sitting. Many women find that the easiest way to feel their breasts is when their skin is wet and slippery, so they like to do this step in the shower.

**Source:** adapted from *breastcancer.org*

# Neoplasms

See Cancer and Pregnancy (**Chapter 3**).

See also **NurseNotes: Medical-Surgical** book for in-depth discussions of these conditions.

I. **Breast**
   A. *Fibrocystic breast disease* (mammary dysplagia, diffuse cystic mastopathy)
      1. *Incidence*: most common of the benign breast lesions. Affects 60% premenopausal women. Peak incidence between 30 and 50 yr.
      2. **Assessment**
         a. *Symptoms*: dull heavy pain, a sense of fullness, tenderness that increases premenstrually.
         b. *Palpation*: cysts are soft, well differentiated, movable. Deeper cysts are harder to palpate; must be differentiated from carcinomas.
         c. *Diagnostic tests/procedures:*
            (1) Surgical biopsy.
            (2) Mammography: visualization of breast tissue by x-ray examination.
            (3) Ultrasonography: can differentiate cysts from solid tumors.
            (4) History.
            (5) Physical examination.
      3. **Management/Intervention**
         a. Conservative: *diet*—limiting dietary fat to 15–20% of total calories; *avoiding* caffeine (while often suggested) has *not* been proven to reduce the incidence.
         b. *Medications*: for severe cases, danazol (*Danocrine*), tamoxifen (*Nolvadex*). Oral contraceptives can alleviate symptoms. (**Pharmacology Box 1.1**)
         c. **Health teaching**: report any changes in breast mass and symptoms; comfort—padded bras.
   B. *Malignant conditions*
      1. *Incidence*: will affect 1:8 -1:9 women during the life span; leading cause of death in women between 35 and 54 years.
      2. **Assessment**
         a. *Symptoms*: pain, nipple discharge—bloody or clear.
         b. *Palpation*: lump or thickening, hard and fixed or soft and spongy, well-defined or irregular borders, usually in the upper outer quadrant. If inflammatory, dimpling, "orange peel"-appearing skin, retraction.
         c. *Diagnostic test/procedures*:
            (1) *BSE* (**Figure 1.4**): recently, a large randomized study showed no benefit from BSE. American Cancer Society no longer recommends BSE as a screening tool for early detection (it is an option if a woman desires).
            (2) Mammography (see **p. 8** text box for schedule).
            (3) Needle aspiration, needle localization, followed by open breast biopsy, (the most definitive test).
      3. **Management/Intervention**
         a. *Medications: estrogens or progestins* (if neoplasm has estrogen or progesterone receptor sites); an *anti-estrogen* such as tamoxifen. See **Pharmacology Box 1.1, p. 7.**
         b. *Surgery*: *lumpectomy* (tylectomy), *quadrectomy* (segmental resection), *total* (*simple*) mastectomy, and *radical* mastectomy. Five-year survival rates for women following lumpectomies are statistically similar to those following total breast removal.
         c. Hormone/surgical procedures in combination.
         d. Chemotherapy and hormonal therapy may improve cytotoxicity of chemotherapy.
         e. Chemotherapy: three classes of agents: anthracyclines (*Adriamycin*, *epirubicin*), taxames (*Taxol, Taxotere*), alkylating agents (*Cytoxam*). In addition to their antineoplastic qualities, these cytotoxins have some immunosuppressive side effects and a higher risk for thrombosis.
         f. *Radiation*: 2 - 3 wk following lumpectomy.
         g. Emotional support!
      4. **Postoperative care**, including discharge planning
         a. Safety: protect arm during hospital stay and at home—due to lack of sensation.
         b. Exercise: to maintain full range of motion; inactivity (secondary to pain, initially) could affect joint action, and alteration in lymphatic drainage → edema formation and further impairment of joint/arm movement.
         c. Woman needs to expect that she will have discomfort and a feeling of tightness in the arm and chest on the affected side.
         d. Explain that axillary node resection leads to edema because lymph flow is interrupted.
         e. Closed self-suction is used to keep the operative site free of fluid so that wound healing with approximation of tissue can occur.

(*continued on p.8*)

## ⬤ PHARMACOLOGY BOX 1.1   NEOPLASMS OF BREAST AND ENDOMETRIUM

| Drug/Dosage | Indication/Action | ◪ Assessment: Side Effects | ◪ Nursing Management |
|---|---|---|---|
| **Danazol** (*Danocrine*) Capsules—50 mg, 100 mg, 200 mg Endometriosis: 400 mg bid for 6-9 mo Fibrocystic breast disease: 100-400 mg/d in 2 divided doses for 3-6 mo | Suppresses release of FSH and LH, inhibiting ovarian function. Complete resolution of endometrial lesions in the majority of cases Symptomatic treatment of severe fibrocystic breast disease Treatment of infertility *secondary* to endometriosis | Anovulation and associated amenorrhea Flushing, sweating Virilization (acne, oily skin, hirsutism, deepening of the voice, decrease in breast size, clitoral hypertrophy), vaginitis, vaginal bleeding, edema, weight gain, nervousness Other effects for which a direct causal relationship has not been established are: loss of hair; changes in libido; pelvic pain; muscle cramps; back, neck, or leg pain; skin rash; nasal congestion; nausea, vomiting, gastroenteritis; dizziness; headache; tremor; paresthesias; and visual disturbances | **Contraindications:** carcinoma of the breast, pregnancy, lactation, undiagnosed vaginal bleeding, and markedly impaired cardiac, hepatic, or renal function Reassure that drug-induced anovulation and amenorrhea are reversible within 60-90 d after termination of therapy Observe for development of ! signs of virilization and advise physician; some of these symptoms may be irreversible |
| **Progestins** *Hydroxyprogesterone caproate(Delalutin)* Injection—125 mg/mL, 250 mg/mL IM—1-7 g/wk | Advanced endometrial carcinoma (Stage III or IV) (DOC) | Stop therapy when relapse occurs or after 12 wk with no objective response Weight gain Mild depression | !Be alert for signs and symptoms of: hypercalcemia (polyuria, polydipsia, weakness, constipation, mental sluggishness or disorientation) in clients with metastatic breast cancer being treated with tamoxifen or progestins; perform periodic *serum calcium* determinations Monitor fluid intake and output |
| *Medroxyprogesterone acetate* (*Provera, Depo-Provera*) Tablets—2.5 mg, 10 mg Oral, IM—400-1000 mg/wk Injection—100 mg/mL, 400 mg/mL Maintenance—400 mg/mo or adjusted to client's needs | Endometrial carcinoma | Recommended only as adjunctive and palliative therapy in advanced inoperable cases; usually well tolerated even in large doses; gluteal abscesses have occurred Weight gain Mild depression | Recommend contraceptive measures for clients receiving ⬤ *estrogens, progestins, tamoxifen,* and *mitotane* Clients with diabetes receiving *progestins* may have a *decreased glucose tolerance*; monitor urine sugar closely and notify physician immediately of any abnormalities |
| *Megestrol acetate* (*Megace, Pallace*) Breast cancer: 40 mg qid Endometrial cancer: 40-320 mg/d in 4 divided doses | Breast and endometrial carcinoma (DOC) | Continue treatment for at least 2 mo to determine efficacy Weight gain Mild depression | |
| **Tamoxifen** (*Nolvadex*)— antiestrogen Tablets—10 mg 10-20 mg bid | Advanced breast carcinoma (DOC) Postmenopausal women respond better than premenopausal women (who get better response from DES) | May *increase serum calcium* levels; transient "flaring" of disease may occur during initial therapy, usually subsides rapidly; ocular toxicity is associated with long-term, high-dose therapy Vaginitis, decreased libido, nausea, or anorexia | Be aware that *tamoxifen* may cause a *transient* flare of the disease with increased tumor and bone pain; advise the client that this is not uncommon, and provide ⬤ additional *analgesics* if needed |

DOC = drug of choice; DES = diethylstilbestrol.

☞ f.  Suture line is cleansed daily with hydrogen peroxide to prevent scar tissue formation and to promote healing.

g.  Recommendations for screening for breast neoplasms:

〰(1)  Women who are at **average** risk:

| Age | Mammography | Clinical Examination |
|---|---|---|
| 29–39 | Not recommended | Included with routine gynecologic examination, or every 3 yr |
| 40 and older | Annually | Annually |

〰(2)  Women who are at **high** risk:

| Age | Mammography | Clinical Examination |
|---|---|---|
| 29–39 | Annually starting at age 35; earlier if breast cancer has occurred | Annually starting at age 35 |
| 40 and older | Annually | Annually |

II.  Uterus

A.  *Endometrial carcinoma*

1.  Women at greatest risk: those who are overweight (> 50 pounds); early menstruation (< 12 years old); late menopause (> 52 years old); nulliparity.

2.  The *most* important sign of endometrial carcinoma is abnormal bleeding, esp. postmenopause bleeding.

⬤ 3.  Oral contraceptive use may protect against such disorders as endometrial and ovarian cancer and other conditions.

B.  *Cervix*

Early detection is usually through regular 〰 cervical cytology (PAP) smears. *Early* stages are treated with cryosurgery. *Later* stages are likely to include a hysterectomy with radiation or chemotherapy.

# Nursing Process

▶ I.  **Assessment**

A.  Health history

1.  Menarche: onset and duration.
2.  Menstrual problems.
3.  Contraceptive use.
4.  Pregnancy history.
5.  Fertility problems.

〰 B.  Physical examination and *laboratory tests:*

1.  External, internal reproductive organs.
2.  Breast examination.
3.  Mammography: if at risk, yearly for 35 yr of

age; annual routine screening for ≥ 40 yr of age.

4.  Periodic Papanicolaou (Pap) smears.
5.  Tests for STD (sexually transmitted diseases).

▶ II.  **Analysis/nursing diagnosis**

A.  *Health-seeking behaviors* related to health promotion.

B.  *Health-seeking behaviors* related to menopause.

▶ III.  **Nursing care plan/implementation**

🏠 A.  Goal: **health teaching**.

1.  Discuss anatomy and physiology of reproductive tract.
2.  Review menstruation, ovulation, fertilization, "fertile" and "safe" days of cycle.
3.  Explain need for periodic Pap smears, annual gynecologic examinations, including mammography.

▶ IV.  **Evaluation/outcome criteria**

A.  Woman displays basic understanding of anatomy and physiology.

B.  Woman understands menstrual cycle and its "fertile" and "safe" days.

C.  Woman understands her chosen method of contraception.

D.  Woman regularly seeks preventive care.

# Decision Making Regarding Reproduction

**General overview:** During the reproductive years, the woman who is sexually active often faces the decision to postpone, prevent, or terminate a pregnancy. The nursing role focuses on assisting her in making an informed decision consistent with individual needs.

## Contraception

▶ I.  **Assessment**

A.  Determine interest in and present knowledge of methods of family planning, e.g., planning for pregnancy, contraception.

B.  Identify factors affecting choice of contraceptive method: cultural and religious objections, contraindications for individual methods, motivation/ability to follow chosen method successfully, financial considerations.

▶ II.  **Analysis/nursing diagnosis:** *knowledge deficit* regarding family planning methods/options.

▶ III.  **Nursing care plan/implementation**

🏠 A.  Goal: **health teaching**. Facilitate informed decision making, selection of option appropriate to individual needs, desires.

1.  Describe, explain, discuss options available and appropriate to the woman.

Include information on advantages and disadvantages of each option (**Table 1.2 p. 10**)

2. Demonstrate, as necessary, method selected.
3. Quick health teaching reminders for missed oral hormone preparations*
   a. One pill should be taken at the same time every day for 21 (or 28) days.
   b. If woman misses one pill, she should take it as soon as she remembers it, and then take the next one at the usual time.
   c. If woman misses two or more pills in a row in the first 2 wk of her cycle, she should take two pills for 2 days, and use a backup method of contraception for at least the next 7 days.
   d. If woman misses two pills in the third wk, or three or more pills anytime
      (1) A *Sunday starter* should keep taking pills until the next Sunday, then start a new pack that Sunday. She should use a backup method of contraception for, at minimum, the next 7 days.
      (2) A *day 1 starter* should throw out the rest of the pack, and start a new pack that day. She should use a backup method of contraception for, at minimum, the next 7 days.
   e. *28-day pill pack*: If woman misses any of the seven pills that do not have any hormones, she should throw out the pills missed and keep taking one pill a day until the pack is empty. She does not need a backup method of contraception.

B. Goal: *alert woman to discontinue use* of *oral hormone contraceptive* preparations if any of the following symptoms occur and to report the symptoms to the physician STAT. Signs of potential problems: "**ACHES**"
   A— Abdominal pain: possible problem with the liver or gallbladder
   C— Chest pain or shortness of breath: possible clot problem within lungs or heart
   H— Headaches (sudden or persistent): possibly caused by a stroke or hypertension
   E— Eye problems: possible vascular problem or hypertension
   S— Severe leg pain: possible thromboembolic process

C. Goal: *alert woman to signs of potential problems related to* **IUD** use: "**PAINS**"†
   P— Period (menstrual) late, abnormal spotting or bleeding
   A— Abdominal pain, pain with coitus (dyspareunia)

I — Infection, abnormal vaginal discharge
N— Not feeling well, fever or chills
S— String missing (nonpalpable on vaginal self-examination, or not seen on speculum examination)

D. Goal: *alert woman to signs/symptoms* of *toxic shock syndrome* (**TSS**)
   1. Fever of sudden onset—over 102°F (38.9°C).
   2. Hypotension—systolic pressure < 90 mm Hg; orthostatic dizziness; disorientation.
   3. Rash—diffuse, macular erythroderma (resembling sunburn).
   4. Sore throat; severe nausea, vomiting.
   5. Copious vaginal discharge.

E. Goal: **heath teaching**. Instructions for prevention of **TSS**:
   1. General
      a. *Avoid* use of tampons, cervical caps, and diaphragms during the postpartum period (6 wk).
      b. Do *not* use any of the above if you have a history of TSS.
      c. Call physician if you experience: sudden onset of a high fever, vomiting, diarrhea, or skin rash.
      d. Insert clean tampons and contraceptive devices with clean hands.
      e. Remove within prescribed time limits.
   2. Tampons
      a. Change tampons every 3-6 hr.
      b. Do *not* use superabsorbent tampons.
      c. For overnight protection, substitute other products such as sanitary napkins or minipads.

IV. **Evaluation/outcome criteria**
   A. Woman avoids or achieves a pregnancy as desired.
   B. Woman expresses comfort and satisfaction with method selected.

# Infertility

I. **Definition**: inability to conceive after 1 yr of unprotected intercourse if < 35 yr of age. If > 35 yr of age, 6 months of unprotected intercourse.

II. **Pathophysiology**: contributing factors—hormonal deficiencies, reproductive system disorders, congenital anomalies, male impotence, sexual knowledge deficit, debilitating disease.

III. **Assessment**
   A. History—general health, reproduction, social history.
      1. Age at menarche
      2. Common menstrual disorders:
         a. Hypogonadotropic *amenorrhea* (absence of menstruation)—problem in central hypothalamic-pituitary axis (most often

(*continued on p.12*)

* Modified from Family Health International. *Using Pill Correctly.* Research Triangle Park, NC: Family Health International.

† Modified from RA Hatcher et al. *Contraceptive Technology*: 2001 17th ed New York: Irving

## TABLE 1.2 CONTRACEPTION

| Type | Use | Benefits | Concerns/Disadvantages |
|---|---|---|---|
| **⬭ Hormonal Contraceptives** | | | |
| Combination of *estrogen* and *progesterone*.<br><br><br><br><br><br><br><br>*Contraceptive patch* | • Suppresses ovulation by suppressing production of FSH and LH<br>• *Most efficient* form of contraception (99.7%) if used consistently | • Convenient<br>• Easy to take<br>• Withdrawal bleeding cycles are predictable<br>• Not related to sex act<br>• Safe for older nonsmoking women until menopause<br>• Many noncontraceptive health benefits<br>• Apply once per week; stays on with showering, bathing, swimming. | • **Absolute contraindications** (e.g., thromboembolic or coronary artery disease, some cancers or liver disease)<br>• **Relative contraindications** (e.g., migraines, hypertension, immobility of 4 wk or more, abnormal genital bleeding)<br>• Some decrease in glucose tolerance<br>• Effectiveness decreased if taken ⬭ during use of barbiturates, phenytoin, antibiotics<br>• **No protection against STDs** |
| *Estrogen* only "Morning-after" pill: *estrogen* (diethylstilbestrol) in very high doses (25 mg) | • Antifertility; taken within 72 hr of unprotected coitus during fertile period | • Available, prn | • Because of *DES* effect on fetus, elective abortion advised if method fails |
| *Progestin* only<br>Minipill (O) qd<br>Depo-Provera (IM) q 3-6 mo | • Impairs fertility<br>• Thickens cervical mucus; decreases sperm penetration<br>• Alters endometrial maturation<br>• *Effectiveness*: undetermined; can reach 100% reliability if used exactly as prescribed | • (O): convenient, easy to take<br>• (IM): 2- 4 times/yr; lactation OK during this time<br>• Not related to sex | • Ovulation may occur<br>• Irregular bleeding<br>• May change glucose and insulin values<br>• **No protection against STDs** |
| **Intrauterine Devices (IUDs)** | | | |
| Small T-shaped device inserted into uterine cavity. Medicated with: Copper Progesterone | • Prevents fertility: damages sperm in transit to fallopian tube (*progesterone* alters cervical mucus and endometrial maturation)<br>• *Effectiveness*: 90-99% | • Can be used by women who cannot use hormonal contraception<br>• Recommended for women who have had at least one child<br>• No disruption of ovulation pattern<br>• *Copper* can be used effectively for 10 yr; *progesterone* effective for 5 years. | • **Contraindications:** history of PID, pregnancy, undiagnosed genital bleeding, genital malignancy, abnormal uterine cavity<br>⚡• *Risks:* uterine perforation, infection (may be followed by PID) in the first 3 mo of insertion; unnoticed expulsion<br>• *Side effects* (especially with *copper T*): heavy flow, spotting between periods, and cramping within first few months of insertion<br>• Must check for string after each menses and before intercourse<br>• **No protection against STDs** |

*(continued)*

## TABLE 1.2  CONTRACEPTION  (continued)

| Type | Use | Benefits | Concerns/Disadvantages |
|---|---|---|---|
| **Mechanical Barriers** | | | |
| *Cervical cap*— 1¼-1½ in. soft, natural rubber dome with a firm but pliable rim | • Physical barrier to sperm <br> • Spermicide inside cap adds a chemical barrier <br> • *Effectiveness*: 94-97% effective with good compliance | • Worn for 8 hr, but *not* longer than 48 hr[a] <br> • *No* need to add spermicide for repeated acts of intercourse | • Need a yearly Pap smear: higher rate of conversion from class I to class III[b] <br> • If in place over 48 hr, it produces an odor, and might be associated with TSS[a] <br> • *Cannot* be worn during menstrual flow (menses), or up to 6 wk postpartum <br> • **Contraindications:** abnormal Pap smear, hard to fit, history of TSS or genital infection, allergy to latex <br> • Change after: genital surgery, vaginal birth <br> • Must be replaced *yearly* <br> • **No protection against STDs** |
| *Diaphragm*— shallow rubber device that fits over cervix | • Barrier preventing sperm from entering cervix (if it is correct size, undamaged, correctly placed, and is used with spermicide) <br> • *Effectiveness*: 83-90%; 99% in highly motivated women | • Does not interrupt sex act, except to add spermicide just before act <br> • Insert up to 6 hr before intercourse and leave in place for 6 hr after last intercourse, but do *not* leave in place longer than 24 hr[a] <br> • Safe: no side effects from well-fitted device, if woman is not allergic to diaphragm or spermicide <br> • Decreased incidence of vaginitis, cervicitis, PID | • Requires careful cleansing with warm water and mild soap; powder with cornstarch and store away from heat <br> • Size/fit needs to be checked after: term birth, 2nd or 3rd trimester abortion, weight gain or loss of 20 pounds or more, and/or 2 yr <br> • Spermicide must be reinserted for additional acts that may follow initial intercourse <br> • **No protection against STDs** |
| *Female condom*— vaginal sheath of natural latex rubber with flexible rings at both the closed and the open ends | • Barrier preventing sperm from entering vagina <br> • *Effectiveness*: similar to other mechanical methods used with spermicide[c] <br> • NOTE: Male and female condoms should *not* be used at the same time | • Apply well in advance of intercourse; spermicide added just before intercourse <br> • Heightens sensation for man <br> • About as satisfying for both woman and man as intercourse without it <br> • **Provides protection from STDs** | • Cost is high <br> • A new one *must* be used for every act of intercourse <br> • Cannot be used if either partner has a latex allergy |
| *Male condom*— thin, stretchable latex sheath to cover penis | • Barrier preventing sperm from entering vagina; is applied over erect penis before loss of preejaculatory drops and is held in place as penis is withdrawn <br> • Spermicidal foam, jelly, or cream is also used[c] <br> • *Effectiveness*: 64-98% when used with spermicide | • Safety—no side effects <br> • **Provides protection from STDs**; with spermicide (0.5 g nonoxynol-9) added to interior or exterior surface, provides protection from STDs including human immunodeficiency virus (HIV) | • Check expiration date <br> • Requires high motivation to use correctly and consistently <br> • Must be properly applied and removed <br> • Sheath may tear during intercourse <br> • Cannot be used if either partner has latex allergy |

[a] Although there is no direct link between *TSS* (*toxic shock syndrome*) and use of the diaphragm or cervical cap, a possible association remains (see **p. 9**).
[b] **Class I** Pap smear: no abnormal cells; **class III** Pap smear: suspicious abnormal cells present.
[c] Spermicide provides lubrication, but if additional lubrication is needed, use only water-based products, e.g., **K-Y Jelly.**

(continued)

## TABLE 1.2 CONTRACEPTION *(continued)*

| Type | Use | Benefits | Concerns/Disadvantages |
|---|---|---|---|
| **Chemical Barriers** | | | |
| *Spermicide*— aerosol foams, foaming tablets, suppositories, creams, and films (V-film) | • Physical barrier to sperm penetration<br>• Chemical action to sperm (kills sperm)<br>• Nonoxynol-9 has a bacteriostatic action<br>• *Effectiveness:* 70–98% when used with diaphragm or condoms | • Increases effectiveness of mechanical barriers<br>• Ease of application<br>• Aids lubrication of vagina<br>• Requires no medical examination or prescription<br>• May be used during lactation<br>• Backup for missed oral contraceptive pills<br>• **May provide some protection from STDs** | • Messy<br>• Some people are allergic to preparations<br>• Tablets or suppositories take 10-5 min to dissolve<br>• If it is the only method being used, each intercourse should be preceded (by 30 min) by a fresh application |
| **Other Methods** | | | |
| *Natural family planning* methods:<br>• Basal body temperature (BBT) each morning before any physical activity<br>• Symptothermal variation—BBT plus cervical mucus changes<br>• Calendar method[d]<br>  Predictor test for ovulation | • Require sexual abstinence during woman's fertile period (4 d before ovulation and for 3 or 4 d after ovulation)<br>• *Effectiveness:* about 80% | • Physically safe to use<br>• No drugs or appliances are used<br>• Meet requirements of most religions | • *Effectiveness:* depends on high level of motivation and diligence<br>• Requires a fairly predictable menstrual cycle<br>• Calendar method also requires knowledge of cycle lengths and formula; formula must be worked for each cycle<br>• **No protection from STDs** |

[d] **Calendar method:** Sperm remain viable in the woman's reproductive tract for approximately **3 days;** they are most capable of fertilizing an egg during the first **24** hr, however. The egg is viable for about **24 hr;** it is most likely to be fertilized during the first **12 hr.** The calendar method considers the life spans of the egg and sperm and that the time of ovulation is unpredictable; the formula that recognizes these variations follows: subtract 18 from the shortest cycle the woman experienced within the last year and subtract 11 from the longest cycle she had during the last year. The difference gives the *"fertile days."* NOTE: *Ovulation takes place 14 days before the next menstrual cycle.*

due to stress or deficit in critical body fat-to-lean ratio).

   **b.** *Dysmenorrhea* (painful menstruation):

     (1) *Primary*—occurs in absence of organic disease.

     (2) *Secondary*—associated with organic pelvic disease, e.g., endometriosis, pelvic inflammatory disease, cervical stenosis, uterine or ovarian neoplasms, and uterine polyps.

   **c.** *Premenstrual syndrome (PMS)*—begins during luteal phase and ends with menses; gives rise to positive symptoms (e.g., heightened sense of creativity), or negative symptoms (e.g., symptoms related to edema or emotional instability).

   **d.** *Endometriosis*—presence and growth of endometrial tissue outside of the uterus; characterized by: secondary amenorrhea, dysmenorrhea, dyspareunia, chronic pelvic pain, abnormal uterine bleeding, and infertility.

   **3.** *Sexually transmitted disease (STD) or pelvic inflammatory disease (PID).*

   **4.** Contraceptive methods used.

   **5.** Obstetric history.

**B.** *Maternal diagnosis:*

   **1.** *Basal body temperature (BBT):* monitored throughout the cycle.

   **2.** Endocrine studies: *FSH, LH;* performed before and following ovulation.

   **3.** *Huhner's* (postcoital) test used to determine: the adequacy of coital technique, cervical mucus, sperm, and degree of sperm penetration through cervical mucus; it is performed within 2 hr *after* ejaculation of semen into the vagina; it is synchronized with the expected time of ovulation.

**4.** *Rubin* test: a transuterine insufflation of the fallopian tubes with carbon dioxide to test their patency; it is performed *before* ovulation.

**5.** *Hysterosalpingogram*: a test to determine patency of fallopian tubes; scheduled before ovulation because there is no chance of an early pregnancy being disrupted by the test.

**6.** *Laparoscopic* examination: to visualize internal structures; can be used in conjunction with tests for tubal patency. Since air is insufflated into the abdominal cavity during this procedure, women can expect some shoulder (referred) pain or subcostal pain following the procedure. This discomfort usually lasts 24 hr and generally can be relieved with mild analgesics.

C. *Diagnosis—Men:*

   **1.** History

     **a.** Parotitis (mumps): acute, communicable viral disease involving chiefly the parotid gland, but frequently affecting tissues such as the gonads, thus impairing male fertility.

     **b.** Tight clothing, sitting for prolonged periods (cross-country truck drivers), or use of a hot tub may affect sperm count until the man changes these behaviors.

     **c.** A large amount of alcohol may affect fertility in that it may affect the libido or erection potential.

   **2.** Physical examination: secondary sex characteristics; anatomy.

   **3.** *Laboratory tests*: especially *semen analysis.* Semen is assessed for sperm: number, morphology, motility; pH; volume. Specimen should be collected in the container provided by the clinic and brought to the clinic *within 2 hr after* ejaculation to support a more accurate semen analysis. If collected in a condom, it must not be coated with nonoxynol–9, which is spermicidal, and it must be delivered to the clinic within 1 hr.

**IV. Analysis/nursing diagnosis:** *Sexuality patterns alteration* related to infertility.

**V. Nursing care plan/implementation**

   A. Goal: *provide emotional support.*

   B. Goal: **health teaching**.

     **1.** Explain testing procedures for diagnosis.

     **2.** Explain ordered drug therapy (**Pharmacology Box 1.2**).

     **3.** Advise woman on use of medication to increase vaginal pH to a neutral or to slightly alkaline pH. Sodium bicarbonate douches help to optimize vaginal pH for sperm motility.

   C. Goal: *assist with referral process* (e.g., adoption agencies).

**VI. Evaluation/outcome criteria**

   A. The couple conceives, or,

   B. If the couple does not conceive, they accept referral for help with adoption, other reproductive alternatives, or childlessness.

## Sterilization

**I. Definition:** process or act that renders a person unable to produce children (e.g., tubal ligation, hysterectomy, vasectomy).

**II.** Sterilization procedures, their effectiveness, advantages and disadvantages, and side effects, are presented in **Table 1.3**.

## Interruption of Pregnancy

Also known as elective, voluntary, or therapeutic abortion. Once the diagnosis of pregnancy and the length of gestation are established, the woman faces the decision to interrupt or to maintain the pregnancy (**Table 1.4**).

**I. Decision-making stage**

**A. Assessment**

   **1.** Health history

     **a.** Determine woman's feelings about the pregnancy, reasons for considering abortion, level of maturity; if decision was already made before she came to clinic, how was decision made?; does she have a support system?

     **b.** Identify factors influencing/ complicating her decisions (religious beliefs, cultural mores, peer and family pressures).

     **c.** Information needs.

   **2.** Physical examination.

   **3.** *Laboratory tests:* blood type, Rh, hemoglobin, hematocrit; urinalysis, pregnancy test, antibody titer, other tests dependent on her health status.

**B. Analysis:** *Some examples of nursing diagnoses*

   **1.** *Individual coping impairment* related to emotional conflicts associated with need for decision to continue/terminate pregnancy.

   **2.** *Family process alteration* related to intrafamily conflict associated with need for/decision to continue/terminate pregnancy.

   **3.** *Anticipatory grieving* related to loss of pregnancy/child.

   **4.** *Self-concept alteration, situational self-esteem disturbance* related to possible guilt feelings, related to pregnancy/termination.

   **5.** *Knowledge deficit* related to available options.

**C. Nursing care plan/implementation**

   **1.** Goal: *emotional support to minimize impact on self-image and self-esteem.*

     **a.** Maintain accepting, nonjudgmental attitude.

## ⬭ PHARMACOLOGY BOX 1.2   THERAPY FOR IMPAIRED FERTILITY

| Drug/Dosage* | Indication/Action | ▶ Assessment: Side Effects | ▶ Nursing Management |
|---|---|---|---|
| **Bromocriptine**<br>*Parlodel*<br>Initial dose: 1.25 -2.5 mg/d; 2.5 mg as tolerated may be added q3 -7d; usual dose: 5 -7.5 mg/d, with a daily range of 2.5 -15 mg | Short-term treatment of amenorrhea/galactorrhea associated with hyperprolactinemia | **Contraindicated** in: presence of hypersensitivity to drug/ergot alkaloids, uncontrolled hypertension<br>CNS: *dizziness, headache,* fatigue, lethargy, epileptiform seizures, nightmares, confusion<br>CV: hypotension, edema, palpitations<br>EENT: nasal congestion, visual disturbances<br>GI: N/V/D,cramps, anorexia, constipation, dyspepsia, dry mouth, metallic taste<br>GU: urinary frequency; other: symptoms of ergotism | Assess for hx of ergot<br>❗ alkaloid hypersensitivity<br>*Avoid* exposure to heat, moisture, light in storage<br>🍎 Administer with *meals/milk*<br>Assess BP for stability before administration<br>🏠 **Health education:** take *with* meals; *avoid* alcohol—may cause dizziness—use caution in potentially hazardous<br>❗ activities; *avoid* changing positions (lying/sitting/standing) rapidly |
| **Clomiphene**<br>*Clomid*<br>*Serophene*<br>*Adults*: 50 mg/24 hr PO for 5 d (if necessary may repeat with 100 mg/24 hr PO for 5 d, *after* at least 30-d rest period)<br>Maximum: 100 mg/24 hr | Induction of ovulation | **Contraindicated** in: abnormal uterine bleeding, severe liver dysfunction, clients with ovarian cysts, and pregnancy<br>May cause multiple pregnancy in approximately 11% of clients; however, over 90% of these are twins<br>Commonly causes abdominal discomfort, visual disturbances, and hot flashes | 🏠 **Health education:**<br>Monitor for abdominal discomfort<br>Observe for hot flashes<br>Observe for visual disturbances |
| **Menotropins**<br>*Pergonal*<br>IM 1 amp (FSH + LH)/day for 9 -12 days (followed by 5000-10,000 U HCG; if ovulation does not occur, repeat with 2 ampules) | Human gonadotropic responses; treatment of secondary anovulation (induces ovulation); stimulation of spermatogenesis | Abortions occur in 25%; failure rate 55-80% of clients; possible multiple births; ovarian enlargement; gynecomastia in men. | Assist in collection of urine 〰 to assess estrogen levels<br>🏠 **Health education:** couple's need to have daily intercourse from day of HCG injection until ovulation |

HCG = human chorionic gonadotropin.
*See **Pharmacology Box 1.1** for danazol.

b. Encourage verbalization of feelings, perceptions, and values.

c. Support woman's decision.

🏠 2. Goal: **health teaching** to facilitate informed decision-making.

a. Explain and discuss available options as applicable (see **Table 1.4**).

b. Describe procedure selected and what to expect after procedure.

3. Goal: *minimize impact on intrafamily relations, family process.* Where applicable, encourage open communication between deciding partners.

▶ **D. Evaluation/outcome criteria**

1. Woman states she understands all information necessary to give consent.

2. Woman expresses comfort and satisfaction with the decision.

II. **Preoperative period**

▶ A. **Assessment**

1. Reassess emotional and physical status and current feelings regarding decision.

2. Determine current knowledge/understanding of authorization form, anticipated procedure, and consequences (informed consent).

3. Monitor physiologic and (if awake) psychological response to procedure.

▶ B. **Analysis:** *some examples of nursing diagnoses*

1. *Anxiety/fear* related to procedure, potential complications.

2. *Knowledge deficit of therapeutic regimen* related to ongoing procedure, sights, sounds, and sensations experienced.

▶ C. **Nursing care plan/implementation**

1. Goal: *provide opportunity to reconsider decision regarding termination of pregnancy.*

## TABLE 1.3    STERILIZATION

| Use | Benefits | Concerns/Disadvantages |
|---|---|---|
| **Men** | | |
| *Vasectomy*: vas deferens is occluded (ligated and severed; bands; clips) to prevent passage of sperm | • Relatively simple surgical procedure<br>• Does *not* affect endocrine function, production of testosterone<br>• Does *not* alter volume of ejaculate<br>• Tubal reconstruction possible (90%) | • Sterility is *not* immediate; sperm are cleared from vas after several ejaculations<br>• Some men develop erectile dysfunction due to psychological response to procedure<br>• Fertility after tubal reconstruction (40-60%) |
| **Women** | | |
| *Tubal ligation*:  Both fallopian tubes are ligated and severed, or occluded with bands or clips to prevent passage of eggs; fulguration of the tubes at the cornu is most effective | • Abdominal surgery utilizing 1-in. incision and laparoscopy<br>• Greater than 99.5% effective | • Major surgery (if done by laparotomy) with possible complications of: anesthesia, infection, hemorrhage, and trauma to other organs; psychological trauma in some |
| *Hysterectomy* and/or *oophorectomy* | • Abdominal or vaginal surgery<br>• Absolute sterility | • Success rate for pregnancy after tubal reanastomosis is about 15% |

a.   Check to ensure all required permission (informed consent) forms have been signed/filed.

b.   Refer to physician if ambivalent or insecure in decision.

2. Goal: *reduce anxiety/fear related to procedure.*

   a.   Explain all anticipated preoperative, operative, and postoperative care.

   b.   Assist with procedure; if awake, explain what is happening, and what she may be experiencing.

3. Goal: *emotional support to facilitate effective coping.*

   a.   Encourage verbalization of feelings, fears, concerns.

   b.   Support woman's decision.

**D. Evaluation/outcome criterion**

   1. Woman experiences no physiologic or psychological problems during procedure.

**III. Postoperative period**

**A. Assessment**

   1. Monitor *physiologic* response to procedure (vital signs, blood loss, uterine cramping).

   2. Determine *psychological* response (happy, relieved; guilt feelings, lowered self-esteem).

   3. Determine desire for family planning information.

   4. Determine need for Rho (D$^u$) immune globulin, *rubella* vaccination.

**B. Analysis**: *some examples of nursing diagnoses*

   1. *Pain* related to procedure.

   2. *Infection risk* related to lack of knowledge of postabortal self-care.

**C. Nursing care plan/implementation**

   1. Goal: *provide and explain postoperative care.*

   a.   Administer IV fluids.

   b.   Administer medications prn for discomfort.

   c.   Administer *oxytocic* for uterine atony, prn.

   d.   If *Rh-negative mother*, 8 or more wk gestation, and laboratory tests indicate no current sensitization (i.e., she is Coombs negative):

     (1)   Explain rationale for post abortion administration of *Rho* (*D$^u$* antigen) immune globulin (*RhoGAM*).

     (2)   Administer *RhoGAM*, as ordered.

   e.   Provide and explain perineal care.

2. Goal: **health teaching** to facilitate active participation in own health maintenance and informed decision making; provide predischarge anticipatory guidance (also provide in written form*).

   a.   Immediately report any cramping, excessive bleeding, signs of infection.

   b.   Provide name and phone number of person to call if she has questions.

   c.   Schedule a postabortal checkup.

   d.   Discuss contraception, if woman indicates interest, or give her place and name to call for information later.

   e.   Discuss resumption of tampon use (3 d-3 wk as ordered) and sexual intercourse (1-3 wk as ordered).

   f.   Discuss need to avoid douching.

**D. Evaluation/outcome criteria**

   1. Woman returns for postabortal appointment.

   2. Woman suffers no adverse physical sequelae to the procedure.

(continued on p.17)

* With attention to woman's level of reading skill and understanding and in her language, whenever possible.

## TABLE 1.4 INTERRUPTION OF PREGNANCY (ELECTIVE/VOLUNTARY ABORTION)

| Procedure | Benefits | Concerns/Disadvantages |
|---|---|---|
| **First-Trimester Procedures** | | |
| *Menstrual extraction*—aspiration of endometrium through undilated cervix | • Performed for women who have not yet missed a menstrual period <br>• 100% effective if implantation site is not missed | ! • Cervical trauma may occur and may lead to incompetent cervix <br>! • Hemorrhage |
| *RU 486 (Mifeprex)*—a progesterone antagonist followed by vaginal insertion of misoprostol (must be less than 63 days since LMP) | • Prevents implantation of fertilized egg <br>• Most effective in early gestation, during luteal phase, within 10 d of first missed period <br>• Softens cervix | • Pain and cramping during period of bleeding, can last 7-14 days. <br>• Uterine aspiration may be needed if RU 486 does not work <br>• Common side effect: nausea, vomiting, headache, diarrhea |
| *Uterine aspiration*(vacuum or suction curettage)—cannula suction under local anesthesia, following cervical dilatation, usually with laminaria tent | • Relatively few complications—minimal bleeding, minimal discomfort <br>• Done on outpatient basis | • Performed after 1 or 2 missed menstrual periods <br>• Cervical and/or endometrial trauma possible |
| *Surgical D & C*—cervix dilated with laminaria tents; endometrium scraped with metal curette or flexible aspiration tip, under local anesthesia (paracervical block) | • After cervix is dilated, procedure time is about 15 min <br>• Outpatient basis <br>• Relatively few complications ($\leq$ 1%)—bleeding like a heavy period, some cramping | • Performed after 1 or 2 missed periods <br>• Possible, but rare: cervical trauma, uterine perforation, infection, hemorrhage |
| **Second-Trimester Procedures** | | |
| *Intraamniotic infusion* between weeks 14 and 16: <br> Transabdominal extraction of 200 mL amniotic fluid and replacement with equal amount of *hypertonic NaCl* (20%; or 30% urea in 5% D/W) (rarely done due to complications) | • Does not require laparotomy <br>• Women may ambulate until labor starts and during early labor <br>• Abortion completed within 36-40 hr; two-thirds of fetuses are aborted in 24 hr <br>• With *urea*: abortion usually occurs within 12 hr <br>• Complications less common or serious than with NaCl | • Complications increase proportionately with weeks of gestation <br>• **Risks:** <br>*Hypernatremia*: tinnitus, tachycardia, and headache <br>*Water intoxication*: edema, oliguria ($\leq$ 200 mL/8 hr), dyspnea, thirst, and restlessness <br>*Hemorrhage* and possible disseminated intravascular coagulation (*DIC*) <br>*Fever with sepsis* <br>• Experiences labor <br>• May require D & C |
| Instillation of 40-45 mg *prostaglandin* $F_2$, $E_2$ | • Labor is usually shorter than with hypertonic *NaCl* <br>• Avoids complications of water intoxication and hypernatremia | • May cause vomiting, diarrhea, nausea <br>! • Fetus may be born alive |
| *D & E (dilation and evacuation)*—extends D & C and vacuum curettage up to 20 wk gestation | • Does not experience labor <br>• Hospitalization is shortened <br>• With a skilled operator, complication rate is lower than with intraamniotic injection methods | • Requires 3 d to dilate cervix; <br>• Procedure done on 3rd day |
| **Second- and Third-Trimester Procedures** | | |
| *Hysterotomy*—cesarean delivery | • Available for gestations more than 14-16 wk <br>• Preferred method if woman wishes a tubal ligation or hysterectomy to follow | ! • *Post*: major surgery complications—hemorrhage and infection possible <br>• Fetus may be born alive, opening ethical, moral, religious, and legal problems |

## TABLE 1.5    SAFER SEX GUIDELINES

*If you are going to have sex, following these guidelines can reduce the risk of HIV transmission.*
- *Always* use a latex or polyurethane condom (rubber) for vaginal, oral or anal sex.
- *Do **not*** get semen or vaginal fluids in your mouth.
- Nonoxynol-9 was previously thought to kill the virus, but it washes away protective cells.
- *Do **not*** use: vaseline, vegetable, mineral oil; hand lotion, massage oil, or Crisco with condoms. They make condoms break more easily. Use water-based lubricants such as *K-Y Jelly* or *Astroglide*.
- *Always* leave some room at the tip of the condom to catch the sperm; be sure no air bubble gets trapped in the tip and use lubricant to reduce friction on the outside of the condom; this will decrease the possibility of the condom breaking.
- Throw the condom away after using it. **Never** use the same condom twice.
- Use a latex square (dental dam) or plastic wrap for oral sex with a woman. Vaginal fluid and menstrual blood can carry the virus.

From *AIDS 101.* San Francisco AIDS Foundation.

3. Woman suffers no adverse psychological sequelae to the procedure.
4. Woman is successful in achieving her goal of either contraception or conception at the time she desires.
5. Postabortion psychological impact
   a. Majority—relieved and happy.
   b. Small number (5-10%)—negative feelings, such as guilt or low self-esteem.

# Preconception Care

Preconception care is care designed for health maintenance for everyone, but especially for women and their potential fetuses. Healthy lifestyles support immune system function and normal cell differentiation in the developing embryo/fetus.

# Components of Preconception Care: Nursing Process

I. **Assessment for risk factors/causes:**
   A. *Medical history*—immune status (e.g., vaccinations, *rubella* titer), infectious illnesses, genetic disorders, current use of medications (including over-the-counter drugs and herbal supplements), medical/surgical conditions.
   B. *Reproductive history*—contraceptive methods used; obstetric.
   C. *Psychosocial history*—family or other support system; spouse/partner situation; assess for domestic violence, use of recreational (mind altering) drugs.
   D. *Reproductive choice*—plans for having children or for childlessness, readiness for pregnancy (e.g., age, life goals, financial resources, stress).
   E. *Environmental* (home/workplace)—safety hazards, toxic chemicals, radiation, noise.

II. **Health promotion: general teaching.**
   A. *Nutrition*—healthy diet; optimum weight.
      1. Important for maximum functioning of the immune system; phagocytosis and humoral and cellular immunity depend on diet.
      2. Deficient or excessive intake of some dietary components, such as vitamins and minerals, can exert negative effects on the immune response.
      3. Protein deficiency alters immune defenses, such as reducing levels of immunoglobulin A (IgA) in secretions and abnormal ratios of lymphocytic white cells.
      4. Breast milk encourages growth of *Lactobacillus bifidus*, which converts lactose into lactic acid.
   B. Exercise and rest.
   C. *Avoidance* of substance abuse.
   D. Practice of "safer sex" (**Table 1.5**).
   E. Family and social needs.
   F. Referrals: genetic counseling, family planning, family and social needs.
   G. Immunizations (e.g., *rubella*, tuberculosis, hepatitis).
   H. Medical/surgical therapy for existing conditions.

# Summary

The nurse needs a basic knowledge of *anatomy and physiology* in order to understand *conception, contraception, impaired fertility, sterilization, interruption of pregnancy*, and lifestyles that support the immune system. *Preconception care* plays an important role in helping people establish a healthy environment for reproduction. Selected conditions that affect the reproductive system are also reviewed: *breast conditions and uterine neoplasias*.

## 💡 Study and Memory Aids

### Menopause—from Greek:

*men* = month
*pausis* = to stop

### Decision–Making Regarding Reproduction

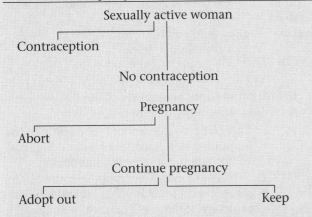

### Oral Contraceptives—Signs of Potential Problems: "ACHES"

**A**bdominal pain
**C**hest pain
**H**eadaches
**E**ye problems
**S**evere leg pain

### IUDs—Signs of Potential Problems: "PAINS"*

**P**eriod late/abnormal
**A**bdominal pain
**I**nfection
**N**ot feeling well
**S**tring missing

* Modified from RA Hatcher et al, *Contraceptive Technology*, New York: Irving Publishers.

### TSS—Key Warning Signs

Sudden fever ( ↑ Fever)
Hypotension ( ↓ BP)
Rash

### Legal Aspects

"Conscience" clauses allow nurses to refuse to assist with procedures that go against their moral, religious, or medical judgment

## Questions

1. A woman asks why she needs to do arm exercises following axillary node dissection. The nurse tells her that the *most important* reason is to:
   1. Strengthen the muscles.
   2. Restore energy levels.
   3. Retain full range of motion.
   4. Provide a diversional activity.

2. Nursing care of the woman with fibrocystic breast disease involves evaluation of a client's response to the nurse's teaching. The client has understood teaching when she eliminates which item from her diet?
   1. Caffeine (methylxanthine): coffee, colas.
   2. Whole grains and legumes.
   3. Cigarettes (nicotine).
   4. Milk and cheese (lactose).

3. The nurse is developing a teaching plan for a woman's health class. The health teaching plan should include explaining that an optional screening procedure for breast cancer is:
   1. Ultrasound imaging.
   2. Monthly breast self-examination (BSE).
   3. Transillumination.
   4. Thermography.

4. The nurse should teach women and their partners that if breast self-examination (BSE) is performed it is best to do:
   1. On the first day of menstruation.
   2. At the time of ovulation.
   3. About the 10th day after menstruation begins.
   4. Just before menstruation begins.

5. The plan of care for a client undergoing therapy for impaired fertility includes a prescription for *Clomid* (clomiphene citrate). The nurse knows that this client's problem is:
   1. Endometriosis.
   2. Endometritis.
   3. Short luteal phase of the menstrual cycle.
   4. Anovulation.

6. The fertility clinic nurse reads the following assessment findings in the chart. Which finding should the nurse recognize as being linked to infertility in men?
   1. Does not take multivitamins or vitamin E supplementation.
   2. Had parotitis (mumps) at the age of 5 yr.
   3. Prefers jockey-type shorts over boxer shorts.
   4. Drinks one to three 12-ounce cans of beer per day.

7. To prepare a woman for tubal ligation, the nurse should include the following information:
   1. The production of estrogen/progesterone will decrease.
   2. Menstrual flow will be much lighter.
   3. Ovulation will continue.
   4. Menopause can be expected soon after the procedure is performed.

8. Predischarge teaching for the man who has just had a vasectomy includes:
   1. Instructing him to avoid sexual intercourse for 4 weeks.
   2. A reminder that he may have hematuria for 12-24 hr.
   3. Explaining that fertility always returns after tubal reanastomosis.
   4. Cautioning him that he is still fertile for several weeks, or until his semen is clear of sperm.

9. If a nurse's religious beliefs do not permit artificial means of family planning, what would be the nurse's most appropriate response to a woman's question about contraceptive methods?
   1. "Personally, I don't believe in contraceptives. Please ask someone else."
   2. "All artificial contraceptives have bad side effects. I recommend 'natural' family planning."
   3. "There are several methods available. I'll tell you about them. Then you and your doctor can decide which is best for you."
   4. "Depoprovera is the most convenient and effective. You can ask for it right away so that you will be protected the next time you have sex."

10. A woman is discussing feminine hygiene with the clinic nurse. Which statement by the woman indicates to the nurse that she correctly understands a concept?
    1. "I should not take a bath and shampoo my hair during my menstrual period."
    2. "I should use a feminine deodorant spray every day to make it effective."
    3. "I need not use a vaginal douche in normal circumstances."
    4. "Superabsorbent tampons need to be changed at least every 24 hr."

11. A woman is admitted to an acute care unit with a diagnosis of toxic shock syndrome (TSS). The nurse knows that the *first* priority of therapy for TSS is:
    1. Fluid resuscitation.
    2. Fever reduction.
    3. Antimicrobial therapy.
    4. Antihypertensive therapy.

12. A nurse is conducting a preconception class on sexuality. A woman states, "Men have it easy to get excited. The tip of the penis is so sensitive." The nurse's response is based on knowledge that the man's glans penis is analogous to the woman's:
    1. Clitoris.
    2. Clitoral hood.
    3. Vaginal meatus.
    4. External cervical os.

13. While teaching a woman's health class, the nurse describes cervical mucus throughout the menstrual cycle, describing the cervical mucus at onset of ovulation as:
    1. Thin, clear, and stretchable.
    2. Decreased in amount.
    3. Pinkish or yellowish in color.
    4. Thickened, cloudy, and viscous.

14. A client in the fertility clinic needs to know when her next fertile period will be. Her menstrual cycles are 30-32 days in length. Her last normal period (LMP) began on August 5. The nurse determines that her next fertile period will be:
    1. August 14-16.
    2. August 19-21.
    3. August 21-23.
    4. August 24-26.

15. A woman is interviewed by the nurse at her 6-wk postpartum check. She expresses a desire to have another child in the future and asks the nurse about birth control methods. Which response by the nurse is true?
    1. "An intrauterine device (IUD) is a safe, reversible form of contraception."
    2. "Birth control pills are completely safe for all women under 40."
    3. "The diaphragm should be removed just after intercourse."
    4. "The basal body temperature (BBT) can help to determine when you ovulate."

16. A woman is admitted for an elective abortion after her second missed menstrual period. For which type of procedure will the nurse assist in preparing her?
    1. Hypertonic salt solution instillation.
    2. Menstrual extraction.
    3. Dilatation and extraction (D & E).
    4. Dilatation and suction (vacuum) curettage (D & C).

17. The nurse knows that intervention with a woman who has been abused has been successful when the woman:
    1. Follows the advice of counselors.
    2. Accepts her marriage vow to be with her husband "in sickness and in health. . . ."
    3. Recognizes which of her behaviors deserve punishment.
    4. Refers to herself specifically using phrases such as "I am. . . ."

18. In preconception counseling of adolescents who are sexually active, when discussing the Papanicolaou (Pap) smear, the nurse should advise them that Pap smears are:
    1. Associated with a low false-negative rate.
    2. Abnormal in 40% of adolescents.
    3. Normal in 10% of women with human papillomavirus (HPV).
    4. Best done annually.

19. After reviewing a woman's chart, the nurse's plan of care would include referral for investigation for endometrial carcinoma if her history shows:
    1. Postmenopausal bleeding.
    2. Use of combined oral hormonal contraceptives between ages of 16 and 30.
    3. Use of an intrauterine device (IUD) for 8 yr.
    4. Menopause that occurred at age 45.

20. The nurse should be alert to the fact that axillary node resection for breast cancer leads to edema because:
    1. The arm is positioned over head during surgery.
    2. Circulation to the arm is interrupted during surgery.
    3. The arm is traumatized during surgery.
    4. Lymph flow is interrupted.

21. A woman who has had breast surgery for cancer is taught to care for the suture line. The nurse knows that she has learned appropriate self-care when the woman:
    1. Covers it with lanolin cream three times per day.
    2. Cleans it every day with hydrogen peroxide ($H_2O_2$) diluted with water or normal saline (NS).
    3. Reapplies a pressure dressing over it once a day for 7 days.
    4. Ignores it.

22. When danazol (*Danocrine*) is prescribed for the management of endometriosis and fibrocystic breast disease, the woman is informed of the side effects. The nurse knows that her chief complaint is not related to danazol therapy when the client describes the following:
    1. Fluid retention.
    2. Hypoestrogenic manifestations.
    3. Dysmenorrhea.
    4. Virilization.

23. After reviewing a woman's diagnostic test results, the nurse explains to her that the pH of the vaginal canal can be a factor in impaired fertility, and that to alter the vaginal pH the physician may order:
    1. Vaginal instillation of clotrimazole (*Gyne-Lotrimin*).
    2. Sodium bicarbonate douches.
    3. Lactic acid douches.
    4. Oral estrogen therapy.

24. The nurse should know that a woman is not a good candidate for using a diaphragm for contraception if she:
    1. Gave birth 6 wk ago.
    2. Did not like using the cervical cap.
    3. Has frequent urinary tract infections (UTIs).
    4. Is planning to go on a diet to lose 10 pounds.

25. A young woman has just been diagnosed with diabetes mellitus. The nurse's teaching plan includes discussion of childbearing and contraception. The contraceptive choice(s) for a woman who is diabetic is/are:
    1. Combined hormonal oral contraceptive pills.
    2. Sterilization.
    3. Intrauterine device (IUD).
    4. Spermicide and diaphragm or condoms.

26. A nurse is conducting an in-service class about contraceptives. One of the group asks how birth control pills affect mucus patterns. The nurse's response is based on knowledge that, under the influence of combination oral hormonal contraception, the dried cervical mucus pattern is:
    1. Dependent on the phase of the menstrual cycle.
    2. Markedly fernlike.
    3. Minimally fernlike.
    4. Amorphous.

# Answers/Rationale

1. **(3)** Inactivity secondary to pain could affect joint action, and alteration in lymphatic drainage leads to edema formation and further impairment of joint/arm movement. Options 1, 2, and 4 are also important, but the *most* important reason for arm exercises at this time is to retain full range of motion of the joint. **PL, COM, 3, HPM, Health promotion and maintenance.**

2. **(1)** Women are advised to reduce their intake of caffeine when they are diagnosed with fibrocystic breast disease. Options 2, 3, and 4 are not items specifically eliminated from the diet of a woman with this disease. **EV, EVL, 4, PhI, Basic care and comfort**

3. **(2)** BSE is the only optional screening method of the procedures listed. Palpation of the breast has an estimated accuracy of 65 -75%; it is considered to be the first step in the diagnostic survey. Options 1, 3, and 4 are not optional screening methods. **IMP, RE/KN, 1, PhI, Reduction of risk potential**

4. **(3)** The best time to perform BSE is about the 10th day after the 1st day of the last menstrual period (LMP), when the hormonal effects on the breast are at the lowest; otherwise stated: about 5 days after menses stop. Options 1, 2, and 4 are all incorrect. Hormonal effect on the breasts is lowest at about the 10th day after the LMP. **IMP, RE/KN, 1, HPM, Health promotion and maintenance**

5. (4) *Clomid*, a nonsteroid estrogen analogue, is used to induce ovulation. Endometriosis (1) requires medications such as danazol or nafarelin that suppress the production of ovarian hormones, estrogen and progesterone. Endometritis (2) requires *antibiotic* therapy. *Clomid* has no effect on the luteal phase of the menstrual cycle (3). **AN, APP, 5, PhI, Pharmacological and parenteral therapies**

6. (2) Parotitis (mumps) is an acute, communicable viral infection involving chiefly the parotid gland, but frequently affects tissues such as the gonads. Vitamins, including E (1), are *not* linked to men's fertility/infertility. Jockey-type shorts (3) are *not specifically* linked to infertility. (Tight clothing, sitting for prolonged periods, or use of a hot tub frequently may affect sperm count, but this is reversed soon after the behavior is changed.) This amount of alcohol (4) may affect the libido or erection potential, but does *not* affect fertility itself. **AN, APP, 5, HPM, Health promotion and maintenance**

7. (3) Ovulation will continue, but the ovum will disintegrate within the abdominal cavity. Ovarian hormone production (1) is unaffected. Menses (2) should not be affected. The woman will experience menopause at the usual time; since ovarian function continues, tubal ligation does not induce menopause (4). **IMP, APP, 5, HPM, Health promotion and maintenance**

8. (4) He is still fertile until all the sperm in his vas deferens above the vasectomy and in the seminal vesicles are emptied. Option 1 is incorrect because he may wish to have sexual intercourse much earlier, after discomfort is past. They should continue to use contraception until his semen contains no sperm. Hematuria (2) is not associated with vasectomy. Option 3 is incorrect because he may develop autoantibodies against his own sperm (as he continues to produce sperm and his body must resorb them), so that he may still be infertile or sterile following the expensive operation for reanastomosis. **IMP, RE/KN, 5, HPM, Health promotion and maintenance**

9. (3) The nurse needs to provide the information about all choices; then the woman (couple) makes the decision along with the physician. In option 1, the nurse gives a personal judgment in what is the client's right to choose; depending on the way it is said, the statement can sound very rude. In option 2, the nurse is giving a personal opinion; the client has the right to choose for herself. In option 4, the nurse is giving a personal opinion without giving the client a chance to review all the options; in addition, the nurse is making an assumption that the woman will have intercourse soon and without protection. **IMP, APP, 5, PsI, Psychosocial integrity**

10. (3) Under normal circumstances, vaginal douching is not necessary. (It should *not* be used during pregnancy.) Bathing and shampooing (1) are *not* contraindicated during the menstrual period. Feminine deodorants (2) are *not* necessary; they can cause an allergic reaction. Superabsorbent tampons (4) should *not* be used; tampons should be changed frequently, and perineal pads are recommended during the night so as to minimize the possibility of developing toxic shock syndrome (TSS). **EV, EVL, 5, HPM, Health promotion and maintenance**

11. (1) The first priority of therapy for TSS is fluid resuscitation to combat hypotension. Reduction of fever (2) is the *second* concern, *then* antistaphylococcal infection therapy (3). *Hypo*tension, not hypertension (4), is characteristic of TSS. **PL, ANL, 6, PhI, Physiological adaptation**

12. (1) The man's glans penis is analogous to the woman's clitoris; each contains the same number of nerve endings, giving these structures an important role in sexual arousal. Options 2, 3, and 4 are all incorrect: The glans penis and *clitoris* are analogous. **IMP, RE/KN, 5, HPM, Health promotion and maintenance**

13. (1) Under estrogen influence, the cervical mucus at about the time of ovulation is thin, clear, and stretchable, like egg white. This mucus promotes sperm viability. The amount of mucus increases, *not* decreases (2), just before ovulation. The mucus is *clear* at this time, not pinkish or yellowish (3). Thick, cloudy, viscous mucus (4) is characteristic of *progesterone* influence *after* ovulation. **IMP, RE/KN, 5, HPM, Health promotion and maintenance**

14. (3) Ovulation occurs 14 days *before* the next menstrual period (30–14 = 16; 32–14 = 18). Adding day 16 to Aug. 5 = Aug. 21; adding day 18 to Aug. 5 = Aug. 23. The client will ovulate between August 21 and 23, depending on whether the next period was to be 30 or 32 days in length. Options 1, 2, and 4 are incorrect: These dates do not take into account the expected date of ovulation based on her LMP. **AS, RE/KN, 5, HPM, Health promotion and maintenance**

---

### Key to Codes

**Nursing process:** AS, assessment; AN, analysis; PL, planning; IMP, implementation; EV, evaluation. (See **Appendix J** for explanation of nursing process steps.)

**Cognitive level:** RE/KN, recall/knowledge; COM, comprehension; APP, application; ANL, analysis; EVL, evaluation; SYN, synthesis. (See **Appendix J** for explanation.)

**Category of human function:** 1, protective; 2, sensory-perceptual; 3, comfort, rest, activity, and mobility; 4, nutrition; 5, growth and development; 6, fluid-gas transport; 7, psychosocial-cultural; 8, elimination. (See **Appendix L** for explanation.)

**Client need:** SECE, safe, effective care environment; HPM, health promotion and maintenance; PsI, psychosocial integrity; PhI, physiological integrity. (See **Appendix M** for explanation.)

**Client subneed:** See **Appendix M** for explanation.

15. **(4)** A slight drop in the BBT, then a sustained rise (for 3 d or more) follows ovulation. The IUD **(1)** may predispose the client to endometritis and pelvic inflammatory disease (PID), which may impair fertility. Birth control pills **(2)** have possible side effects for some women (e.g., smokers). A diaphragm **(3)** should be left in place for 6 - 8 hr after intercourse. **IMP, RE/KN, 5, HPM, Health promotion and maintenance**

16. **(4)** The woman is in her first trimester; the procedure of choice is dilatation and suction (vacuum) curettage (D & C). Hypertonic salt solution via amniocentesis **(1)** is not possible during the *first* trimester, when the uterus is a *pelvic* structure; it is done during the *second* trimester when the uterus becomes an *abdominal* structure. Menstrual extraction **(2)** is best done around the time of the first missed period. D & E **(3)** is done during the second trimester. **PL, ANL, 1, PhI, Reduction of risk potential**

17. **(4)** Goals have been met when the woman can use phrases such as "*I am. . . ,*" which indicate a developing self-esteem, feelings of worth and personal adequacy, and independence. Options **1**, **2**, and **3** reflect a continuation of learned helplessness, submissiveness, passivity, and dependence. **EV, EVL, 1, PsI, Psychosocial integrity**

18. **(4)** Because HPV-related lesions will not otherwise be detected at a manageable stage, the Pap smear must be done annually. Option **1** is incorrect because Pap results have a recognized false-negative rate of 8–50%. Option **2** is incorrect because between 3 and 20% of adolescents will have an abnormal Pap smear. Option **3** is incorrect because the Pap smear will be normal in 30% of women with HPV. **IMP, RE/KN, 1, HPM, Health promotion and maintenance**

19. **(1)** The most important sign of endometrial carcinoma is abnormal bleeding, e.g., reappearance of "menstrual bleeding" after 6 mo of menopause. Oral contraceptives **(2)** may protect against such disorders as endometrial and ovarian cancer and other conditions. *Neither* use of the IUD **(3)** *nor* menopause at age 45 **(4)** is associated with endometrial carcinoma. **AS, ANL, 1, HPM, Health promotion and maintenance**

20. **(4)** Axillary lymph node resection for breast cancer often leads to edema because lymph flow is interrupted. None of the conditions in options **1**, **2**, and **3** should occur and interrupt lymph flow. **AN, RE/KN, 6, PhI, Physiological adaptation**

21. **(2)** Cleaning it every day with $H_2O_2$ diluted with water or NS prevents scar tissue formation and promotes healing. (Some physicians order Betadine or nothing at all.) *None* of the actions in options **1**, **3**, and **4** are appropriate for the care of the incision site. **EV, EVL, 1, HPM, Health promotion and maintenance**

22. **(3)** When the woman describes dysmenorrhea, the nurse knows that this is *not* a side effect of danazol. Fluid retention **(1)**, hypoestrogenic manifestations **(2)**, and virilization **(4)** *are* all side effects of danazol therapy. **EV, ANL, 3, PhI, Pharmacological and parenteral therapies**

23. **(2)** Sperm motility is increased as vaginal pH approaches neutral or is slightly alkaline; sodium bicarbonate douches help to optimize vaginal pH for sperm motility. Vaginal instillation of clotrimazole **(1)** does *not* raise the pH to support sperm motility; this is an excellent treatment of infection with *Candida albicans*. Lactic acid douches **(3)** make the vaginal fluids more acid, a condition that does *not* optimize vaginal pH for sperm motility. Estrogen therapy **(4)** does *not* alter the vaginal pH. **IMP, RE/KN, 5, PhI, Pharmacological and parenteral therapies**

24. **(3)** The diaphragm may place pressure on the urethra, preventing complete emptying and leading to UTI recurrence. She *can* be fitted for a diaphragm 6 wk after giving birth **(1)**. Her experience with the cervical cap **(2)** is not a contraindication (unless she did not like touching herself). A 10-pound loss **(4)** is not likely to cause a problem; she needs to have the diaphragm refitted after the gain or loss of *20* pounds. **AN, RE/KN, 5, HPM, Health promotion and maintenance**

25. **(4)** Spermicide and a diaphragm or condoms do not affect metabolism and are not associated with infection. Combined hormonal contraceptive pills **(1)** may affect metabolism. Diabetes mellitus usually can be controlled by client compliance to her planned care; therefore, this condition should not keep a woman from having children if she so chooses **(2)**. Infection is possible during the first 3 mo after insertion of an IUD **(3)**, and this can compromise the diabetic condition. **IMP, RE/KN, 5, HPM, Health promotion and maintenance**

26. **(4)** The combination of estrogen and progesterone gives an amorphous appearance in dried cervical mucus, a condition that prevents sperm penetration and mobility. There is no "phase of the menstrual cycle" **(1)**; the bleeding that occurs is known as withdrawal bleeding—it is *not* menstrual flow. Fernlike patterns **(2 and 3)** occur in response to estrogen alone; combination hormone contraception includes progesterone, which inhibits formation of this pattern. **AN, RE/KN, 5, HPM, Health promotion and maintenance**

# Normal Pregnancy

**2**

## Chapter Outline

- Key Points
- Key Words
- General Aspects of Nursing Care
- Genetics, Conception, and Embryonic and Fetal Development
  - Basic Genetic Components
  - Sex Determination
  - Fertilization and Implantation
  - Stages of Prenatal Development
- Biophysical Foundations of Pregnancy
  - Anatomic and Physiologic Modifications
  - Alterations Affecting Fluid-gas Transport
    - Cardiovascular System
    - Respiratory system
  - Alterations Affecting Elimination
    - Urinary System
    - Gastrointestinal System
  - Alterations Affecting Nutrition
    - Gastrointestinal System
    - Endocrine System
    - Metabolism
  - Alterations Affecting Protective Functions
    - Integumentary System
  - Alterations Affecting Comfort, Rest, Mobility
    - Musculoskeletal System
- Psychosocial-Cultural Alterations
  - Emotional Changes
  - Physical Bases of Changes

- Prenatal Management
  - Initial Assessment Goal
  - Objectives
  - Assessment: *History*
  - Assessment: *Initial Physical Aspects*
    - Validation of Pregnancy:
      - Presumptive Symptoms
      - Presumptive Signs
      - Probable Signs
      - Positive Signs
  - Assessment: *Nutritional Status*
  - Assessment: *Psychosocial Aspects*
- Antepartal Experience and Management
  - General Aspects of Prenatal Management
  - Common Minor Discomforts During Pregnancy
  - Nutrition During Pregnancy and Lactation
    - Nutrient Needs
      - Ethnic Food Patterns
      - Religious Considerations in Food Planning
      - Food List for Ready Reference in Menu Planning
  - Childbirth Preparation/Parent Education
    - Grantly Dick-Read
    - Lamaze Method
    - Bradley
  - Warning Signs of Potential Problems
- Summary
- Study and Memory Aids
- Questions
- Answers/Rationale

---

## 🔑 Key Points

- The prenatal period is a preparatory one; both physically, in terms of fetal growth and maternal adaptations, and psychologically, in terms of anticipation of parenthood.

- Nutritional risk factors that compromise the well-being of the mother and her fetus include adolescent pregnancy; bizarre or faddist food habits; other risk factors include: abuse of nicotine, alcohol, or drugs; a low weight for height; and frequent pregnancies.

- The expected outcome of preparation for childbirth and parenting is "education for choice" and enhanced coping skills.

- Every woman/couple needs to know the warning signs of potential problems (e.g., preterm labor) and how and to whom to report these signs.

## Key Words

Amniotic fluid

Birth plan

Conception

Expected date of birth

Fertilization

Fetal membranes:

    Amnion

    Chorion

Gate control theory

Implantation

Kegel's exercises

Physiologic anemia

Placenta

Signs of pregnancy:

    Presumptive

    Probable

    Positive

Supine hypotension

**General overview:** This review of the normal physiologic and psychosocial changes occurring during each trimester of pregnancy provides essential components of the database for accurate nursing judgments and anticipatory guidance during the prenatal period.

# General Aspects of Nursing Care

**I. Assessment**—based on nursing knowledge of:
   A. Biophysical and psychosocial aspects of conception and gestation.
   B. Parameters of normal pregnancy.
   C. Risk factors, signs, symptoms, and implications of deviations from normal patterns of maternal and fetal health.

**II. Analysis/nursing diagnosis**
   A. *Knowledge deficit* related to normal pregnancy-related alterations (physiologic and emotional alterations/trimester).
   B. *Pain* related to normal physiologic alterations in pregnancy.
   C. *Bowel elimination and renal alteration* related to normal physiologic changes during pregnancy (polyuria, constipation).
   D. *Nutrition alteration* related to increased metabolic needs due to pregnancy.
   E. *Adjustment impairment* related to altered self-image; anticipated role change; resurgence of old, unresolved conflicts.

**III. Nursing care plan/implementation**
   A. Goal: *emotional support*.
      1. Encourage verbalization of feelings, fears, concerns.
      2. Validate normalcy of behavioral response to pregnancy.
   B. Goal: *anticipatory guidance*.
      1. Facilitate achievement of developmental tasks.
      2. Strengthen coping techniques for pregnancy, labor, birth. Suggest appropriate resources (preparation for childbirth classes).
   C. Goal: **health teaching.** Describe, explain, discuss:
      1. Normal physiologic alterations during pregnancy.
      2. Common discomforts of pregnancy, management.

**IV. Evaluation/outcome criteria**
   A. Woman takes an active, informed part in her pregnancy-related care.
   B. Woman copes effectively with common alterations associated with pregnancy (physiologic, psychological, role change).
   C. Woman successfully carries an uneventful pregnancy to term.

# Genetics, Conception, and Embryonic and Fetal Development

**I. Basic genetic components**
   A. *Chromosomes*—elements within the cell nucleus carrying genes and composed of DNA and proteins. The diploid number of 46 (23 pairs) in each cell: 22 pairs of autosomes (somatic cells) and 1 pair of sex chromosomes.
   B. *Genes*—factors on a chromosome responsible for hereditary characteristics of offspring.

**II. Sex determination**
   A. Established at time of fertilization by the male sex chromosome.
   B. Mature ovum: contains haploid number of 23 chromosomes, one of which is always an X.
   C. Mature spermatozoon: contains haploid number of 23 chromosomes, one of which is either an X or a Y type.
      1. If spermatozoon contains an X, a female results (XX).
      2. If spermatozoon contains a Y, a male results (XY).

**III. Fertilization and implantation**
   A. *Before fertilization*
      1. *Ovum* (egg) life span: approximately 24 hr after ovulation.
      2. *Spermatozoon* life span: approximately 72 hr after ejaculation into female reproductive tract.
         a. *Acrosome reaction*—release of proteolytic enzymes that enable the sperm to digest the cumulus cells and penetrate the zona pellucida (a thin layer of proteins and polysaccharides that surrounds the ovum and provides protection during transport in fallopian tubes).
         b. *Capacitation*—process that enables sperm to bind to the ovum.
         c. After one sperm has entered, changes occur within the zona pellucida that prevent other sperm from entering.
   B. *Conception* (fertilization) usually occurs within 12–24 hr after ovulation, in the outer third (ampulla) of fallopian tube. With fertilization, the diploid number of chromosomes is reestablished; egg and sperm unite to form the single cell known as the *zygote*.
   C. *Implantation* (nidation) usually occurs within 7 days after conception, or about day 21 of a 28-day menstrual cycle.

D. *Placenta*
 1. Functions:
  a. Endocrine gland: human chorionic gonadotropin (HCG), human placental lactogen (HPL), progesterone, estrogens.
  b. Metabolism: respiration, nutrition, excretion, and storage.
 2. Methods of exchanging nutrients, etc.:
  a. *Diffusion*: Oxygen diffuses from the maternal blood across the placental membrane into the fetal blood; carbon dioxide diffuses in the opposite direction.
  b. *Facilitated* and *active transport*: assist in the transfer of glucose, amino acids, calcium, iron, and substances with higher molecular weight.
  c. *Pinocytosis*: mechanism used for transferring large molecules, such as albumin and gamma globulins, across the placental membrane.
 3. A thin membrane, only one cell thick, separates maternal and fetal circulation; occasionally breaks occur, allowing fetal red blood cells to leak into the maternal circulation.
 4. Placental function depends on the maternal blood pressure.
 5. Placental "barrier" resembles other membranes. Small molecules, and lipid-soluble substances diffuse readily but water-soluble substances either do not diffuse or diffuse poorly. Examples:
  a. Heparin replaces use of warfarin (*Coumadin*) in treatment of coagulation problems during pregnancy.
  b. Anesthetics and analgesics readily cross both the blood-brain and placental barriers; e.g., morphine-induced respiratory depression and miosis (constriction of pupils) may occur in both the mother and her newborn.
  c. Newborns of narcotic-addicted mothers will be born with dependence on narcotics.
E. *Fetal membranes*
 1. *Chorion*: develops from the trophoblast and contains the chorionic villi on its surface.
 2. *Amnion*: develops from interior cells of blastocyst; forms a fluid-filled sac; covers umbilical cord and covers the chorion on fetal surface of the placenta.
F. *Amniotic fluid*
 1. *Composition*: albumin, urea, uric acid, creatinine, lecithin, sphingomyelin, bilirubin, fructose, fat, leukocytes, epithelial cells, enzymes, and lanugo hair.

 2. Forms initially by diffusion from maternal blood; fetus urinates into fluid, greatly enhancing its volume.
 3. *Volume*: normally between 800 and 1200 mL; slightly transparent, yellow liquid.
 4. *Functions*: cushions fetus, allows freedom of movement, keeps embryo from tangling with the membranes, helps maintain constant body temperature, acts as source of oral fluid as well as a waste repository, assists in lung development.

IV. **Stages of prenatal development**
 A. *Ovum* (preembryonic)—period until primary villi have appeared, usually about 12–14 d; embryonic membranes (chorion and amnion) and germ layers (ectoderm, mesoderm, and endoderm) form.
 B. *Embryo*—period from end of ovum stage until measurement reaches approximately 3 cm: 54–56 d (8 wk).
 C. *Fetus*: week 9 to birth.
 D. Summary of development:
  1. **First trimester**
   a. Susceptible to teratogens; malformation possible.
   b. Heart functions at 3–4 wk.
   c. Eye formation at 4–5 wk.
   d. Arm and leg buds at 4–5 wk.
   e. Recognizable face at 8 wk.
   f. Brain: rapid growth.
   g. External genitalia at 8 wk.
   h. Placenta formed at 12 wk.
   i. Bone ossification at 12 wk.
  2. **Second trimester**
   a. Less danger from teratogens after 12 wk; dysfunction possible, however.
   b. Fetal heartbeat heard by 10–12 wks with a doppler.
   c. Quickening at 18–20 wk.
   d. Length: 10 in., weight: 8–10 ounces.
   e. Vernix: present.
   f. Lanugo: present.
  3. **Third trimester**
   a. Iron stored.
   b. Surfactant production begins in increasing amounts.
   c. Size: 15 in., 2–3 pounds at 28–32 wk.
   d. Calcium stored at 28–32 wk.
   e. Reflexes present at 28–32 wk.
   f. Subcutaneous fat deposits at 36 wk.
   g. Lanugo shedding at 38–40 wk.
   h. Average size: 18-22 in., 7.5–8.5 pounds at 38–40 wk.

# Biophysical Foundations of Pregnancy

## Anatomic and Physiologic Modifications

I. **Bases of functional alterations:**
   A. *Hormonal*: **Table 2.1** explains the effects of estrogen and progesterone during pregnancy. Nursing implications provide the knowledge base for:
      1. Anticipatory guidance regarding normal maternal adaptations.
      2. Early identification of deviations from normal patterns.
   B. *Mechanical*: enlarging uterus → displacement and pressure; increased weight of uterus and breasts → changes in center of gravity, posture and pressure.

II. **Reproductive organs**
   A. *Uterus*
      1. Amenorrhea. Occasional spotting common, especially at time of first missed menstrual period.
      2. Increased vascularity adds to increase in size and softening of the lower uterine segment (*Hegar's sign*).
      3. Growth is due to hypertrophy and hyperplasia of existing muscle cells and connective tissue.
      4. *Fundal height measurement landmarks*:

| Uterus | Nonpregnant | Pregnant (at term) |
|--------|-------------|--------------------|
| Length | 6.5 cm | 32 cm |
| Width | 4 cm | 24 cm |
| Depth | 2.5 cm | 22 cm |
| Weight | 50 g | 1000 g |

   B. *Cervix*
      1. Increased vascularity → softening (*Goodell's sign*) and deepened blue-purple coloration (*Chadwick's sign*).
      2. Edema, hyperplasia, thickening of mucous lining, and increased mucus production; formation of mucous plug by end of second month.
      3. Becomes shorter, thicker, and more elastic.
   C. *Vagina*
      1. Hyperemia deepens color (*Chadwick's sign*).
      2. Hypertrophy and hyperplasia thicken vaginal mucosa.
      3. Relaxation of connective tissue.
      4. pH acidic (4.0–6.0).
      5. Leukorrhea—nonirritating.

   D. *Perineum*
      1. Increases in size—hypertrophy of muscle cells, edema, and relaxation of elastic tissue.
      2. Deepens color—increases vascularization/hyperemia.
   E. *Ovaries*
      1. Ovum production ceases.
      2. Corpus luteum persists; produces hormones to week 10–12 until placenta "takes over."

## Alterations Affecting Fluid–Gas Transport

### Cardiovascular System

I. **Physiologic changes**
   A. Heart displaced upward and to the left.
   B. Circulation
      1. Cardiac volume *increases* by 20–30%.
      2. Labor—cardiac output *increases* by 20–30%.
   C. Hemoglobin and hematocrit values remain between 10–14 g and 35–42%; normal drop is 10% during second trimester (**Table 2.2, p. 28**).
   D. Hypercoagulability—*increased* levels of blood factors VII, IX, and X.
   E. Nonpathologic increased sedimentation rate—due to 50% increase in fibrinogen level.
   F. Blood pressure should remain stable, with drop in second trimester due to decreased peripheral resistance.
   G. Heart rate often *increases* 10–15 beats/min at term.
   H. Compression of pelvic veins → stasis of blood in lower extremities.
   I. Compression of inferior vena cava when supine → bradycardia → reduced cardiac output, faintness, sweating, nausea (*supine hypotension*). *Fetal response*: marked bradycardia due to hypoxia secondary to decreased placental perfusion.

II. **Assessment**
   A. Apical systolic murmur.
   B. Exaggerated splitting of first heart sound.
   C. Physiologic anemia.
   D. Dependent edema in third trimester (**Table 2.3, p. 28-29**).
   E. *Vena cava syndrome* (*supine hypotension*)—drop in systolic blood pressure may occur due to compression of descending aorta and inferior vena cava when supine.
   F. Varicosities (vulvar, anal, leg) (**Table 2.1, p. 27** and **Table 2.3, p. 29**).

III. **Nursing care plan/implementation**
   A. Goal: **health teaching.**
      1. *Elevate* lower extremities frequently.
      2. Apply support hose.
      3. Assume *side lying position* at rest.
      4. Learn signs and symptoms of pre-eclampsia-eclampsia.

*(continued on p. 30)*

## TABLE 2.1   HORMONES OF PREGNANCY

| *Primary Action* | *Clinical Indications for Nursing Actions* |
| --- | --- |
| **Estrogen** | |
| Level rises in serum and urine | Basis of test for maternal/placental/fetal well-being |
| Uterine development | *Probable* sign of pregnancy |
| Breast development | *Probable* sign of pregnancy; increased tingling, tenderness |
| Genital enlargement: increased vascularization, hyperplasia | Vaginal growth facilitates vaginal birth |
| Softens connective tissue | Results in back and leg ache; relaxes joints to increase size of birth canal and rib cage |
| *Alters nutrient metabolism:* | *GI and metabolic changes:* |
| *Decreases* HCl and pepsin | Digestive upsets |
| Antagonist to insulin—makes glucose available to fetus | Anti-insulin effect challenges maternal pancreas to produce more insulin; failure of beta cells to respond leads to "gestational" diabetes |
| | For the woman who is insulin-dependent, insulin requirements increase by an average of 67% during the second half of pregnancy |
| Supports fat deposition | Protect source of energy for fetus |
| Sodium and water retention; edema of lower extremities (nonpitting) | Meet increased plasma volume needs and maintain fluid reserve |
| *Hematologic changes:* | |
| *Increased* coagulability | *Increased* tendency to thrombosis |
| *Increased* sedimentation rate (SR) | SR loses diagnostic value for heart disease |
| Vasodilation: *spider nevi; palmar erythema* | Resolves spontaneously after birth |
| Increased production of melanin-stimulating hormone | Resolves spontaneously after birth |
| **Progesterone** | |
| Development of decidua | High levels result in tiredness, listlessness, and sleepiness |
| Reduces uterine excitability | Protection against abortion/early birth |
| Development of mammary glands | Prepares breasts for lactation |
| *Alters nutrient metabolism:* | *Nutritional significance:* |
| Antagonist to insulin | Diabetogenic |
| Favors fat deposition | Energy reserve |
| *Decreases* gastric motility and relaxes sphincters | Favors heartburn and constipation |
| *Increases* sensitivity of respiratory center to $CO_2$ | Increases depth, some dyspnea, increased sighing |
| *Decreases smooth muscle tone:* | *Decreased tone can lead to:* |
| Colon | Constipation |
| Bladder, ureters | Stasis of urine with infection |
| Veins | Dependent edema; varicosities |
| Gallbladder | Gallbladder disease |
| *Increases basal body temperature* (BBT) by 0.5°C | Discomfort from hot flashes and perspiration |
| **Human Chorionic Gonadotropin** | |
| Maintains corpus luteum during early pregnancy | Placenta must "take over" after a few weeks |
| Stimulates male testes | Increases testosterone in male fetuses |

*(continued)*

## TABLE 2.1 HORMONES OF PREGNANCY (continued)

| Primary Action | Clinical Indications for Nursing Actions |
|---|---|
| May suppress immune response | May inhibit response to foreign protein, for example, fetal portion of placenta |
| | *Diagnostic value* |
| | Biologic marker for pregnancy test |
| | Decreased level with threatened abortion |
| | Increased level with multifetal pregnancy, H. mole |
| **Human Placental Lactogen** | |
| Antagonizes insulin | Diabetogenic; may → gestational diabetes or complicate management of existing diabetes |
| Mobilizes maternal free fatty acids | Increased tendency to *ketoacidosis* if pregnant and diabetic |
| **Prolactin** | |
| Suppressed by estrogen and progesterone | No milk produced before birth |
| Increased level after placenta is delivered | Milk production 2–3 d after birth |
| **Follicle Stimulating Hormone** | |
| Production suppressed during pregnancy; level returns to prepregnant levels within 3 wk after birth | No ovulation during pregnancy; ovulation usually returns: within 6 wk for 15%, within 12 wk for 30% |
| **Oxytocin** | |
| Causes uterus to contract when the oxytocin levels exceed those of estrogen and progesterone | Labor induction or augmentation; treatment for postpartum uterine atony |
| **Melanotropin** | |
| Increases after 8 wk gestation; activity increased by increase in adrenocorticotropic hormone (ACTH) during pregnancy | Responsible for chloasma ("mask of pregnancy"), linea nigra, deeper color of areola (around nipple) and genitalia |
| Deepens pigmentation | Women with histories of melanoma should delay pregnancy for about 3 yr following surgical excision |

## TABLE 2.2 BLOOD VALUES

| Consist of : | Non-Pregnant | Pregnant | Postpartum* |
|---|---|---|---|
| WBC | 4–11,000 | 9–16,000 (25,000 labor) | 20,000–25,000 within 10–12 d of birth, then returns to normal |
| RBC volume | 1600 mL | 1900 mL | Prepregnant level of 1600 mL |
| Plasma volume | 2400 mL | 3700 mL | Prepregnant level of 2400 mL |
| Hct (PCV) | 37–47% | 32–42% | At 72°, returns to prepregnant level of 37–42% |
| Hgb (at sea level) | 12–16 g/dL | 10–14 g/dL | At 72°, returns to prepregnant level of 12–16 g/dL |
| Fibrinogen | 250 mg/dL | 400 mg/dL | At 72°, returns to prepregnant level of 250 mg/dL |

*Postpartum values depend on factors of amount of blood loss, mobilization, and physiologic edema (excretion of extravascular water). Normal blood loss for vaginal birth of one fetus is 300–400 mL.

## TABLE 2.3 COMMON DISCOMFORTS DURING PREGNANCY

| Discomfort and Cause | Health Teaching |
|---|---|
| **Ankle edema**—normal and nonpitting; gravity | Rest legs often during day with legs and hips *raised* |
| **Backache**—increased elasticity of connective tissue, increased weight of uterus, and increased lumbar curvature | Correct posture, low-heeled, wide-base shoes; do pelvic rock often; maternity support belt, apply warm heat, rest |
| **Constipation**—decreased motility (hormones, enlarging uterus) and increased reabsorption of water; iron therapy (oral) | *Diet*—prunes, fruits, vegetables; drink plenty of water, ↑ fiber, exercise; *avoid:* enemas, mineral oil, laxatives. |

*(continued)*

## TABLE 2.3  COMMON DISCOMFORTS DURING PREGNANCY (continued)

| *Discomfort and Cause* | 🏠 *Health Teaching* |
|---|---|
| **Cramp in side or groin**—round ligament pain; stretching of round ligament with cramping | To get out of bed, turn to side, use arm and upper body and push up to sitting position |
| **Fainting (syncope)**—*early* pregnancy: due to slightly decreased arterial blood pressure; *late* pregnancy: due to venous stasis in lower extremities | *Elevate* feet; sit down when necessary; when standing, do *not* lock knees; *avoid* prolonged standing, fasting |
| **Fatigue (sleep hunger)**—first 3 mo; *cause:* possibly hormones; often returns in late pregnancy when physical load is great | Iron supplement if anemic—foods high in *iron, folic acid,* and *protein*; adequate rest, warm bath before bed; *avoid* eating large meals within two hours of bedtime; take naps |
| **Flatulence**—altered digestion from enlarging uterus and hormones | Maintain regular bowel habits, *avoid* gas-forming foods; antiflatulent may be prescribed |
| **Headache**—cause unknown; possibly blood pressure change, nutritional, tension (unless associated with pre-eclampsia) | If pain relief needed, consult physician (*avoid* over-the-counter drugs without prescription); reduce tension; eat frequent, small meals; drink plenty of fluids. |
| **Heartburn**—enlarging uterus and hormones slow digestion; progesterone → reverse peristaltic waves → reflux of stomach contents into esophagus | Physician may prescribe an *antacid; "flying exercise"; avoid* use of antacids containing sodium; do *not* lie down directly after eating; *limit fatty and fried* foods in diet; small, frequent meals |
| **Hemorrhoids**—varicosities around anus; aggravated by pushing with stool and by uterus pressing on blood vessels supplying lower body | As above, *avoid* constipation; use refrigerated witch hazel pads applied externally; use any other preparation with physician's advice |
| **Hot flashes**—heat intolerance, due to increased metabolism → diaphoresis | Alter clothing, bathing, and environmental temperature prn |
| **Insomnia**—fetal movements, fears or concerns, and general body discomfort from heavy uterus | Medication by prescription only; exercise; *side-lying positions* with pillow supports; change position often; back rubs, ventilate feelings |
| **Leg cramps**—pressure of enlarging uterus on nerve supplying legs; possible *causes:* lack of calcium, fatigue, chilling, and tension | Stretch affected muscle and hold until it subsides; *do not rub* (may release a blood clot, if present) |
| **Morning sickness**—first 3 mo; nausea and vomiting; may occur anytime, day or night; *cause:* hormonal, psychological, and empty stomach | Alternate dry carbohydrate and fluids hourly; take dry carbohydrate before rising, stay in bed 15 more minutes; *avoid:* empty stomach, offending odors, and food difficult to digest (food high in fat, for example) |
| **Nasal stuffiness**—due to increased vascularization; allergic rhinitis of pregnancy | Antihistamines and nasal sprays by *prescription only* |
| **Pelvic joint pain**—hormones relax connective tissue and joints and allow movement within joints | Rest; good posture; will go away after giving birth, in 6-8 wk |
| **Shortness of breath**—enlarging uterus limits expansion of diaphragm | Good posture; cut down/stop smoking; *position—supine* and upright |
| **Urinary frequency**—enlarging uterus presses on bladder, turgescence of structures from hormone stimulation; relieved somewhat as uterus rises from pelvis; recurs with lightening | *Kegel's exercises;* rule out urinary tract infection |
| **Vaginal discharge**—months 2–9, mucus, acid, and increases in amount (leukorrhea) | Cleanliness important; treat only if infection sets in; douche *contraindicated* in pregnancy |
| **Varicose veins**—lower legs, vulva, pelvis; pressure of heavy uterus; relaxation of connective tissue in vein walls; hereditary | Progressively worse with subsequent pregnancies and obesity; *elevate* legs above level of heart; support hose may help |

## Respiratory System

I. **Physiologic changes**

A. *Increased* tidal volume, vital capacity, respiratory reserve, oxygen consumption, production of $CO_2$.

B. Diaphragm elevated by approximately 3 cm, increased substernal angle → flaring of rib cage allowing for increase in tidal volume.

C. Uterine enlargement prevents maximum lung expansion in third trimester.

II. **Assessment**

A. Shortness of breath or dyspnea on exertion and when lying flat in third trimester (**Table 2.3**).

B. Nasal stuffiness due to estrogen-induced edema (**Table 2.3, p.29**).

C. Deeper respiratory excursion.

III. **Nursing care plan/implementation**

A. Goal: **health teaching.**

1. Sit and stand with good posture.

2. When resting assume *semi-Fowler's position.*

3. *Avoid* overdistention of stomach.

# Alterations Affecting Elimination

## Urinary System

I. **Physiologic changes**

A. Relaxation of smooth muscle results in conditions that can persist 4–6 wk after birth:

1. Dilatation of ureters.

2. *Decreased* bladder tone.

3. Increased potential for urinary stasis and *infection* (urinary tract infection [UTI]).

B. *Increased* glomerular filtration rate (50%) during last two trimesters.

C. *Increased* renal plasma flow (25–50%) during first two trimesters; returns to near normal levels by end of last trimester.

D. *Increased* renal-tubular reabsorption rate—compensates for increased glomerular activity.

E. Glycosuria common—reflects kidney's inability to reabsorb all glucose filtered by glomeruli (urine glucose *not* reliable index of diabetic status during pregnancy).

F. *Increased* renal clearance of urea and creatinine (creatinine clearance used as test of renal function during pregnancy).

G. Hormone-induced turgescence of bladder and pressure on bladder from gravid uterus (**Table 2.3, p.29**).

II. **Assessment**

A. Urinary frequency, first and third trimesters (**Table 2.3, p.29**).

B. Nocturia.

C. Stress incontinence in third trimester.

III. **Nursing care plan/implementation**

A. Goal: **health teaching.**

1. Void with urge, to prevent bladder distention.

2. Learn signs and symptoms of UTI.

3. Perform *Kegel's* exercises to reduce incontinence (**p. 39**).

## Gastrointestinal System

I. **Physiologic changes**

A. General *decrease* in smooth muscle tone and motility due to actions of progesterone (**Table 2.1**).

B. *Intestines*: slowed peristalsis, *increased* water reabsorption in bowel.

C. *Stomach*

1. Gastric emptying time is delayed (e.g., 3 hr vs. 1 ½ hr).

2. Gastric secretion of HCl and pepsin *decreases.*

3. *Decreased* motility delays emptying; *increased* acidity.

D. *Cardiac sphincter* relaxes.

E. Increasing size of *uterus* and displacement of *intraabdominal organs.*

F. *Gallbladder*: decreased emptying.

II. **Assessment (Table 2.3, p.28-29)**

A. Nausea and vomiting in first trimester.

B. Constipation and flatulence.

C. Hemorrhoids.

D. Heartburn, reflux esophagitis, indigestion.

E. Hiatal hernia.

F. Epulis—edema and bleeding of gums.

G. Ptyalism—excessive salivation.

H. Jaundice.

I. Gallstones.

J. Pruritus due to increased retention of bile salts.

III. **Nursing care plan/implementation**

A. Goal: **health teaching.** (see **Table 2.3, p.28-29**

1. *Nausea and vomiting*

a. *Avoid* fatty food; *increase* carbohydrates.

b. Eat small, frequent meals.

c. Eat dry unsalted crackers in a.m.

d. *Decrease* liquids with meals.

e. *Avoid* odors that predispose to nausea.

2. *Constipation and flatulence*

a. *Increase* fluids (6–8 8 oz. glasses/d).

b. Maintain exercise regimen.

c. *Add fiber* to diet.

d. *Avoid* mineral oil laxatives.

e. *Avoid* gas-producing foods (i.e., beans, cabbage).

3. *Heartburn and indigestion*

a. *Eliminate* fatty or spicy foods.

b. Eat small, frequent meals (6/d).

c. Eat slowly.

d. *Avoid* gastric irritants (i.e., alcohol, coffee).

e. Perform "flying exercises."

f. *Avoid* lying flat.

g. Take antacids *without sodium* or *phosphorus*.

h. Sip milk or eat yogurt with heartburn.

i. *Avoid* sodium bicarbonate.

4. *Hemorrhoids*

a. Increase *fluid and fiber* intake.

b. Maintain exercise regimen.

c. *Avoid* constipation and straining to defecate.

d. Take warm sitz baths.

e. Apply witch hazel pads (refrigerate).

f. *Elevate* hips and legs frequently.

g. Use hemorrhoidal ointments only with advice of health care provider.

# Alterations Affecting Nutrition (see also **p. 34, 36–39**)

I. **Physiologic changes**

A. *Gastrointestinal system*

1. Gingivae soften and enlarge due to *increased* vascularity.

2. *Increased* saliva production.

B. *Endocrine system*

1. *Increased* size and activity of pituitary, parathyroids, adrenals.

2. *Increased* vascularity and hyperplasia of thyroid.

3. Pancreas: *increased* insulin production during second half of pregnancy, needed to meet rising maternal needs; placental HPL and insulinase deactivate maternal insulin; may precipitate *gestational diabetes* in susceptible women.

C. *Metabolism*

1. *Basal metabolic rate (BMR): increases* 25% as pregnancy progresses, due to increasing oxygen consumption; protein-bound iodine (PBI) *increases* to 7–10; mcg/dL; metabolism returns to normal by sixth postpartal week.

2. *Protein*: need *increased* for fetal and uterine growth, maternal blood formation.

3. *Water retention: increased*.

4. *Carbohydrates*: need *increases* in order to spare protein stores.

a. *First half of pregnancy*—glucose rapidly and continuously siphoned across placenta to meet fetal growth needs; may lead to hypoglycemia and faintness.

b. *Second half of pregnancy*—placental production of anti-insulin hormones; normal maternal hyperglycemia; affects coexisting diabetes.

5. *Fat: increased* plasma-lipid levels.

6. *Iron*: supplements recommended to meet *increased* need for red blood cells by maternal/placental/fetal unit.

II. **Assessment**

A. Weight gain: 20–30 pounds (average gain, 24 pounds).

B. Normal pattern: first trimester, 1 pound/mo; remainder of gestation, 0.9–1 pound/wk.

III. **Nursing care plan/implementation**

A. Goal: **health teaching.**

1. Evaluate diet for adequacy of nutrient and caloric intake.

2. Evaluate cultural, religious, and economic influences on diet.

3. Review dietary recommendation for pregnancy with woman.

4. *Avoid* dieting in pregnancy (even if obese).

5. Supplement diet with *vitamins, iron*, or *folic acid* on advice of health care provider.

6. Ptyalism

a. Suck hard candies.

b. Perform frequent oral hygiene.

c. Maintain adequate oral intake (6–8 8 oz. glasses/d).

d. Use lip balm to prevent chapping.

7. Epulis

a. Frequent oral hygiene.

b. Use soft toothbrush.

c. Floss gently.

d. See dentist regularly.

# Alterations Affecting Protective Functions

## Integumentary System

I. **Physiologic changes**—estrogen-induced vascular and pigment changes.

II. **Assessment** (see **Table 2.1**)

A. *Increased* pigmentation (**p. 28**).

B. Striae gravidarum (stretch marks).

C. *Increased* sebaceous and sweat gland activity.

D. Palmar erythema (**p. 27**).

E. Angiomas—vascular "spiders" (**p. 27**).

III. **Nursing care plan/implementation**

A. Goal: **health teaching.**

1. Bathe or shower daily.

2. Reassure woman that skin changes decrease after pregnancy.

# Alterations Affecting Comfort, Rest, Mobility

## Musculoskeletal System

I. **Physiologic changes**

A. Progesterone, estrogen, and relaxin-induced relaxation of joints, cartilage, and ligaments.

B. Function in childbearing: increases anterior-posterior diameter of rib cage and enlarges birth canal.

**II. Assessment**

A. Complaint of pelvic "looseness."

B. Duck-waddle walk.

C. Tenderness of symphysis pubis.

D. Lordosis (exaggerated lumbar curve)—*increased* weight of pelvis tilts pelvis forward; to compensate, woman throws head and shoulders backward; complaint of leg and back strain and fatigue.

**III. Nursing care plan/implementation**

A. Goal: **health teaching.** (see **Table 2.3**, p.28-29)

1. Good body alignment—tuck pelvis under; tighten abdominal muscles.

2. Pelvic-rock exercises.

3. Squat; bend at knees, *not* at waist.

4. Wear low-heeled, sturdy shoes.

5. Advise against tight-fitting clothing interfering with circulatory return in legs.

6. *Modify exercise programs* during pregnancy. Calisthenic exercise in water is encouraged; however, swimming in water that is too cold or too hot (above 85-90°F) is to be *avoided*. The serious jogger may jog with her physician's permission. The pregnant woman should *not* exercise if the temperature and/or humidity is *high*. Women should *avoid* exercising on hard surfaces. Maternal arrhythmia is not associated with maximal exercise; exercise is safe up to 148 beats/min (approximately 70% of maximal aerobic power).

7. Travel during pregnancy is safest during the second trimester.

   a. During the *first* trimester: susceptible women may suffer *spontaneous abortion* if traveling to high altitudes or flying in unpressurized aircraft (some private planes).

   b. During the *third* trimester: susceptible women may experience *preterm labor* if traveling to high altitudes or flying in unpressurized aircraft (some private planes).

# Psychosocial–Cultural Alterations

I. **Emotional changes**—affected by age, maturity, support system, amount of current stresses, coping abilities, physical and mental health status. *Developmental tasks of pregnancy*:

A. Accept the pregnancy as real: "I am pregnant"; progress from symbiotic relationship with the fetus to perception of the child as an individual.

B. Seek and ensure acceptance of child by others.

C. Seek protection for self and fetus through pregnancy and labor ("safe passage").

D. Prepare realistically for the coming child and for necessary role change: "I am going to be a parent."

II. **Physical bases of changes**

A. *Increased* metabolic demands may result in anemia and fatigue.

B. *Increased* hormone levels (steroids, estrogen, progesterone) affect mood as well as physiology.

III. *Characteristic behaviors*: **Table 2.4** describes behaviors commonly exhibited in each trimester.

IV. *Sexuality and sexual expression*: Feelings and expressions of sexuality may vary during pregnancy as a result of maternal adaptations.

V. *Intrafamily relationships*

A. Pregnancy a maturational crisis for the family.

B. Requires changes in lifestyle and interactions

1. Increased financial demands.

2. Changing family and social relationships.

3. Adapting communication patterns.

4. Adapting sexual patterns.

5. Anticipating new responsibilities and needs.

6. Responding to reactions of others.

# Prenatal Management

I. **Initial assessment goal**: establish baseline for health supervision, teaching, emotional support, and/or referral.

II. **Objectives**

A. Determine woman's present health status and validate pregnancy.

B. Identify factors affecting and/or affected by pregnancy.

C. Describe current gravidity and parity.

D. Identify present length of gestation.

E. Establish an estimated date of delivery (EDD); **Naegele's** determination of EDD—subtract 3 mo, add 7 days to date of last menstrual period (LMP).

F. Determine relevant knowledge deficit.

III. **Assessment**: *history*

A. *Family*: inheritable diseases, reproductive problems.

B. *Personal*: medical, surgical, gynecologic, past obstetric, average nonpregnant weight.

1. *Gravida*—a pregnant woman.

   a. *Nulligravida*—woman who has *never* been pregnant.

   b. *Primigravida*—woman with a *first* pregnancy.

   c. *Multigravida*—woman with a *second or later* pregnancy.

## TABLE 2.4 BEHAVIORAL CHANGES IN PREGNANCY

| ► Assessment/Characteristics | ► Nursing Care Plan/Implementation |
|---|---|
| **First Trimester** | |
| Emotional lability (mood swings) | Encourage verbalization of feelings, concerns |
| Displeasure with subjective symptoms of early pregnancy (nausea, fatigue, etc.) | Validate normalcy of feelings, behaviors |
| Feelings of ambivalence | 🏠 **Health teaching**: diet, rest, relaxation, diversion |
| **Second Trimester** | |
| Accepts pregnancy (usually coincides with awareness of fetal movement, i.e., "quickening") | Encourage exploration of feelings of dependency, introspection, mood swings |
| Becomes introspective: resolves old conflicts (feelings toward mother, sexual intimacy, masturbation) | Discuss childbirth preparation and preparation for parenthood classes; refer, as necessary |
| Reevaluates self, lifestyle, marriage<br>Daydreams, fantasizes self as "mother"<br>Seeks out other women who are pregnant and new mothers | |
| **Third Trimester** | |
| Altered body image | Encourage verbalization of concerns, discomforts of late pregnancy |
| Fears body mutilation (stretching of body tissues, episiotomy, cesarean birth) | Help meet dependency needs; reassurance, as possible |
| Distress over loss of control over body functions (ptyalism, colostrum leakage, leukorrhea, urinary frequency, constipation, stress incontinence) | 🏠 **Health teaching**: *Kegel's* exercises; preparation for labor; anticipatory guidance and planning for needs of self, baby, and family in early postpartum |
| Anxiety for baby (deformity, death)<br>Fears pain, loss of control in labor<br>Acceptance of impending labor during last 2 wk (ready to "move on") | |

2. *Para*—refers to *past pregnancies* (not number of babies) that reached ≥ 20 wks gestation whether or not born alive).
   a. *Nullipara*—woman who has *not* carried a pregnancy to ≥ 20 wks; e.g., may have had one or more abortions.
   b. *Primipara*—woman who has carried *one* pregnancy ≥ 20 wks.
   c. *Multipara*—woman who has had *two or more* pregnancies that reached ≥ 20 wks.
   d. *Grandmultipara*—woman who has had *six or more* pregnancies that reached ≥ 20 wks.
3. Methods of recording gravidity/parity— several methods of describing gravidity and parity are in common use.
   a. One method—*GTPAL*—describes the number of **G**ravida (pregnancies), **T**erm (full-term) infants, **P**reterm infants, **A**bortions, and number of **L**iving children. Examples:
      (1) A woman who is pregnant for the *first* time and is currently *undelivered* is designated as 1-0-0-0-0. *After* giving birth to a full-term living neonate, she becomes 1-1-0-0-1.
      (2) If a woman's second pregnancy ends in abortion and she has a living child from a previous pregnancy, born at term, she is designated as 2-1-0-1-1.
      (3) A woman who is pregnant for the fourth time and whose previous pregnancies yielded one full-term neonate, premature twins, and one abortion (spontaneous or induced), and who now has three living children, may be designated as 4-1-1-1-3.
   b. Others record as follows: number gravida/number para. Applying this system to the examples given above, those mothers would be designated as follows:
      (1) G1P1
      (2) G2P1
      (3) G4P2
   c. Others include recording of abortions; based on above examples:
      (1) G1P1 Ab0
      (2) G2P1 Ab1
      (3) G4P2 Ab1.

IV. **Assessment**: initial *physical* aspects
  A. Height and weight.
  B. Vital signs.
  C. *Blood* work—hematocrit (Hct) and hemoglobin (Hgb) for anemia; type and Rh factor; tests for sickle cell trait, syphilis, rubella antibody titer, and Hepatitis B antibody (see also **Table 2.2**).
  D. Urinalysis—glucose, protein, acetone, signs of infection, and pregnancy test (HCG).
  E. Breast examination.
  F. Pelvic examination:
    1. Signs of pregnancy.
    2. Adequacy of pelvis and pelvic structures.
    3. Size and position of uterus.
    4. Papanicolaou smear.
    5. Smears for monilial and trichomonal infections.
    6. Signs of pelvic inflammatory disease.
    7. Tests for sexually transmitted diseases (STD): gonorrhea/chlamydia.
  G. *Validation of pregnancy*—physician or midwife makes differential diagnosis between presumptive/probable signs/symptoms of early pregnancy and other signs.
    1. **Presumptive symptoms**—*subjective* experiences:
      a. Amenorrhea—more than 10 days past missed menstrual period.
      b. Breast tenderness, enlargement.
      c. Nausea and vomiting ("morning sickness").
      d. Quickening (week 16–18).
      e. Urinary frequency.
      f. Fatigue.
      g. Constipation (50% of women).
    2. **Presumptive signs:**
      a. Striae gravidarum, linea nigra, chloasma (after week 16).
      b. Increased basal body temperature (BBT).
    3. **Probable signs**—examiner's *objective* findings:
      a. Positive pregnancy test.
      b. Enlargement of abdomen/uterus.
      c. Reproductive organ changes (after sixth week)
        (1) *Goodell's sign*—cervical softening.
        (2) *Hegar's sign*—softening of lower uterine segment.
        (3) Vaginal changes (*Chadwick's sign*): purple hue in vulvar/vaginal area.
      d. Ballottement (after 16–20 wk).
      e. *Braxton Hicks* contractions.
    4. **Positive signs:**
      a. Fetal heart tones.
        (1) Doppler: week 10–12.
        (2) Fetoscope: week 18–20.
      b. Examiner visualizes and feels fetal movements (usually after week 24).
      c. Sonographic examination

V. **Assessment**: *nutritional status*
  A. Physical findings suggesting poor nutritional status:
    1. Skin: rough, dry, scaly.
    2. Lips: lesions in corners.
    3. Hair: dull, brittle.
    4. Mucous membranes: pale.
    5. Dental caries.
  B. **Risk factors** at *onset* of pregnancy:
    1. Age: 15 yr or younger or 35 yr or older.
    2. Weight: less than 85% of standard weight for height or more than 120% of standard weight.
    3. Frequent pregnancies: three or more during a 2-yr period.
    4. Therapeutic diet required for a chronic disorder.
    5. Abuse of nicotine, alcohol, or drugs.
    6. Low socioeconomic status.
  C. **Risk factors** occurring *during* pregnancy:
    1. Low hemoglobin and /or hematocrit
      a. Hemoglobin less than 11 g.
      b. Hematocrit less than 33 mg/dL.
    2. Inadequate or excessive weight gain (see **p. 38**).
  D. Nutrition history.
  E. **Analysis/nursing diagnosis**
    1. *Nutrition deficit (less than body requirements)* related to anemia, vitamin/mineral deficit.
    2. *Nutrition excess (more than body requirements)* related to obesity.
  F. **Nursing care plan/implementation**
    1. Goal: **health teaching.** Nutritional counseling for diet in pregnancy and/or lactation.
  G. **Evaluation/outcome criteria**
    1. Woman's weight gain and pattern of weight gain are within normal limits.
    2. Woman's hemoglobin and hematocrit remain within normal limits.

VI. **Assessment**: *psychosocial aspects*
  A. Pregnancy: planned or not; desired or not.
  B. Present plans:
    1. Continue pregnancy, keep baby.
    2. Continue pregnancy, adopt baby out.
    3. Elective abortion.
  C. Cultural, ethnic influences on decisions: will influence range of activities, types of safeguarding actions, diet, and health-promotion behaviors.
  D. Parenting potential: actively seeking medical care and information about pregnancy, childbirth, parenthood.
  E. Family readiness for childbearing/child rearing:
    1. Physical maintenance.
    2. Allocation of resources: identify support system.
    3. Division of labor.
    4. Socialization of family members.

5. Reproduction, recruitment, launching of family members into society.
6. Maintenance of order (relationships within family).

F. Perceptions of present and projected family relationships.

G. Review lifestyle for smoking, drugs, ETOH (alcohol), attitudes to pregnancy, and health care practices.

**H. Analysis/nursing diagnosis**
1. *Role performance alteration* related to stress imposed by developmental tasks.
2. *Coping: individual, family impairment* related to stress caused by developmental tasks/crises.
3. *Family process alteration* related to developmental tasks. First baby may precipitate individual or family developmental crisis.

**I. Nursing care plan/implementation**
1. Goal: *provide anticipatory guidance/support.*
   a. Discuss mood swings, ambivalent feelings, negative feelings.
   b. Reinforce "normalcy" of such feelings.
2. Goal: *increase individual/family coping skills, reduce intrafamily stress.*
   a. Reinforce family strengths (both partners), sense of family identity.
      (1) Encourage open communication between partners; share feelings and concerns.
      (2) Increase understanding of mutual needs, encourage mutuality of support.
      (3) Increase tendency of mother to turn to partner as most significant person (as opposed to physician).
      (4) Enhance bond, success of childbirth preparation classes.
   b. Promote understanding/acceptance of role change.
      (1) Facilitate/support achievement of developmental tasks.
      (2) Reduce probability of postpartal psychological problems.
      (3) Promote family bonding.
3. Goal: **health teaching.**
   a. *Siblings:*
      (1) Alert parents to sibling needs for security, love.
      (2) Include sibling in pregnancy experience.
      (3) Provide clear, simple explanations of happenings.
      (4) Continue demonstrations of love.
      (5) Describe increased status ("big sister/brother").
      (6) Discuss possible misbehavior to gain attention.

   b. *Relatives*: alert parents to possible negative feelings of in-laws.
   c. Referral to childbirth preparation/parenting classes.
   d. Appropriate community referrals for financial assistance to decrease stress and provide aid.

**J. Evaluation/outcome criteria: The woman:**
1. Actively participates in pregnancy-related decision making.
2. Expresses satisfaction with decisions made.
3. Demonstrates growth and development in parenting role.
4. Prepares for the birth and for early parenthood.

# Antepartal Experience and Management

I. **General aspects of prenatal management**
   A. *Scheduled visits*
      1. Once monthly—until week 32.
      2. Every 2 wk—weeks 32–36.
      3. Weekly—week 36 until labor.

II. **Assessment**
   A. General well-being, signs of deviations, concerns, questions.
   B. Weight gain pattern.
   C. Blood pressure.
      1. By midpregnancy, diastolic and systolic blood pressure normally *falls* by 10–15 mm Hg.
      2. NOTE: For women who are obese, use thigh cuff to obtain accurate readings.
   D. Abdominal palpation:
      1. Fundal height; tenderness, masses, hernia.
      2. Fetal heart rate (FHR).
      3. *Leopold's* maneuvers for presentation.
   E. *Laboratory tests:*
      1. *Urinalysis*—for protein, sugar, ketones, signs of asymptomatic infection.
      2. *Venous blood*—for Hgb, Hct (done initially: VDRL, anti-Rh titer, sickle cell), hepatitis B antibody, human immunodeficiency virus (HIV) testing recommended for high-risk groups.
      3. Cultures (vaginal discharge; cervical scrapings, for *Chlamydia trachomatis*) prn.
      4. Tuberculosis screening.
      5. Maternal alpha-fetoprotein screen, 16–18 wk optimum time.
      6. Serum glucose screen, 24–28 wk.
   F. Follow-up on medications (*vitamins, iron*) and nutrition.

## TABLE 2.5 🍎 NUTRIENT NEEDS DURING PREGNANCY

| Nutrient | Maternal Need | Fetal Need | Food Source |
|---|---|---|---|
| **Calories** | Increased BMR | Primary energy source for growth of fetus | Carbohydrates: 4 Kcal/g<br>Proteins: 4 Kcal/g<br>Fats: 9 Kcal/g |
| **Minerals** | | | |
| Calcium (and phosphorus) | Increase in maternal Ca²⁺ metabolism | Skeleton and tooth formation | Milk and milk products, especially Swiss cheese* |
| Iron | Increase in RBC mass<br>Prevent anemia<br>Decrease infection risk | Liver storage (especially in *third* trimester) | Organ meats—liver, animal meat; egg yolk, whole or enriched grains; green leafy vegetables; nuts |
| **Protein** | Maternal tissue growth: uterus, breasts, blood volume, storage | Rapid fetal growth | Milk and milk products; animal meats—muscle, organs; grains, legumes; eggs, tofu, nuts |
| **Vitamins** | | | |
| A | Tissue growth | Cell development—tissue and bone growth and tooth bud formation | Butter, cream, fortified margarine; green and yellow vegetables |
| B's | Coenzyme in many metabolic processes | Coenzyme in many metabolic processes | Animal meats, organ meats; milk and cheese; beans, peas, nuts; enriched grains |
| Folic acid | Meet increased metabolic demands in pregnancy<br>Production of blood products | Meet increased metabolic demands, including production of cell nucleus material | Liver; deep-green, leafy vegetables |
| C | Tissue formation and integrity<br>Increase iron absorption | Tissue formation and integrity | Citrus fruit, berries, melons; peppers; green, leafy vegetables; broccoli; potatoes |
| D | Absorption Ca²⁺, phosphorus | Mineralization of bone tissue and tooth buds | Fortified milk and margarine |
| E | Tissue growth; cell wall integrity; RBC integrity | Tissue growth; cell integrity; RBC integrity | Widely distributed: meat, milk, eggs, grains, leafy vegetables |

*Swiss cheese contains twice the amount of calcium as 8 oz. of whole milk but only 0.09 as much lactose; therefore, it is a good source for those with lactose intolerance. Tofu (soybean curd) is also high in calcium, and contains *no* lactose.

III. **Common minor discomforts during pregnancy**
  ▶ (For **Assessment**, see **Table 2.3**).
  A. **Etiology**: normal maternal physiologic/psychological alterations in pregnancy.
  ▶ B. **Nursing care plan/implementation**
    1. Goal: *anticipatory guidance*. Discuss the importance of adequate rest, exercise, diet, and hydration in minimizing symptoms.
    🏠 2. Goal: **health teaching.** (see **Table 2.3**)
  ▶ C. **Evaluation/outcome criteria**: avoids, minimizes, and/or copes effectively with minor usual discomforts of pregnancy.
🍎 IV. **Nutrition during pregnancy and lactation**
  A. **Nutrient needs** (**Table 2.5** and **Figure 2.1**).
    1. **Milk group**—important for calcium, protein of high biologic value, and other vitamins and minerals.
      a. *Pregnancy*—three to four servings.

  b. *Lactation*—four to five servings.
  c. *Count as one serving*—1 cup milk, ½ cup undiluted evaporated milk, ¼ cup dry milk, 1¼ cups cottage cheese, 2 cups low fat cottage cheese, 1½ cups cheddar or Swiss cheese, or 1½ cups ice cream.
  2. **Meat group**—important for protein, iron, and many B vitamins.
    a. *Pregnancy*—three servings.
    b. *Lactation*—two servings.
    c. *Count as one serving* (12–14 g protein)—6–8 ounces lean meat, fish, or poultry; two eggs; two frankfurters; 4 tbsp peanut butter; or 1 cup cooked dry beans, dry peas, or lentils.
  3. **Vegetable and fruit groups**—vitamins and minerals (especially A and C) and roughage.
    a. *Pregnancy*—five to six servings.

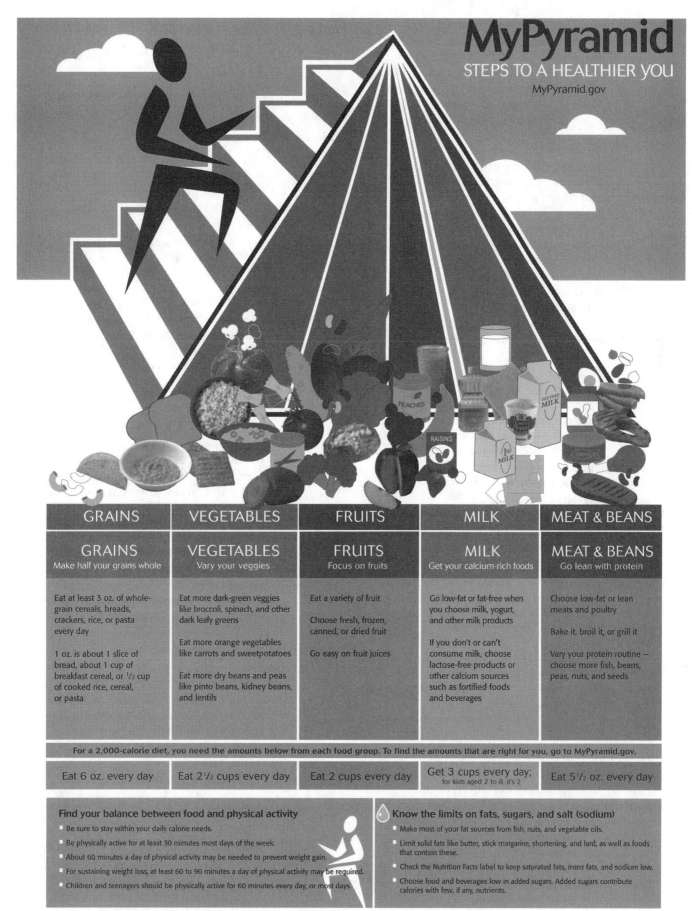

**FIGURE 2.1   FOOD GUIDE PYRAMID: A GUIDE TO DAILY FOOD CHOICES**

(United States Department of Agriculture). *Source*: http://www.mypyramid.gov

b. *Lactation*—five to six servings.
c. *Count as one serving*—one-half medium grapefruit; one medium apple, banana, or orange; ¾ cup fruit juice.
d. *Good sources (vitamin C)*—citruses, cantaloupe, mango, papaya, strawberries, broccoli, and green and red bell peppers.
e. *Fair sources (vitamin C)*—tomatoes, honeydew melon, asparagus tips, raw cabbage, collards, kale, mustard greens, potatoes (white and sweet), spinach, and turnip greens.
f. *Good sources (vitamin A)*—dark green or deep yellow vegetables and a few fruits (apricots, broccoli, pumpkin, sweet potato, spinach, cantaloupe, carrots, and winter squash).
g. *Good sources of folic acid*—dark-green foliage-type vegetables.

4. **Bread and cereal group**—good for thiamine, iron, niacin, and other vitamins and minerals.
   a. *Pregnancy*—10 servings.
   b. *Lactation*—10 servings.
   c. *Count as one serving*—one slice bread, 1 ounce ready-to-eat cereal, ½ to ¾ cup cooked cereal, cornmeal, grits, macaroni, noodles, rice, or spaghetti.
5. **Water** (fluids)—six to eight 8 oz. glasses (1500–2000 mL)/d.
6. **Energy**—increase per day
   a. Pregnancy—300 calories (e.g., 1 cup low fat milk, 2 slices bread, and an orange).
   b. Lactation–500 calories (for each child).
7. **Weight gain**
   a. Average overall gain: 24–30 pounds; total of gain depends on prepregnancy weight for height (body mass index ), nutritional state (**Table 2.6**).
   b. Pattern:

| Trimester | Gain | Site |
|-----------|------|------|
| 1 | 1–2 kg (2–4 pounds) | Maternal tissues |
| 2 | Almost 0.4 kg (1 pound) per wk | Primarily in mother |
| 3 | Almost 0.4 kg (1 pound) per wk | Primarily in fetus |

c. *Consequences* of deviations from expected weight gain.
   (1) *Underweight before* pregnancy: low-birth-weight (LBW) infant.
   (2) *Inadequate* gain: LBW infants and intrauterine growth restriction (IUGR).
   (3) *Overweight before* pregnancy: gestational diabetes, large baby, hypertension, and pre-eclampsia.
   (4) *Excessive* gain: may indicate fluid retention and development of pre-eclampsia.

**TABLE 2.6   GUIDELINES FOR TOTAL WEIGHT GAIN RANGES FOR WOMEN WHO ARE PREGNANT**

| Pre-pregnancy BMI* | Recommended Weight Gain | |
|--------------------|-------|------|
| | Pounds | Kg |
| **Underweight** (BMI < 19.8) | 28–40 | 12.5–18 |
| **Normal Weight** (BMI 19.8–26.0) | 25–35 | 11.5–16 |
| **Overweight** (BMI > 26.0) | 15–25 | 7.0–11.5 |

If a **multiple** pregnancy (twins, triplets or more): will need to gain more weight during pregnancy, depending on the number of fetuses.
*BMI - body mass index

**V. Assessment** (see also **p. 34**)
  A. Interview—history including diet history and evaluation, food practices, living situation; access to food; inclusion or exclusion of any foods that could be problematic, such as adherence to a strict vegetarian diet, cultural, ethnic, religious food practices, or fad diets.
  B. Physical examination:
    1. General appearance, including height and weight, posture, muscle tone, nervous control, general vitality.
    2. Signs of *malnutrition*: dull, dry, brittle hair that is thin and sparse; rough, dry, scaly, pale skin; spongy, bleeding, or receding gums; unfilled caries, absent teeth; eye membranes dull; enlarged thyroid; rapid heart beat, abnormal heart rhythm; spoon-shaped, brittle nails.
    3. *Laboratory tests*—hemoglobin and hematocrit, serum folacin and $B_{12}$, serum albumin and total serum protein, glucose (urine and serum).

**VI. Analysis/nursing diagnosis**
  A. *Nutrition excess (more than body requirements)* related to a poor understanding of nutritional needs and optimal weight gain, cultural patterns, use of unneeded dietary supplements.
  B. *Nutrition alteration (high risk for more than body requirements)* related to same factors as for preceding diagnosis.

**VII. Nursing care plan/implementation**
  A. Goal: *discuss dietary needs and assist in developing a dietary plan with input relating to preferences.*
    1. *Ethnic* food patterns: **Table 2.7**.
    2. *Religious* considerations in meal planning.
      a. Orthodox Jews
        (1) Kosher meat and poultry.
        (2) *No* shellfish or pork products.
        (3) Milk and dairy products *cannot* be consumed with meat or poultry; requires separate utensils.

b. Conservative and Reform Jews: dietary practices may vary from religious laws.

c. Muslims: *no* pork or alcohol.

d. Hindus: vegetarians (cows are sacred).

e. Seventh-day Adventists
   (1) Vegetarianism is common (lacto-ovo).
   (2) *No* shellfish or pork products.
   (3) *Avoid* stimulants (coffee, tea, other caffeine sources).
   (4) *No* alcohol.

f. Mormons: *no* caffeinated coffee, tea, or alcohol.

3. Food list for ready reference in menu planning.

   a. **High cholesterol foods**—over 50 mg/100-g portion: beef, butter, cheese, egg yolks, fish, kidney, liver, pork, veal.

   b. **High sodium foods**—over 500 mg/serving: bacon—cured, Canadian; baking powder; beef—corned, cooked, canned, dried, creamed; biscuits, baking powder; bouillon cubes;cereal (dry), soup (canned), macaroni and cheese, cheese—cheddar, parmesan, Swiss, pasteurized American; olives—green, ripe; pickles; salad dressing—blue, Roquefort, French, Thousand Island; sausages—bologna, frankfurters; ham, salami, pizza; soy sauce; tomato catsup; tuna in oil.

   c. **High potassium foods**—more than 225mg/serving: all meats, poultry and fish; apricots, cantaloupe; avocado, spinach; banana, kiwi; lima beans; milk, potatoes; prunes, oranges, orange juice.

   d. **Foods high in B vitamins**
      (1) *Thiamine*: whole-grain cereals, bread, red meat, green leafy vegetables, legumes.
      (2) *Riboflavin*: milk, meat, eggs, cheese and peas.
      (3) *Niacin*: meats, fish, milk, eggs, legumes, nuts, potatoes.

   e. **Foods high in vitamin C**—oranges, strawberries, dark green leafy vegetables, potatoes, grapefruit, tomato, cabbage, broccoli, melons.

   f. **Foods high in iron, calcium, and residue**
      (1) *Iron*: breads; fish, tuna; poultry; organ meats; whole-grain cereals; shellfish; egg yolk; fortified cereal and flour; dried fruits—dates, prunes, apricots, peaches, raisins; vegetables—dark-green leafy, potatoes; dried beans and peas; peanut butter.

      (2) *Calcium*: milk—dry, skim, whole, evaporated, buttermilk; cheese—American, Swiss, hard; vegetables—kale; turnip greens; mustard greens; collards.

      (3) *Residue*: whole-grain cereals—oatmeal, bran, shredded wheat; breads—whole-wheat, cracked wheat, rye, bran muffins; vegetables—lettuce, spinach, Swiss chard, raw carrots, raw celery, corn, cauliflower, eggplant, sauerkraut, cabbage; fruits—bananas, figs, apricots, oranges.

B. Goal: make referrals as necessary—WIC (women, infants, and children) program or food stamps, etc.

C. Goal: **health teaching.** Supplementation, if ordered (e.g., take iron with vitamin C [citrus fruits, tomatoes, melons] when stomach is empty [take between meals]); *avoid:* bran, tea, coffee, milk, oxalates (in spinach and Swiss chard) and egg yolk when taking iron; keep this and all medications in a childproof container out of the reach of any children in the household. *Caution* against taking excessive amounts of vitamins.

VIII. **Evaluation/outcome criteria**

A. Woman remains healthy during pregnancy, shows adequate weight gain, and carries the pregnancy to term.

B. Fetus is of adequate weight for age and shows no signs of maternal malnutrition.

# Childbirth Preparation/Parent Education

Most programs are a combination of the following methods.

I. **Methods:**

A. *Grantly Dick-Read*: Childbirth is viewed as a natural event; education decreases fear and tension, and therefore pain; exercises improve *muscle* tone, increase relaxation; emphasis is on *slow* breathing, muscle relaxation, and *pushing* techniques.

B. *Lamaze method (psychoprophylactic childbirth)*: Focus is on developing a conditioned response to stimuli that then occupies nerve pathways, dulling pain perception; this is known as the **gate control theory.** This conditioned response combines: relaxation, concentration on a focal point, and complex breathing patterns.

C. *Bradley ("father-coached")*: Similar to the Dick-Read method with the *addition* of a coach; emphasis is on *slow* breathing and *deep* relaxation.

II. Content

A. **General**: prenatal care, nutrition, labor and birth including cesarean birth, postpartum care, coping strategies: self-care, relaxation, breathing, and exercise. Most include asking the expectant parent(s) to develop a birth plan, which includes choice of attendant at labor and birth, birthing environment, type of pain control desired, etc.

## TABLE 2.7 🍎 ETHNIC FOOD PATTERNS—SELECTED EXAMPLES

| Ethnic Group | Cultural Food Patterns | Dietary Excesses or Omissions |
|---|---|---|
| African American | Milk with coffee; pork, poultry, eggs; fish; fruit: strawberries, watermelons; okra, collard greens, turnip greens, mustard greens, kale; sweet potatoes; cereals (including grits, hominy); corn bread; hot breads; molasses (dark molasses is especially good source of calcium, iron, vitamins $B_1$ and $B_2$, and niacin) | *Limited* use of milk group (lactose intolerance); extensive use of frying, "smothering," simmering for cooking; *large* amounts of fat: salt pork, bacon drippings, lard, gravies; may have *limited* use of citrus and enriched breads |
| Chinese (mostly Cantonese) | Cheese, soybean curd (tofu), many meats, chicken and pigeon eggs; nuts; legumes; many different vegetables, leaves, bamboo sprouts; rice and rice-flour products; wheat, corn, millet seed; green tea; mixtures of fish, pork, and chicken with vegetables—bamboo shoots, broccoli, cabbage, onions, mushrooms, pea pods | Tendency among some immigrants to use *excess* grease in cooking; may be *low* in protein, milk, and milk products (the latter may be due to lactose intolerance); often wash rice before cooking; large amounts of soy and oyster sauces, both of which are *high in salt* |
| Filipino (Spanish-Chinese influence) | Most meats, eggs, nuts, legumes; many different kinds of vegetables; large amounts of rice and cereals | May *limit* meat, milk, and milk products (the latter may be due to lactose intolerance); tend to prewash rice; tend to fry many foods |
| Italian | Staples are pasta with sauces; bread; eggs; cheese; tomatoes and vegetables such as artichokes, eggplant, greens, and zucchini; only small amount of meat is used | *Limited* use of whole grains; *insufficient* servings from milk group; tendency to overcook vegetables; enjoy sweets |
| Mexican (native) | Basic sources of protein—dry beans, flan, cheese, most meats, fish, eggs; chili peppers and many deep-green and yellow vegetables; fruits include: zapote, guava, papaya, mango, citrus; tortillas (corn, flour); sweet bread; fideo; tacos, burritos, enchiladas | *Limited* meats, milk, and milk products; some are using flour tortillas more than the more nutritious corn tortillas; *excessive* use of lard (manteca), sugar; tendency to boil vegetables for long periods of time |
| Middle Eastern (Greek, Syrian, Armenian) | Yogurt; predominantly lamb, nuts, dried peas, beans, lentils; deep-green leaves and vegetables; dried fruits; dark breads and cracked wheat | Tend to use *excessive* sweeteners, lamb fat, olive oil; tend to fry meats and vegetables; *insufficient* milk and milk products (almost no butter—use olive oil); *deficiency* in fresh fruits |
| Middle European (Polish) | Many milk products; pork, chicken; root vegetables (potatoes); cabbage; fruits; wheat products; sausages, smoked and cured meats; noodles, dumplings; bread; cream with coffee | Tend to use *excessive* sweets and to overcook vegetables; *limited* amounts of fruits (citrus), raw vegetables, and meats |
| Native American (American Indian—much variation) | If "Americanized," use milk and milk products; variety of meats: game, fowl, fish; nuts, seeds, legumes; variety of vegetables, some wild; variety of fruits, some wild, rose hips; roots; variety of breads, including tortillas, cornmeal, rice | *Nutrition-related problems*: obesity, diabetes, dental problems, iron-deficiency anemia; alcoholism; *limited* quantities of high protein foods depending on availability (flocks) and economic situation; *excessive* use of sugar |
| Puerto Rican | Milk with coffee; pork, poultry, eggs, dried fish; beans (habichuelas); viandas (starchy vegetables; starchy ripe fruits); avocados, okra, eggplant, sweet yams; rice, cornmeal | Utilize *large* amounts of lard for cooking; *limited* use of milk and milk products; *limited* amounts of pork and poultry |

B. Relaxation methods.
   1. Imagery, aroma therapy, music therapy, effleurage, biofeedback, hypnosis, yoga.
   2. **Kegel's exercises:** Woman locates the correct (pubococcygeal) muscles by stopping her flow of urine. Then she can perform the exercises in one of the following ways. *Slow:* tighten the muscle, hold it for the count of three, and relax it. *Quick:* tighten the muscle, and relax it as rapidly as possible. *Push out, pull in:* Pull up the entire pelvic floor as though trying to suck up water into the vagina. Then *bear down* as if trying to push the imaginary water out. This version uses abdominal muscles as well. Exercises should be practiced 10 times in a row, at least 5 times or more per day.

C. Programs offered during *different trimesters*:
   1. *First*: anatomy/physiology, fetal development, nutrition, sexuality, early discomforts.
   2. *Second* and *third*: same as above, and preparation for labor and birth, infant care, parenting.
D. *Family* programs: siblings and grandparents.
E. *Birthing environments*:
   1. Hospital: traditional; LDR (labor-delivery-recovery) rooms and/or LDRP (labor-delivery-recovery-postpartum rooms), with homelike accommodations.
   2. Freestanding birth center.
   3. Home birth.

**III. Assessment**
A. Knowledge of available resources, prenatal care, nutrition.
B. Available support system: who will coach?
C. Cultural and ethnic variations that apply.

**IV. Analysis/nursing diagnosis**
A. *Knowledge deficit* related to resources available, self-care during pregnancy and labor and birth.
B. *Individual coping impairment* related to lack of knowledge of childbirthing environment, comfort measures available.

**V. Evaluation/outcome criteria**
A. Parent(s) verbalizes satisfaction with information given regarding available childbirthing methods and environments.
B. Parent(s) verbalizes satisfaction with choices she/he made.
C. Parent(s) learn relaxation techniques, breathing patterns.
D. Parent(s) express feeling more confident and having less anxiety about the coming experiences.

## Warning Signs of Potential Problems

I. **Etiology**: Specific disease processes are discussed in Chapter 3.

**II. Nursing care plan/implementation**
A. Goal: **health teaching**: Safeguard status. Signs to report **immediately**:

| *Signs/Symptoms* | *Possible Causes* |
|---|---|
| Persistent vomiting beyond first trimester, or severe vomiting any time | Hyperemesis gravidarum |
| Fluid discharge from vagina—bleeding or amniotic fluid (anything other than leukorrhea) | Placental problem, rupture of membrane (ROM) |
| Severe or unusual pain: abdominal | Abruptio placentae |
| Chills or fever | Infection |
| Burning on urination | UTI |
| Absence of fetal movements after quickening | Intrauterine fetal death |
| Visual disturbances (blurring, double vision, "spots before eyes") | Pre-eclampsia |
| Swelling of fingers or face | Pre-eclampsia |
| Severe, frequent, or continual headache | Pre-eclampsia |
| Muscle irritability or convulsions | Pre-eclampsia |
| Uterine contractions > 6 per hour, menstrual-like cramping, pelvic pressure, low backache, or bloody spotting or leaking of fluid from vagina | Preterm labor |

**III. Evaluation/outcome criteria**: The woman/family:
A. Actively participates in own health maintenance/pregnancy management.
B. Identifies early signs of potentially serious complications during the antepartal period.
C. Promptly reports signs/symptoms and seeks medical attention.

# Summary

The prenatal period is one of growth and change in the woman and the fetus. Prenatal visits are scheduled to provide the maximum supervision during this critical period. The woman (family) needs to learn about the *alterations* in the body systems, some *common discomforts* and how to cope with them, *emotional changes, warning signs* that need to be reported immediately to the physician/midwife/nurse practitioner, *nutrition*, and *childbirth preparation resources*. This period presents the nurse with an ideal time to teach health maintenance because of the parents' heightened readiness to learn.

## 💡 Study and Memory Aids

### Sex Determination—Sex Chromosomes

| | |
|---|---|
| Female | XX |
| Male | YY |

### Stages of Prenatal Development

Ovum
↓
Embryo
↓
Fetus

### Prenatal Development by Trimester

| | |
|---|---|
| 1st | Organogenesis |
| 2nd | Growth |
| 3rd | Storage |

### Laboratory Values—General Effects of Pregnancy

↓ Blood values (dilution due to ↑ blood volume)
↑ Sedimentation rate
↑ WBC

### Recording Gravidity/Parity

**G**—**G**ravida
**T**—**T**erm
**P**—**P**reterm
**A**—**A**bortions
**L**—**L**iving children

### Validation of Pregnancy—"3 P's"

**P**resumptive signs and symptoms
**P**robable signs
**P**ositive signs

## Questions

1. The nurse is assessing the adequacy of the diet of a 30-year-old gravida 3, para 2, who is 4 wk pregnant. The woman has been a vegan-vegetarian (eats no eggs or dairy products) for 8 yr. To which food group(s) should the nurse pay particular attention?
   1. Grains.
   2. Protein foods.
   3. Vitamin C-rich foods.
   4. Fruits and vegetables.

2. The nurse is planning to do diet teaching for a 17-year-old primigravida at 30 wk gestation, who is diagnosed with iron-deficiency anemia. She takes her iron and vitamin supplements sporadically because of unacceptable gastrointestinal side effects, but eats many foods that are high in iron. Which nutrient will the nurse emphasize to promote heme production?
   1. Niacin.
   2. Vitamin A.
   3. Vitamin D.
   4. Folic acid.

3. The nurse knows additional nutrition counselling is needed when a woman states that her need for additional vitamin C intake increases if she:
   1. Smokes.
   2. Drinks more than 2 cups of caffeinated coffee each day.
   3. Uses oral hormonal contraceptives.
   4. Drinks more than 8 oz. of alcohol every day.

4. The nurse's health teaching about self-care related to "morning sickness" during pregnancy should include instructions to:
   1. Eat dry carbohydrates.
   2. Use antiemetics per physician's directions.
   3. Eat three large meals per day.
   4. Eat highly seasoned foods to increase taste appeal.

5. At midpregnancy, the nurse expects a woman's blood pressure (BP) to:
   1. Fall by 10–15 mm Hg.
   2. Increase by 10–15 mm Hg.
   3. Remain the same.
   4. Fall below her baseline, then rise above her baseline by the end of pregnancy.

6. During which time period in pregnancy should the nurse first expect a woman to experience physiologic anemia, relaxation of the ureters, linea nigra, and increasing introspection?
   1. First trimester.
   2. Second trimester.
   3. Third trimester.
   4. Postpartum.

7. In planning care with a woman who is pregnant, the nurse needs to consider that normal cardiovascular adaptations to pregnancy include:
   1. A 30–50% increase in blood volume.
   2. A decrease in sedimentation rate.
   3. A gradual increase in blood pressure.
   4. An immediate increase in hematocrit.

8. During a childbirth education class, a woman in her 6th month of pregnancy expresses concern that she is "short of breath," feels her uterus up under her ribs, and wonders if she gets enough air for herself and her baby. To ease her anxiety, the nurse bases a response on knowledge that maternal adaptation allows for an increase in volume of tidal air, because:
   1. The diaphragm is displaced upward by about 3 cm.
   2. The heart is displaced upward and to the left of the midclavicular line.
   3. Expansion of lower ribs increases.
   4. Blood volume is increased by about one-third.

9. In preparing childbirth education classes, the nurse knows that one characteristic of the third trimester of pregnancy is that:
   1. Quickening occurs.
   2. The uterus becomes an abdominal organ.
   3. It is the best time to learn relaxation and breathing for labor.
   4. The mother experiences increased concern about acceptance of coming baby by husband and other children.

10. In the tenth week of pregnancy, a woman is concerned about her dark nipples and the dark line beginning from her symphysis pubis in the midline. The nurse explains that these pregnancy changes are temporary and are due to hyperactivity of the:
    1. Ovaries.
    2. Pituitary gland.
    3. Adrenal gland.
    4. Thyroid gland.

11. Ferrous sulfate, 300 mg every day, has been ordered for an adolescent who is pregnant. The nurse can best evaluate client compliance by:
    1. Asking her if her stools are black.
    2. Asking her if she is taking it as ordered.
    3. Assessing fundal height for fetal growth.
    4. Assessing hemoglobin and hematocrit.

12. The nurse instructs an expectant couple that travel during pregnancy is safest during which trimester(s)?
    1. First.
    2. Second.
    3. Third.
    4. All trimesters, equally.

13. The nurse is planning a preconception counseling class for a group of women who enjoy an active lifestyle that includes a great deal of exercise, such as jogging. The nurse needs to include in the plan teaching that maximal exercise during pregnancy has been associated with:
    1. Maternal arrhythmia.
    2. Maternal bradycardia.
    3. Fetal bradycardia.
    4. Fetal tachycardia.

14. To plan care for an adolescent who is pregnant, the nurse should ask her:
    1. "How are your parents taking your being pregnant?"
    2. "Did you get along with your mother when you were growing up?"
    3. "When did you become sexually active?"
    4. "Why did you become pregnant?"

15. A couple who is expecting request prenatal classes because they want "everything to go just right with this pregnancy."' The nurse knows that the primary purpose of prenatal classes is to:
    1. Prepare for childbirth.
    2. Experience childbirth without tension or fear in order to decrease the perception of pain.
    3. Minimize amount of analgesia and/or anesthesia the mother will need.
    4. Minimize the possibility of dystocia and/or medical/surgical intervention.

16. A prenatal nurse's intake interview must include an obstetric history as a basis for risk management. A woman who is pregnant with a history of one pregnancy that ended in a miscarriage at 11 wk should be recorded as a:
    1. Primigravida.
    2. Multipara.
    3. Gravida 1, para 1.
    4. Gravida 2, para 0.

17. A woman has had her initial clinic visit for a pregnancy of 8 wk duration. Before she leaves, the nurse tells her that at each prenatal visit she can expect to have:
    1. Finger stick for hemoglobin and hematocrit.
    2. Measurement of fundal height.
    3. Collection of urine for culture.
    4. An ultrasound test.

18. While giving her diet history, a woman who is pregnant indicates she cannot tolerate milk and does not eat meat. The nurse can suggest alternate protein-rich foods, such as:
    1. Pasta, cereal, and bread made with fortified flour.
    2. Broccoli, green beans, potatoes.
    3. Cooked dry beans, tofu, and peanut butter.
    4. Eggs, yogurt, nuts.

19. At the end of a prenatal class, the nurse evaluates the women's (couples') understanding of warning signs/symptoms during pregnancy. Which statement by a woman would indicate a need for further evaluation/intervention?
    1. "I will report any burning on urination and urinary frequency to my midwife."
    2. "I will see my eye doctor if I have a bad headache and blurred vision."
    3. "I will report severe vomiting to my doctor."
    4. "If I cough and have to sit up to breathe, I will call the doctor."

20. A woman's LMP started March 23; she "spotted a little" on April 23. The nurse tells her that she can expect to give birth on:
    1. January 16.
    2. January 30.
    3. December 16.
    4. December 30.

21. The nurse notes the following physiologic changes in the chart of a woman who is pregnant. Which changes are *abnormal*?
    1. Hgb ↑, sedimentation rate ↓, respirations 28, BMR ↓ 25%.
    2. Hct ↓, glucosuria, BP ↓, palpitations.
    3. Vaginal pH 6.5, pulse 92, urinary frequency, leukorrhea.
    4. Montgomery's tubercles, audible $S_1$–$S_2$ split, slightly ↓ clotting time, funic souffle.

22. The nurse knows intervention is required when a woman who is pregnant states that she relieves:
    1. Morning sickness by eating dry toast before getting out of bed.
    2. Leg cramps by plantar-flexing her foot to point her toes.
    3. Heartburn by bending at the knees instead of leaning over.
    4. Constipation by eating raw fruits, vegetables, and wheat bread.

23. To prevent heartburn, the nurse advises the woman who is pregnant to:
    1. Sleep lying flat in a lateral position.
    2. Eat dry, unsalted carbohydrates at bedtime.
    3. Bend from the waist.
    4. Avoid coffee or cigarette smoke.

24. A woman of standard weight for height (BMI [body mass index] 19.8–26) at the start of her pregnancy is encouraged by the nurse to gain:
    1. No more than 10 pounds.
    2. 10–20 pounds.
    3. 25–35 pounds.
    4. Just enough to keep her Hgb at a minimum of 12 g.

25. The nurse should counsel a woman who is pregnant that the lunch menu that provides the most calcium is:
    1. One cup low fat yogurt, rhubarb pie.
    2. Turkey on white toast, orange juice.
    3. Bagel with peanut butter, one ear of corn.
    4. Spaghetti and meatballs with tomato sauce.

26. The nurse should advise a woman who is pregnant that the snack that provides the most iron is:
    1. One ounce cheddar cheese and crackers.
    2. One cup tapioca pudding.
    3. One-half cup tuna salad and water wafers.
    4. One-half cup dried peaches or apricots.

27. A pregnant woman's obstetric history reveals one elective abortion and one child at home. The nurse determines her gravidity and parity to be:
    1. G-2, P-1001.
    2. G-3, P-1011.
    3. G-3, P-1111.
    4. G-3, P-0121.

28. During a childbirth education class for couples, a spouse/partner of a woman who is pregnant asks how to be of most assistance during the pregnancy. The nurse-led discussion identifies that the most helpful response would be to:
    1. Give sympathy regarding the discomforts of pregnancy.
    2. Assist with household duties.
    3. Meet the expectant mother's needs for affection and support.
    4. Encourage the expectant mother to keep her weight within prescribed limits.

29. In planning the care of a 16-year-old who is pregnant, the nurse should set goals based on the knowledge that the teen will most likely be:
    1. Self-centered.
    2. In need of instant gratification.
    3. Realistic in coping with stress.
    4. Emotionally independent from her parents.

30. Which finding needs further assessment to rule out cardiac decompensation in a woman who is pregnant?
    1. Exaggerated splitting of the first heart sound.
    2. Heart rate increased by 10–15 beats/min.
    3. Respirations: 25/min.
    4. Occasional shortness of breath at rest.

31. The nurse knows intervention is required when a woman who is pregnant states that she relieves:
    1. Morning sickness by eating dry toast before going to bed at night.
    2. Leg cramps by dorsiflexing her foot to point her heel.
    3. Heartburn by assuming the knee-to-chest position.
    4. Backache by wearing a maternity bra and low-heeled shoes.

32. A woman who is pregnant states that she has lactose intolerance and cannot drink milk, but knows how important calcium is during pregnancy. The nurse counsels her that a food source high in calcium and low in lactose is:
    1. Cottage cheese.
    2. Swiss cheese.
    3. Eggs.
    4. Yogurt.

# Answers/Rationale

1. (2) Vegetarians who omit dairy foods may be unable to meet the requirement for an additional 30 g protein per day over their nonpregnant needs. Individuals who have been vegetarians for some time usually have evolved diets adequate in grain intake (1), along with a wide variety of vitamin C-rich fruits and vegetables (3 and 4), which meet pregnancy requirements not only for vitamin C, but also for fiber and other nutrients. **AS, RE/KN, 4, PhI, Basic care and comfort**

2. (4) Folic acid (folacin) is essential for increased heme production for hemoglobin and prevention of megaloblastic anemia. Niacin (1) has no direct or indirect role in erythropoiesis or heme production. Vitamin A (2) is essential for *fetal bone growth* and tooth development. Vitamin D (3) is essential for *mineralization of bone tissue* and calcium and phosphorus absorption. **PL, COM, 4, PhI, Basic care and comfort**

3. (2) Since coffee does not increase one's need for additional vitamin C, additional counseling is needed. The actions in options 1, 3, and 4 *do* increase one's need for additional vitamin C. **EV, ANL, 4, PhI, Basic care and comfort**

4. (1) Eating dry carbohydrates, such as unbuttered toast, crackers, or popcorn, before arising slowly is one preventive measure. Others include avoiding unpleasant odors or greasy foods. Medications (2) are generally not prescribed for this discomfort of pregnancy. She should eat six small meals, rather than three large meals (3). Highly seasoned foods (4) can contribute to this discomfort. **IMP, RE/KN, 4, PhI, Basic care and comfort**

5. (1) At midpregnancy, the healthy woman's BP drops by about 10-15 mm Hg. If it remains at her baseline, she is observed for possible pre-eclampsia in her third trimester. The BP decreases *rather than* increasing (2) or remaining the same (3). The BP should rise to the woman's normal range, *not* above (4), by term. **EV, COM, 5, HPM, Health promotion and maintenance**

6. (2) Physiologic anemia, relaxation of ureters, linea nigra, and increasing introspection are usually seen first in the second trimester. The time periods in options 1, 3, and 4 are all incorrect: The maternal adaptations listed all appear first during the *second* trimester. **AN, RE/KN, 5, HPM, Health promotion and maintenance**

7. (1) There is a 30-50% increase in blood volume during pregnancy; therefore, the nurse can expect physiologic anemia, altered laboratory test results, altered response to blood loss, and increased stress on the cardiovascular system. An increase, *not* a decrease (2) is seen in the sedimentation rate, due to the increase in globulins and fibrinogen products. There is a small *drop* in BP, not increase (3), at midpregnancy, with a gradual rise to within the woman's normal range at term pregnancy. Initially, there seems to be a *drop* in hematocrit, not an increase (4), due to physiologic anemia. **AN, RE/KN, 6, HPM, Health pomotion and maintenance**

8. (3) The lower ribs expand; thus, tidal air volume can increase. Women can be reassured that although respiratory rate increases only slightly (2/min), they do breathe deeper. A feeling of shortness of breath is normal. Because of rib expansion plus breast development, a maternity bra is needed. Although the diaphragm is displaced upward by 3 cm (1), that adaptation does *not* result in an increase in volume of tidal air. Although the heart is displaced upward and to the left of the midclavicular line (2), that adaptation does *not* result in an increase in volume of tidal air. Although the blood volume is increased (4), that adaptation does *not* result in an increase in volume of tidal air. **IMP, RE/KN, 6, HPM, Health promotion and maintenance**

9. (3) The third trimester is the best time to learn relaxation and breathing for labor. The expectant mother experiences ambivalence in first trimester and introspection in second trimester. Thoughts of labor become foremost as the expected date of delivery approaches (e.g., she becomes ready to learn). Quickening, or feeling of life (1), is characteristic of the *second* trimester. The uterus becomes an abdominal organ (2) between the end of *first* and start of the *second* trimester. The feelings in option 4 usually surface during the *second* trimester. **AN, RE/KN, 5, HPM, Health promotion and maintenance**

---

**Key to Codes**

**Nursing process: AS,** assessment; **AN,** analysis; **PL,** planning; **IMP,** implementation; **EV,** evaluation. (See **Appendix J** for explanation of nursing process steps.)

**Cognitive level: RE/KN,** recall/knowledge; **COM,** comprehension; **APP,** application; **ANL,** analysis; **EVL,** evaluation; **SYN,** synthesis. (See **Appendix J** for explanation.)

**Category of human function: 1,** protective; **2,** sensory-perceptual; **3,** comfort, rest, activity, and mobility; **4,** nutrition; **5,** growth and development; **6,** fluid-gas transport; **7,** psychosocial-cultural; **8,** elimination. (See **Appendix L** for explanation.)

**Client need: SECE,** safe, effective care environment; **HPM,** health promotion and maintenance; **PsI,** psychosocial integrity; **PhI,** physiological integrity. (See **Appendix M** for explanation.)

**Client subneed:** See **Appendix M** for explanation.

10. (2) The melanotropin from the anterior pituitary gland increases during pregnancy; this hormone is responsible for increased pigmentation. Because of the feedback mechanism, the ovaries (1) are *quiescent* during pregnancy. Hyperactivity of the adrenal gland (3) results in symptoms of Cushing's syndrome, which are *not* seen during pregnancy. Hyperactivity of the thyroid gland (4) would manifest as increased temperature, pulse, and respirations. **IMP, RE/KN, 5, HPM, Health promotion and maintenance**

11. (4) Assessing hemoglobin and hematocrit provides evidence of compliance with prescribed therapy. Black stools (1) may or may not mean that she is taking the medication; they could also indicate internal GI bleeding. If asked about compliance (2), the adolescent will probably answer the way she thinks the nurse wants her to; in addition, she may feel threatened if asked whether she has "obeyed." Assessing fundal height (3) does not provide the data needed to evaluate client compliance with the medication. **EV, EVL, 6, HPM, Health promotion and maintenance**

12. (2) Travel during pregnancy is safest during the second trimester. If traveling to high altitudes or flying in unpressurized airplanes (some private planes), women who are susceptible may experience spontaneous abortion in the first trimester (1) and preterm labor in the third trimester (3). Therefore, travel is safest during the *second* trimester, not all trimesters (4). **IMP, RE/KN, 1, HPM, Health promotion and maintenance**

13. (3) Maximal exercise during pregnancy has been associated with fetal bradycardia. Maternal arrhythmia (1) is not associated with maximal exercise. Maternal exercise is safe up to 148 beats/min (approximately 70% of maximal aerobic power); at this level there is little risk of fetal bradycardia (2). Fetal bradycardia, *not* tachycardia (4), follows maximal exercise. **IMP, COM, 3, HPM, Health promotion and maintenance**

14. (1) To develop a therapeutic plan of care for the adolescent who is pregnant, it is important to know how the parents are reacting to the pregnancy. In addition, this tells the adolescent that the nurse understands that this is an emotionally-charged area. The questions in options 2, 3, and 4 are irrelevant and may sound judgmental and condescending to the adolescent. **IMP, COM, 7, PsI, Psychosocial integrity**

15. (1) Prenatal classes prepare parents for labor and childbirth, and possible unexpected outcomes. They also clarify misconceptions, and suggest various means of self-help (e.g., relaxation techniques). No one type of method can guarantee that all tension or fear will be *eliminated* (2), although the perception of pain may be decreased. Childbirth preparation does help the woman to cope better with the labor and may be one factor in minimizing the amount of pharmacologic pain relief she will need (3), but that is *not* the *primary* purpose of childbirth classes. Childbirth preparation may have a positive effect on the course of labor and the ability to cope with dystocia (4), but it *cannot* eliminate dystocia for some women, and *cannot* guarantee a labor/birth without medical/surgical intervention. **PL, COM, 5, HPM, Health promotion and maintenance**

16. (4) This is her second pregnancy; she is gravida 2. She has carried no pregnancy past the age of viability; she is para 0. She is a secunda gravida (pregnant for the second time), not a primigravida (1 and 3). She is a nullipara since she has not yet retained a pregnancy past the age of viability at 22 wk, *not* a multipara (2) or primipara (3). NOTE: Using the five-digit system (GTPAL), this woman is 2-0-0-1-0. This is her second pregnancy (2), she has carried no pregnancy to term (T), she has had no preterm births (P), she has had one abortion (A), and she has no living children (L). **AN, APP, 5, SECE, Management of care**

17. (2) She can expect fundal height to be measured at each clinic visit as one means of assessing the growth of the fetus. Hgb and Hct (1) are done at the initial visit and then repeated at about 30 - 32 wk in most cases. Urine cultures (3) are done only if there is an indication of urinary tract infection. An ultrasound (4) is not done for every woman. Some women may have one to determine fetal age and growth and development, or to rule out possible hydramnios, etc. **PL, COM, 5, HPM, Health promotion and maintenance**

18. (3) Cooked dry beans, tofu (a soybean product), and peanut butter all contain vegetable protein. Bread products alone (1) do *not* provide sufficient protein. The vegetables in option 2 are *not* high in protein. Yogurt (4) is a milk product, which she *cannot* tolerate. **IMP, APP, 4, PhI, Basic care and comfort**

19. (2) The nurse will need to intervene if the woman thinks that headache with blurred vision is reportable to an *eye* doctor; these symptoms may be indicative of pre-eclampsia, and should be reported to the woman's health care provider (physician/midwife). Women *should* report possible UTIs (1), hyperemesis gravidarum (3), or cardiac decompensation (4) to the physician or midwife, and therefore no intervention is needed. **EV, EVL, 2, HPM, Health promotion and maintenance**

20. (4) To determine the expected date of delivery (EDD), identify the start of the LMP, count forward 9 mo, and add 7 days. March 23 is the correct LMP, since about 25% of women "spot" during the time of their first missed period following conception. (Naegele's rule is used to calculate the due date; however, counting forward 9 mo from the LMP and adding 7 days is the easier method.) Options 1, 2, and 3 are all incorrect: None follows the known methods of calculating the expected date of delivery. NOTE: If the woman's cycles are extremely short or extremely long, the EDD is adjusted accordingly. **AN, APP, 5, HPM, Health promotion and maintenance**

21. **(1)** This list includes abnormal changes. Hgb normally *decreases* in pregnancy secondary to increased plasma volume (physiologic anemia); sedimentation rate normally *increases* (therefore, it cannot be used in evaluating for infection); respirations usually remain at the same rate; BMR *increases* by 25%. The other options list *normal* changes. Option 2: Hct *does* decrease as a result of physiologic anemia during pregnancy; glucosuria is *normal*; BP *does* decrease by 10-15 mm Hg during the second trimester; palpitations are *normal*. Option 3: Vaginal pH *is* less acidic (6.5) during pregnancy (making the woman more vulnerable to vaginal infections); pulse *does* increase about 10 beats/min; urinary frequency *is* common; leukorrhea (whitish, watery vaginal discharge in increased amounts) *is* common. Option 4: Montgomery's tubercles *do* become more prominent around the areola during pregnancy; the increased cardiac output and plasma volume *do* result in the audible $S_1$-$S_2$ split; the tendency to coagulate *increases*; the funic souffle is the sound of blood in the fetal umbilical cord (the souffle is the same as the FHR). **AN, ANL, 5, PhI, Reduction of risk potential**

22. **(2)** The nurse must intervene because plantar-flexing the foot will aggravate the cramp; the woman should *dorsiflex* her foot to point the *heel*, thus stretching the gastrocnemius muscle and relieving the cramp. For the other options, the nurse does not need to intervene; the woman who is pregnant *is* using the *correct* methods to prevent/relieve morning sickness (1), heartburn (3), and constipation (4). **EV, EVL, 3, HPM, Health promotion and maintenance**

23. **(4)** Coffee and cigarette smoke can increase the risk for heartburn because of their irritating effect on the stomach lining. She should sleep propped up on pillows, *not* flat (1); this position helps to keep the stomach from being compressed by the growing uterus, thus preventing stomach contents from entering the esophagus through the pregnancy-caused relaxed pyloric sphincter. Eating dry unsalted carbohydrates (2) before getting *out* of bed is a preventative measure for "*morning sickness*." Bending from the waist (3) encourages stomach contents to re-enter the esophagus through the relaxed pyloric sphincter; she should bend at the *knees*, not from the waist.

   ☼ The question asks for an intervention that *prevents* heartburn, not one that *treats/relieves* it (4). **IMP, APP, 3, HPM, Health promotion and maintenance**

24. **(3)** To meet energy needs for normal pregnancy, an adequate weight gain is necessary: for this woman, 25-35 pounds. The amounts in options 1, 2 and 4 are *not* within the range of weight gain recommended by the National Academy of Sciences. **IMP, ANL, 4, HPM, Health promotion and maintenance**

25. **(1)** One cup yogurt has 415 mg calcium; rhubarb pie has 211 mg. Calcium needs during pregnancy increase from 800 mg/d to 1200 mg/d. The other menus provide less calcium. Option 2: Turkey = 7 mg; orange juice = 27 mg. Option 3: Bagel = 9 mg; peanut butter = 9 mg; one ear of corn = 2 mg. Option 4: Spaghetti and meatballs with tomato sauce = 20 mg. NOTE: Calcium, HCl, and ascorbic acid are needed for the absorption of iron. **IMP, APP, 4, PhI, Basic care and comfort**

26. **(4)** Dried peaches have 5 mg iron; apricots have 3.6 mg. The other foods contain less iron: 1 ounce cheddar cheese (1) = 0.2 mg, 1 cup tapioca pudding (2) = 0.7 mg, and ½ cup tuna salad (3) = 1.4 mg. NOTE: The iron effect in the body is increased with vitamin C, and is decreased with milk (and other dairy foods), eggs, whole-grain bread and cereal, and tea. Iron supplements are to be taken 1 hr before or 2 hr after meals, with liquid (water, orange juice— but not with milk or tea). The nurse should caution women that their stools may appear black. **IMP, APP, 4, PhI, Basic care and comfort**

27. **(2)** This woman has been pregnant three times; therefore, she is a G3; she has had one full-term pregnancy, no preterm births, one elective abortion, and one living child. The numbers in options 1, 3, and 4 do not match her status. **AN, ANL, 5, HPM, Health promotion and maintenance**

28. **(3)** The mother who is pregnant needs affection and support to assist her transition to the mothering role. Although expressing sympathy (1) may help somewhat, it is a *less* active form of support than meeting her needs for affection. Assisting with household duties (2) is a definite "plus," but meeting her needs for affection and support takes priority at this time. Encouraging her about her weight (4) can be seen as controlling or scolding, and could be seen by her as nonsupportive. **IMP, COM, 7, PsI, Psychosocial integrity**

29. **(1)** Self-centeredness is characteristic of adolescence. Option 2 reflects a characteristic of a *younger* age (e.g., toddlers), although some adults may occasionally demonstrate this trait. Option 3 is incorrect since at this stage of psychosocial development, she has not developed cognitively to the point of being realistic in coping with stress. Option 4 is incorrect since she is only now learning how to become independent from her parents; pregnancy interrupts this developmental phase. **PL, RE/KN, 5, PsI, Psychosocial integrity**

30. **(3)** Rapid respirations, 25 breaths per minute or more, may suggest cardiac decompensation; further assessment is needed. The findings in options 1, 2, and 4 are *normal* manifestations of adaptations to pregnancy. NOTE: The woman should also be assessed for other symptoms of cardiac decompensation (increasing fatigue or dyspnea, or both, with usual activities; frequent coughing and feeling of smothering; palpitations), and for other

signs (irregular, weak, rapid pulse [100 beats per/min or more]; progressive, generalized edema; crackles [rales] at base of lungs; orthopnea; moist, frequent cough; cyanosis of lips and nail beds).
**EV, ANL, 6, PhI, Reduction of risk potential**

31. **(1)** The nurse must intervene since a dry, unsalted carbohydrate (toast, cracker, popcorn) should be taken before getting *out* of bed in the *morning*. For the other options, the nurse will *not* have to intervene because the woman who is pregnant *is* using the correct methods to prevent/relieve leg cramps (2), heartburn (3), and backache (4). NOTE: The knee-to-chest position also helps to expel burps and flatus. **EV, EVL, 4, HPM, Health promotion and maintenance**

Read the *entire* option.

32. **(2)** Swiss cheese is high in calcium and low in lactose, and therefore an excellent food source during pregnancy. The foods in options **1, 3,** and **4** are high in calcium *and* lactose.
**IMP, APP, 4, PhI, Basic care and comfort**

# High-Risk Conditions and Complications During Pregnancy

## Chapter Outline

- Key Points
- Key Words
- High-Risk Conditions
  — General Aspects
  — Disorders Affecting Fluid-Gas Transport: *Cardiac Disease*
  — Disorders Affecting Fluid-Gas Transport in Fetus: *Rh Incompatibility*
  — Disorders Affecting Nutrition: *Diabetes Mellitus*
    Antepartal Hospitalization
    Anticipatory Planning—Management of Labor
    Anticipatory Planning—Management of Postpartum Period
  — Disorders Affecting Psychosocial-Cultural Behaviors:
    *Substance Abuse*
  — Disorders Affecting Protective Function: *Infections:*
    Vaginitis
    Gonorrhea
    *Chlamydia Trachomatis*
    *Herpes Genitalis*
    Syphilis
    Pelvic Inflammatory Disease (PID)
    HIV-Positive Status and AIDS
      Woman who is HIV-Positive
      Newborn or Neonate with AIDS
    *Other Infections:*
    TORCH
    Chickenpox
    Tuberculosis
    Human Papillomavirus (HPV)
  — Age-Related Risk Factors:
    The Adolescent Who is Pregnant
    Mothers who are Older: Primigravida over Age 35
    Mothers who are Older: Multipara over Age 40
  — Other Medical-Surgical Conditions Placing Pregnancy at Risk:
    Asthma
    Sickle Cell Disease
    Systemic Lupus Erythematosus (SLE)
    Women Who Have Had Phenylketonuria (PKU)
    Cystic Fibrosis
    Hyperthyroidism
    Epilepsy
    Spinal Cord Injury (SCI)
    Life-threatening Situations
    Surgical Emergencies
  — Cancer and Pregnancy
    Breast Cancer
    Malignant Melanoma
    — Violence
      Rape: Sexual Assault
      Assault and Battery
      Trauma
- Common Complications: First Trimester
  — Emergency Conditions
  — Complications Affecting Fluid-Gas Transport: *Hemorrhagic Disorders*
    General Aspects
    Spontaneous Abortion
    Hydatidiform Mole (Complete)
    Ectopic Pregnancy
  — Complications Affecting Nutrition/Elimination: *Hyperemesis Gravidarum*
- Common Complications: Second Trimester
  — Emergency Conditions
  — Complications Affecting Comfort, Rest, Mobility: *Incompetent Cervix*
  — Complications Affecting Protective Functions: *Preterm Labor*
- Common Complications: Third Trimester
  — Emergency Conditions
  — Complications Affecting Sensory/Perceptual Functions:
    *Pre-eclampsia/Eclampsia* and *HELLP Syndrome*
  — Pharmacology: Hypertension in Pregnancy and Labor
  — Complications Affecting Fluid-Gas Transport:
    *Placenta Previa*
    *Abruptio Placentae*
  — Complications Affecting Comfort, Rest, Mobility:
    *Polyhydramnios*
- Diagnostic Tests To Evaluate Fetal Growth and Well-Being
  — Daily Fetal Movement Count (DFMC)
  — Nonstress Test (NST)
  — Contraction Stress Test (CST); Oxytocin Challenge Test (OCT)
  — Biophysical Profile (BPP)
  — Ultrasound
  — Amniocentesis
  — Analysis of Amniotic Fluid
  — Chorionic Villous Sampling (CVS)
- Summary
- Study and Memory Aids
- Questions
- Answers/Rationale

## 🔑 Key Points

- Risk factors affecting the pregnancy and fetus/neonate include *anatomic, physiologic, therapeutic, environmental*, and *idiopathic* events.
- *Hypertensive* disorders, *infections*, and *hemorrhage* are leading causes of maternal and perinatal morbidity and mortality worldwide.
- Effects of *alcohol* and *substance abuse, sexually transmitted diseases (STDs)*, and *genital and perigenital infections* are biologic events, for which all individuals have a right to expect objective, compassionate, and effective health care.
- Preexistent and concurrent endocrine, cardiovascular, and medical-surgical problems are *affected* by pregnancy, and *affect* the pregnancy and its outcome.
- Nurses skilled in home care can significantly affect the outcome of the pregnancy and the newborn.

# Key Words

Cardiac decompensation

Cerclage

Cullen's sign

Fomites

Gestational trophoblastic disease (GTD)

Glycosylated hemoglobin (HgbA$_{lc}$)

Kehr's sign

Learned helplessness

Phosphatidylglycerol

Rape trauma syndrome

Rh incompatibility

    Isoimmunization

    Coombs test

# High-Risk Conditions

## General Aspects

I. **Etiology**
   A. Normal alterations and increasing physiologic stress of pregnancy affect status of coexisting medical disorders.
   B. Conditions affecting mother's general health also affect ability to adapt successfully to normal physiologic stress of pregnancy.
   C. Aberrations of normal pregnancy.

II. **General goal:** *reduce incidence of health problems affecting maternal/fetal health and pregnancy outcome.*
   A. Identify presence of risk factors and signs and symptoms of complications early.

   B. Treat emerging complications promptly and effectively.
   C. Minimize effects of complications on pregnancy outcome.

III. **Assessment of** *risk factors:*
   A. *Age:*
      1. Adolescent, $\leq$ 17 yr.
      2. Primigravida, age 35 or older.
      3. Multigravida, age 40 or older.
   B. *Socioeconomic* level: lower.
   C. *Ethnic group/race*: higher perinatal/newborn mortality and morbidity among nonwhite groups.
   D. Previous pregnancy *history:*
      1. Habitual abortion.
      2. Multiparity greater than 5.
      3. Previous stillbirths.
      4. Previous cesarean birth.
      5. Preterm labor.
   E. *Multifetal pregnancy.*
   F. *Prenatal* care:
      1. Enters health care system late in pregnancy.
      2. Irregular/episodic prenatal care visits.
      3. Noncompliance with medical/nursing recommendations.
   G. *Pre- or coexisting medical disorders:*
      1. *Cardiovascular*: hypertension, heart disease (e.g., women who have taken methyldopa for hypertension for more than 1 yr may have direct and indirect Coombs'-positive hemolytic anemia).
      2. *Diabetes.*
      3. Other: *renal, respiratory, infections,* acquired immunodeficiency syndrome (*AIDS*).
   H. *Substance abuse.*

IV. **Nursing care plan/implementation**
   A. Goal: **health teaching** (discussed under specific health problem).
   B. Goal: *early identification/treatment of emerging health problems* (if any).
      1. Monitor status and progress of pregnancy.
      2. Refer for medical management, as necessary.
   C. Goal: *emotional support.*

V. **Evaluation/outcome criteria**. The woman (family):
   A. Understands present health status, interactions of coexisting disorder and pregnancy.
   B. Accepts responsibility for own health maintenance.
   C. Makes informed decisions regarding pregnancy.
   D. Minimizes potential for complications of coexisting disorder/pregnancy.
      1. Avoids factors predisposing to health problems.
      2. Understands and implements therapeutic management of coexisting disorder/pregnancy.

3. Increases compliance with medical/nursing recommendations.

E. Carries uneventful pregnancy to successful termination.

# Disorders Affecting Fluid–Gas Transport

## Cardiac Disease

I. **Pathophysiology**: cardiac overload → cardiac decompensation → right-sided failure → pulmonary edema.

II. **Etiology/risk factors**:
A. Congenital heart defects.
B. Valvular damage—due to rheumatic fever; most common lesion is mitral stenosis, which can lead to pulmonary edema and emboli.
C. Increased circulating-blood volume and cardiac output—exceeds cardiac reserve. Greatest risk: *after 28 wk gestation*—reaches maximum (30–50%) volume increase; *postpartum*—due to diuresis.
D. Secondary to treatment (e.g., tocolysis and betamethasone).
E. Pregnancy after valve replacement.

III. **Normal physiologic alterations** during pregnancy that *mimic cardiac disorders:*
A. Systolic murmurs, palpitations, tachycardia, and hyperventilation with some dyspnea on normal moderate exertion.
B. Edema of lower extremities.
C. Cardiac enlargement.
D. *Elevated* sedimentation rate near term.

IV. **Assessment**
A. Medical evaluation of cardiac status. Classification of severity of cardiac involvement:
1. *Class I*—least affected; asymptomatic with ordinary activity.
2. *Class II*—activities somewhat limited; ordinary activities cause fatigue, dyspnea, angina.
3. *Class III*—moderate/marked limitation of activity; common activities result in *severe* symptoms of fatigue, etc.
4. *Class IV*—most affected; symptomatic (dyspnea, angina) at rest; should *avoid* pregnancy.
B. **Emergency: cardiac decompensation**
1. **Subjective symptoms:**
a. Palpitations; feeling that her heart is "racing."
b. Increasing fatigue or difficulty in breathing, or both, with her usual activities.
c. Feeling of smothering and/or frequent cough.
d. Periorbital edema; edema of face, fingers (e.g., rings do not fit anymore), feet, legs.

2. **Objective signs:**
a. Irregular, weak, rapid pulse (≥ 100 beats/min).
b. Rapid respirations (≥ 25 breaths/min).
c. Progressive, generalized edema.
d. Crackles (rales) at base of lungs, after two inspirations and exhalations.
e. Orthopnea; increasing dyspnea on minimal physical activity.
f. Moist, frequent cough.
g. Cyanosis of lips and nail beds.

V. **Analysis/nursing diagnosis**
A. *Fluid volume excess* related to inability of compromised heart to handle increased workload (decreased cardiac reserve → heart failure).
B. *Gas exchange impairment* related to pulmonary edema secondary to heart failure (HF).

VI. **Nursing care plan/implementation**
A. *Medical management*
1. *Diuretics*, electrolyte supplements.
2. Digitalis
a. Dose may need to be higher because of dilution in the increased blood volume of pregnancy.
! b. *Alert*: shortens the length of labor.
3. *Antibiotics*: prophylaxis against rheumatic fever; treatment of bacterial infections during pregnancy.
4. *Anticoagulants*: **heparin** is preferred since its large molecule cannot easily cross placenta. Occasionally, sequelae may include maternal hemorrhage, preterm birth, stillbirth.
5. *Narcotics-antagonists* may be needed: naloxone hydrochloride (*Narcan*) or naltrexone hydrochloride (*Trexan*):
! a. Physical and emotional stress stimulate the production of endorphins, which have a depressive effect on the cardiovascular system and blood pressure; therefore, narcotics-antagonists may be needed.
6. Oxygen, as needed.
7. Mitral valvotomy for mitral stenosis often brings dramatic relief.
8. If woman is a transplant recipient:
a. Transplant recipients can become pregnant, but they need to postpone conception for 1–2 yr so that graft function stabilizes and immuno-suppressive agents can be given at maintenance levels.
b. Women with cardiac transplantation can have a successful pregnancy, but they are at increased risk for complications such as heart failure.

B. **Nursing management**: *home care*

🏠 1. Goal: **health teaching**.

    a. Need for compliance with therapeutic regimen, medical/nursing recommendations.

    b. Drug actions, dosage, necessary self-care actions (how to take own pulse, reportable signs/symptoms).

    c. Methods for *decreasing work of heart*:

        (1) Adequate *rest*—minimum 10 hr sleep each night; half-hr nap after each meal.

        (2) *Avoid* heavy physical *activity* (including housework), fatigue, excessive weight gain, emotional stress, infection.

        (3) *Avoid situations* of reduced ambient oxygen, such as smoking, exposure to pollutants, flight in unpressurized small planes.

🍎 2. Goal: *nutritional counseling*.

    a. Well-balanced *diet*; adequate protein, fresh fruits and vegetables, water.

    b. *Avoid* "junk food," stimulants (caffeine), excessive salt intake.

C. **Management of labor**: *anticipatory planning*

    1. Goal: *minimize physiologic and psychological stress*.

    2. *Medical management*:

        a. Reevaluation of cardiac status before estimated date of delivery (EDD) and labor.

        b. Regional anesthesia for labor/birth.

        c. Low-outlet forceps birth or vacuum extraction: episiotomy.

📧 3. **Assessment**: continuous

    a. Physiologic response to labor stimuli—frequent vital signs (*heart rate* most sensitive and reliable indicator of impending HF).

    b. Color, respiratory effort, diaphoresis.

    c. Contractions, etc.—same as for any mother in labor.

📧 4. **Nursing care plan/implementation**: *labor*

    a. Goal: *safeguard status*.

        (1) Report *promptly*: pulse rate over 100; respirations ≥ 25 between contractions.

      ☞ (2) Oxygen at 6 liters, as needed.

    b. Goal: *emotional support*—to reduce anxiety, facilitate cooperation.

        (1) Encourage verbalization of feelings, fears, concerns.

        (2) Explain all procedures.

    c. Goal: *promote cardiac function*.

        (1) *Position*—semirecumbent; support arms and legs.

    d. Goal: *promote relaxation/control over labor discomfort*. Encourage prepared childbirth breathing/relaxation techniques.

    e. Goal: *reduce stress on cardiopulmonary system*. Discourage bearing-down efforts.

    f. Goal: *relieve stress of pain, eliminate bearing-down*. Prepare for regional anesthesia.

    g. Goal: *maintain effective cardiac function*.

        (1) Administer medications, as ordered

💊 (e.g., digitalis, diuretics, antibiotics).

D. **Postpartal management**: *anticipatory planning*

    1. Factors increasing risk of cardiac decompensation:

        a. Birth → rapid, decreased intra-abdominal pressure → vasocongestion and rapid rise in cardiac output.

        b. Loss of placental circulation.

        c. Normal diuresis increases circulating blood volume → cardiac overload.

📧 2. **Assessment**

 ❗ a. Observe for tachycardia and/or respiratory distress.

 ❗ b. Monitor blood loss, I&O—potential hypovolemic shock, cardiac overload due to diuresis.

 ❗ c. Pain level—potential neurogenic shock.

    d. Same as for any mother who is postpartum (fundus, signs of infection, etc.).

📧 3. **Nursing care plan/implementation**: *postpartum*

    a. Goal: *minimize stress on cardiopulmonary system*.

        (1) Methods:

            (a) Rest, dangle, ambulate with aid.

            (b) Gradual increase in activity—as tolerated without symptoms.

            (c) *Position*: semi-Fowler's if needed.

            (d) Extra help with newborn care.

📧 VII. **Evaluation/outcome criteria**: The woman:

    A. Successfully carries uneventful pregnancy to term.

    B. Experiences no cardiopulmonary embarrassment during labor, birth, or postpartum.

# Disorders Affecting Fluid–Gas Transport in Fetus

## Rh Incompatibility

I. **Pathophysiology**—in a mother who is *Rh-negative*: Rh-positive fetal red blood cells enter the maternal circulation → maternal antibody formation → antibodies cross placenta and enter fetal bloodstream → attack fetal red blood cells → hemolysis → anemia, hypoxia.

A. The *pregnant mother who is Rh-positive* carries her infant (Rh negative or positive) without incident.

B. The *pregnant mother who is Rh-negative* carries an *infant who is Rh-negative* without incident.

C. The *pregnant mother who is Rh-negative usually* carries her *first child who is Rh-positive* without problems *unless* she has been sensitized by inadvertent transfusion with Rh-positive blood. NOTE: Fetal cells do not usually enter the maternal bloodstream until placental separation (at abortion, abruptio placentae, amniocentesis, or birth).

II. **Etiology**

A. The Rh factor is an antigen on the red blood cells of some people (these people are *Rh positive*); the Rh factor is dominant; a person may be homozygous or heterozygous for Rh factor.

B. A person who is *Rh-negative* is homozygous for this recessive trait—does *not* carry the antigen; develops antibodies when exposed to Rh-positive red blood cells (**isoimmunization**) via transplacental (or other) transfusion.

C. Following birth of an infant who is Rh-positive, if fetal cells enter the mother's bloodstream, maternal antibody formation begins; antibodies remain in the maternal circulation.

D. At time of next pregnancy with a fetus who is Rh-positive, antibodies cross placenta → hemolysis. NOTE: *Degree* of hemolysis depends on amount (titer) of maternal antibodies present.

III. Possible serious complication (fetal)—rare today.
**!** **Hydrops fetalis**—most severe hemolytic reaction: severe anemia, cardiac decompensation, hypoxia, edema, ascites, hydrothorax; may be stillborn.

IV. **Assessment**

A. *Prenatal—diagnostic procedures*:
1. Maternal blood type and Rh factor.
2. **Indirect Coombs' test**—to determine presence of Rh sensitization (titer indicates amount of maternal antibodies).
3. **Amniocentesis**—as early as 26 wk gestation—amount of bilirubin by-products indicates severity of hemolytic activity.
4. Rho (Du antigen) immune globulin (RhoGAM) given between 28 and 32 wk to prevent maternal antibody formation.

B. *Intrapartal* observation of amniotic fluid (on membrane rupture):
1. Straw-colored fluid—mild disease.
2. Golden fluid—severe fetal disease.

C. *Postnatal*—see II. A. **Rh Incompatability, in Chapter 9, p. 201.**

V. **Nursing care plan/implementation**

A. Goal: *prevent isoimmunization in women who are Coombs'-negative.*
1. *Postabortion*—if no evidence of Rh sensitization (antibody formation) in the mother who is Rh-negative, administer RhoGAM.

2. *Prenatal*—if no evidence of sensitization, administer RhoGAM at 28 wk gestation, as ordered, to all women who are Rh-negative.

3. *Postpartum*—if no evidence of sensitization, administer RhoGAM to a mother who is Rh-negative within 72 hr of birth of a baby who is Rh+.

4. An injection of RhoGAM results in artificial passive immunity; it contains high concentrations of antibodies produced by another person. The new mother will have temporary benefit for as long as these antibodies are present.

B. Goal: **health teaching.**
1. Explain, discuss that RhoGAM suppresses antibody formation in susceptible women who are Rh-negative carrying a fetus who is Rh-positive. NOTE: Cannot reverse sensitization if already present.
2. RhoGAM required during and after each pregnancy, with fetus who is Rh+.

VI. **Evaluation/outcome criteria**: The woman:
A. Successfully carries pregnancy to term.
B. Shows no evidence of Rh isoimmunization.
C. Gives birth to viable infant.

# Disorders Affecting Nutrition

## Diabetes Mellitus

I. **Pathophysiology**: increased demand for insulin exceeds pancreatic reserve → inadequate insulin production; enzyme (insulinase) activity breaks down circulating insulin → further reduction in available insulin; increased tissue resistance to insulin; glycogenolysis/gluconeogenesis → ketosis.

II. **Etiology**: increased metabolic rate; action of placental hormones (see below), enzyme (insulinase) activity.

III. **Normal physiologic** alterations during pregnancy that may affect management of the woman who has *diabetes*, or *precipitate gestational diabetes* in women who are susceptible

A. Hormone production:
1. Human placental lactogen (hPL).
2. Progesterone.
3. Estrogen.
4. Cortisol.

B. *Effects of hormones and insulinase*:
1. *Decreased* glucose tolerance.
2. *Increased* metabolic rate.
3. Increased production of adrenocortical and pituitary hormones.
4. Decreased effectiveness of insulin (increased resistance to insulin by peripheral tissues).
5. Increased gluconeogenesis.
6. Increased size and number of islets of Langerhans to meet increased maternal needs.

7. Increased mobilization of free fatty acids.
8. Decreased renal threshold, increased glomerular filtration rate; *glycosuria* common.
9. Decreased carbon dioxide combining power of blood; higher metabolic rate increases tendency to *acidosis*.

C. *Effect of pregnancy on diabetes*:
1. Nausea and vomiting—predispose to ketoacidosis.
2. Insulin requirements—relatively stable or may decrease in first trimester; rapid *increase* during second and third trimesters; rapid *decrease* in postpartum to prepregnant level.
3. Pathophysiologic progression (nephropathy, retinopathy, and arteriosclerotic changes) may appear; existing pathology may worsen.

D. *Effect of poorly controlled diabetes on reproduction/ pregnancy*—increased incidence of:
1. Infertility.
2. Urinary tract infection (UTI).
3. Vaginal infections (moniliasis).
4. Spontaneous abortion.
5. Congenital anomalies (3 times as prevalent).
6. Pre-eclampsia/eclampsia.
7. Polyhydramnios.
8. Preterm labor and birth.
9. Fetal macrosomia—cephalopelvic disproportion (CPD).
10. Stillbirth.

IV. **Assessment**: *gestational diabetes mellitus*
A. History:
1. Family history.
2. Previous infant 4200 g or more.
3. Unexplained fetal wastage—abortion, stillbirth, or early neonatal death.
4. Obesity with very rapid weight gain.
5. *Polyhydramnios* (excessive amniotic fluid).
6. Previous infant with congenital anomalies.
7. Increased tendency for intense vaginal and/ or urinary tract infections.
B. Symptoms: *three "P's"—polydipsia, polyphagia, polyuria*—and weight loss.
C. *Abdominal assessment*:
1. Fetal heart rate.
2. Excessive fundal height
   a. Polyhydramnios.
   b. Large-for-gestational-age (LGA) fetus. *Note*: With vascular pathology, small-for-gestational-age (SGA) fetus.
D. *Diagnostic procedures*:
1. Abnormal glucose tolerance test (GTT): two or more of the following findings are not within normal limits (normal values follow).
   a. Fasting blood sugar (FBS)—under 95 mg/dL.
   b. One hr—under 180 mg/dL.
   c. Two hrs—under 155 mg/dL.
   d. Three hrs—under 140 mg/dL.

2. *Diabetic classification criteria*
   a. *Class A*—gestational or chemical diabetes (abnormal GTT).
   b. *Class B*—overt diabetes, onset after age 20, duration less than 10 yr, no vascular involvement.
   c. *Class C*—overt diabetes, onset before age 20, duration 10-20 yr, no vascular involvement.
   d. *Class D*—overt diabetes, onset before age 10, duration longer than 20 yr, vascular involvement, benign retinopathy, calcification of leg vessels.
   e. *Class E*—renal impairment.

3. *Glycosylated hemoglobin* (Hgb$_{Alc}$) provides a measurement of glycemic control over the past 90 days; < 6.5% = good glycemic control, > 8% = poor glycemic control. High levels are associated with spontaneous abortion and congenital anomalies.

E. *Assessment: Woman with known diabetes*—all classes.
1. Knowledge and acceptance of disease and its management.
   a. Signs and symptoms of hyperglycemia/ hypoglycemia (see **Table 3.1, p. 56**).
   b. Appropriate behaviors (e.g., skim milk for symptoms of hypoglycemia).
2. Skill and accuracy in monitoring serum glucose.
3. Skill and accuracy in preparing and administering insulin dosage; site rotation; subcutaneous injection.
4. Close monitoring—prenatal status assessment every 2 wk until 30 wk, then weekly until birth. Alert to signs of emerging problems (need for insulin adjustment, polyhydramnios, macrosomia).
5. Other—as for any woman who is pregnant.

V. **Analysis/nursing diagnosis**
A. *Knowledge deficit* related to pathophysiology, interactions with pregnancy, management (e.g., insulin administration).
B. *Nutrition alteration, more or less than body requirements*, related to weight gain.
C. High-risk pregnancy at *high risk for*: infection, ketosis, perinatal wastage, fetal macrosomia, cephalopelvic disproportion, polyhydramnios, preterm labor and birth, congenital anomalies.

VI. **Nursing care plan/implementation**
A. Goal: **health teaching.**
1. Pathophysiology of diabetes, as necessary; effect of pregnancy on management.
2. Signs and symptoms of hyperglycemia, hypoglycemia; appropriate management of symptoms.
3. Hygiene—to reduce probability of infection.
4. Exercise—needed to control serum-glucose levels, regulate weight gain, and for feeling of well-being.

5. Need for close monitoring during pregnancy.

6. Insulin regulation:

   a. Requirements vary through pregnancy: *first trimester*—may *decrease* with some periods of hypoglycemia due to fetal drain; *second trimester*—*increased* need for insulin; *third trimester*—needs may be triple prepregnant dose; *acidosis* more common in late pregnancy (precipitated by emotional stress, infection).

   b. Serum-glucose testing—dextrometer, acucheck, or other.

   c. Preparation and self-administration of insulin injection, as necessary.

   d. Prompt reporting of fluctuating serum-glucose levels.

7. *Diagnostic testing*/hospitalization:

   a. Nonstress test.
   b. Sonography.
   c. Amniocentesis.
   d. Amniotic fluid index (AFI).

B. Goal: *dietary counseling.*

   1. Optimal weight gain—about 24 pounds.
   2. > 1800 Kcal in at least six meals and snacks throughout the day.
   3. Protein: 0.8 gm/kg+10 gms.
   4. Carbohydrates: > 40% Kcal in complex form (milk, bread).
   5. Fats—unsaturated < 40% Kcal (< 10% saturated).

C. *Medical management*: hospitalize woman for:

   1. Regulation of insulin (oral hypoglycemics **contraindicated** in the 1st trimester of pregnancy, due to teratogenicity). Glyburide (oral agent) is being used in gestational diabetes (minimally crosses placenta).
   2. Control of infection.
   3. Determination of fetal jeopardy and/or indications for early termination of pregnancy.

VII. **Evaluation/outcome criteria**: The woman:

A. Understands and accepts diagnosis of diabetes.

B. Actively participates in effective management of diabetes and pregnancy.

C. Maintains serum-glucose levels within acceptable parameters (e.g., 60–90 mg/dL after fasting; 2 hr postprandial, less than 120 mg/dL).

   1. Monitors serum-glucose levels accurately (dextrometer, acucheck).
   2. Prepares and self-administers insulin appropriately.
   3. Demonstrates compliance with dietary regimen.

# Diabetes—Antepartal Hospitalization

I. **Assessment**

A. *Medical evaluation—procedures:*

   1. Serum-glucose levels (≤ 120 mg).
   2. Sonography for fetal growth: biophysical profile (BPP) evaluates fetal physical well-being and volume of amniotic fluid.
   3. Nonstress testing/contraction stress testing.
   4. Amniocentesis for fetal maturity (NOTE: lecithin-sphingomyelin [L/S] ratio may be *elevated* in women with diabetes); *phosphatidylglycerol* (*PG*) more accurate for women with diabetes.

B. **Nursing assessment**

   1. Daily weight, vital signs, fetal heart rate (FHR) q4h, I&O.
   2. Fundal height and Leopold's maneuvers on admission.

II. **Nursing care plan/implementation:**

A. Goal: *emotional support*—to reduce anxiety and tension, which contribute to insulin imbalance

   1. Explain all procedures.
   2. Assist with tests for fetal status.
   3. Prepare for possibility of preterm or cesarean birth.

# Diabetes: Anticipatory Planning—Management of Labor

I. **Assessment**: continuous

A. Signs and symptoms of hypoglycemia, ketoacidosis (hyperglycemia) (**Table 3.1**).

B. *Electronic fetal monitoring*—to identify signs of fetal distress.

C. Other—as for any woman in labor.

II. **Nursing care plan/implementation**

A. Goal: *safeguard maternal/fetal status.*

   1. *Position*: lateral Sims'—to reduce compression of inferior vena cava/aorta due to hydramnios or LGA baby. (*Supine hypotensive syndrome* results from compression; reduced placental perfusion increases incidence of fetal hypoxia/anoxia.)

III. *Medical management of labor*—varies widely.

A. Timing—*amniocentesis* to determine PG (phosphatidyl glycerol) and phosphatidylinositol levels (estimate fetal pulmonary surfactant).

B. Maintain maternal blood glucose between 70–110 mg/dL. Initiate insulin drip if blood glucose > 110. Use only short acting insulin. Initiate infusion of $D_5LR$ at 125 mL/hr if blood sugar < 70. *Avoid* rapid infusion (bolus) of $D_5LR$—can cause fetal acidemia. $D_5LR$ needed to prevent hypoglycemia that may lead to maternal ketoacidosis; hyperglycemia may result in newborn hypoglycemia.

C. Ultrasound to identify *macrosomia*; suggest delivery by cesarean section if estimated fetal weight > 4050 gms on ultrasound at 38 weeks.

*continued on p.57*

## TABLE 3.1 COMPARISON OF DIABETIC COMPLICATIONS

| | *Hypoglycemia* | *Ketoacidosis/Hyperglycemia* |
|---|---|---|
| **Pathophysiology** | Major metabolic complication when too little food or too large dose of insulin or hypoglycemic agents administered; interferes with oxygen consumption in nervous tissue | Major metabolic complication in which there is insufficient insulin for metabolism of carbohydrates, fats, and proteins; seen most frequently with clients who are *insulin dependent*; precipitated in the person with known diabetes by stressors (such as infection, trauma, major illness) that increase insulin needs |
| **Risk factors/causes** | Too little food<br>Emotional or added stress<br>Vomiting or diarrhea<br>Added exercise | Insufficient insulin or oral hypoglycemics<br>Noncompliance with dietary instructions<br>Major illness/infections<br>Therapy with steroid administration<br>Trauma, surgery |
| ◄ **Assessment** | **Behavioral change:**<br>*Subjective data*—nervous, irritable, anxious, confused, disoriented<br>*Objective data*—abrupt mood changes, psychosis<br><br>**Visual:**<br>*Subjective data*—blurred vision, diplopia<br>*Objective data*—dilated pupils<br><br>**Skin:** *Objective data*—diaphoresis, **pale**, cool, clammy, goose bumps (piloerection), tenting<br><br>**Vital signs:** *Objective data*—tachycardia; palpitations, thready pulse<br><br>**Gastrointestinal:**<br>*Subjective data*—hunger, nausea<br><br>*Objective data*—diarrhea, vomiting<br><br>**Neurologic:**<br>*Subjective data*—headache; lips/tongue: tingling, numbness<br>*Objective data*—fainting, yawning; speech: incoherent; convulsions; coma<br><br>**Musculoskeletal:**<br>*Subjective data*—weak, fatigue<br>*Objective data*—trembling | **Behavioral change:**<br>*Subjective data*—irritable, confused<br><br>*Objective data*—drowsy<br><br>**Visual:**<br><br>*Objective data*—eyeballs: soft, sunken<br><br>**Skin:** *Objective data*—loss of turgor, **flushed face**, pruritus vulvae<br><br>**Vital signs:** *Objective data*—respirations: Kussmaul's breath: fruity; BP: hypovolemic shock<br><br>**Gastrointestinal:**<br>*Subjective data*—increased thirst and hunger, abdominal pain, nausea<br>*Objective data*—vomiting, diarrhea, dry mucous membrane; lips, tongue: red, parched<br><br>**Neurologic:**<br>*Subjective data*—headache; irritability; confusion; lethargy, weakness<br><br><br><br>**Musculoskeletal:**<br>*Subjective data*—fatigue; general malaise.<br><br>**Renal:** *Objective data*—polyuria |
| | **Blood sugar: < 60mg/dL** | **Blood sugar: >180 mg/dL** |
| ◄ **Analysis/nursing diagnosis** | *Injury risk* related to deficit of needed glucose<br>*Knowledge deficit* related to proper dietary intake or proper insulin dosage<br>*Nutrition deficit* related to glucose deficiency | *Injury risk* related to glucose imbalance<br>*Knowledge deficit* related to proper balance of diet and insulin dosage |
| ◄ **Nursing care plan/ implementation** | Goal: *provide adequate glucose to reverse hypoglycemia*: administer simple sugar **STAT**, PO or IV; glucose paste absorbed in mucous membrane; monitor blood sugar levels: identify events leading to complication | Goal: *promote normal balance of food and insulin*: **regular** insulin as ordered; IV saline, as ordered; bicarbonate and electrolyte replacements, as ordered; potassium replacements once therapy begins and urine output is adequate |

*(continued)*

**TABLE 3.1   COMPARISON OF DIABETIC COMPLICATIONS** (*continued*)

| *Hypoglycemia* | *Ketoacidosis/Hyperglycemia* |
|---|---|
| ⌂ Goal: **health teaching**. Prevent further episodes; importance of careful monitoring of balance between glucose levels and insulin dosage | ⌂ Goal: **health teaching**. Diet instructions; desired effects and side effects of prescribed insulin or hypoglycemic agent (onset, peak, and duration of action); importance of recognizing signs of imbalance |
| ⊨ **Evaluation/ outcome criteria**    Adheres to diet and correct insulin dosage<br>Adjusts dosage when activity is increased<br><br>Target glucose level: 70–110 mg/dL | Avoids serious complications<br>Accepts prescribed diet<br>Takes medication (correct dose and time)<br>Target glucose level: 70–110 mg/dL |

Source: ©Lagerquist, S. *Davis's NCLEX-RN® Success*, Philadelphia, 2006.

## Diabetes: Anticipatory Planning—Management of Postpartum Period

I. **Risk factors** influencing serum-glucose levels:

   A. Loss of placental hormones that degrade insulin.

   B. Lower metabolic rate. Woman requiring large doses of insulin may need to triple caloric intake and decrease insulin by one-half.

⊨ II. **Assessment**

!   A. Observe for:

     1. Hypoglycemia.

     2. Infection.

     3. Pre-eclampsia/eclampsia (higher incidence in women who are diabetic).

     4. Hemorrhage (associated with polyhydramnios, macrosomia, induction of labor, forceps birth, vacuum-assisted, or cesarean birth).

   B. Monitor healing of episiotomy/abdominal incision.

⊨ III. **Nursing care plan/implementation**

   A. *Medical management*: insulin calibration—requirement may *drop* to one-half or two-thirds pregnant dosage on first postpartum day if woman is on full diet (due to loss of human placental lactogen and conversion of serum glucose to lactose).

   B. **Nursing management.**

☞   1. Goal: *euglycemia*. Acucheck, insulin as ordered.

     2. Goal: *avoid trauma, reduce risk of UTI. Avoid* catheterization, where possible.

⌂   3. Goal: **health teaching**. Nipple care—to prevent fissures and possible mastitis.

     4. Goal: *reduce serum-glucose and insulin needs*. Encourage/support breastfeeding → antidiabetogenic effect. NOTE: If *acetonuria* occurs, stop breastfeeding while physician readjusts diet/insulin balance; may pump breasts to maintain lactation. If *hypoglycemic*, adrenaline level rises → decreased milk supply and letdown reflex.

   C. *Anticipatory guidance*—**discharge planning.**

     1. Goal: *counseling*. Reinforce recommendations of physicians/genetic counselors.

       a. Risk of infant inheriting gene for diabetes is greater if mother has early-onset disease.

       b. Increased risk of congenital disorders.

     2. Goal: *family planning*.

       a. Oral contraceptives *not* recommended since they decrease carbohydrate tolerance; intrauterine device (IUD) *not* recommended—due to impaired response to infection. Barrier contraceptives (diaphragm or condoms with spermicides) recommended.

       b. Tubal ligation: if mother has vascular involvement, i.e., retinopathy or nephropathy, increased risk with later pregnancies.

⌂   3. Goal: **health teaching**.

       a. Self-care measures.

       b. Importance of eating on time, even if infant must wait to breast- or bottlefeed.

       c. Importance of adequate rest and exercise to maintain insulin/glucose balance.

       d. Organize schedule to care for infant, other children, and her diabetes. Allow time for self.

⊨   4. **Evaluation/outcome criteria**: The woman:

       a. Successfully completes an uneventful pregnancy, labor, and birth of a normal, healthy newborn.

       b. Makes informed judgments regarding parenting, family planning, management of her diabetes.

# Disorders Affecting Psychosocial–Cultural Behaviors:

## Substance Abuse

⊨ I. **Assessment** of **risk factors**: *pregnant substance abuser*

   A. *Medical history*:

     1. Infections: human immunodeficiency virus (HIV)-positive status, AIDS, STDs, hepatitis, cirrhosis of liver, cellulitis, endocarditis, pancreatitis, pneumonia.

2. Psychiatric illness: depression, paranoia, irritability.
3. Trauma related to violence.
B. *Obstetric history:*
   1. Spontaneous abortions.
   2. History of abruptio placentae.
   3. Preterm labor.
   4. Premature rupture of membranes.
   5. Fetal death.
   6. Low-birth-weight (LBW) infants.
C. *Current pregnancy:*
   1. Preterm labor contractions.
   2. Hypoactivity—hyperactivity in fetus.
      a. Maternal withdrawal from cocaine puts fetus at risk for intrauterine *asphyxia*. Its significant and agonizing withdrawal is felt as violent movements in utero.
      b. Maternal episodes of vasospastic hypertension cause numerous small strokes in the fetus.
   3. Poor or decreased weight gain.
   4. Sexually transmitted disease.
   5. Undiagnosed vaginal bleeding.
   6. Drugs being used and methods of self-administration.
D. *Psychosocial history:*
   1. Attitudes re: pregnancy.
   2. Current support system: lacking.
   3. Current living arrangements; lifestyle.
   4. History of psychiatric illness.
   5. History of physical, sexual abuse.
   6. Involvement with legal system.
E. *Physical examination.*
F. *Commonly abused substances:*
   1. Nicotine.
   2. Alcohol (fetal alcohol syndrome [FAS] or fetal alcohol effects [FAE]).
   3. Marijuana.
   4. Stimulants—cocaine, crack, ice.
   5. Opiates—heroin, methadone, propoxyphene hydrochloride (*Darvon*), oxycodone.
   6. Sedatives, hypnotics.
   7. Caffeine.

II. **Analysis/nursing diagnosis**
   A. *Nutritional excess* with weight gain related to poor nutritional choices.
   B. *Nutritional deficit* with slow fetal growth related to slow gain in weight.
   C. *Placental function alteration* related to high risk for abruptio placentae.
   D. *Noncompliance* with health care protocols related to persistent drug use.
   E. *Parenting alteration* related to psychological illness (substance dependence).

III. **Nursing care plan/implementation**
   A. Early identification of substance abuser.
   B. Urge consistent obstetric care.

C. Stabilize physiologic status.
D. Refer to substance abuse programs.
E. Refer for social services.
F. Surveillance of *neonatal outcomes:*
   1. LBW (low birth weight), small heads.
   2. Irritable, difficult to console.
   3. Disorganized suck-swallow reflex.
   4. Motor development: impaired
   5. Congenital anomalies: genitourinary, gastrointestinal, limb anomalies.
   6. Cerebral infarctions (strokes).
   7. Breastfeeding is **contraindicated** in women who are HIV positive, allowed in other substance abuse.
   8. Weight: poor, slow gain; failure to thrive.

IV. **Evaluation/outcome criteria**: The woman:
   A. Seeks out and utilizes social services and drug treatment program.
   B. Abstains from illicit substances during pregnancy.
   C. Successfully completes an uneventful pregnancy, labor, and birth of normal healthy infant.

# Disorders Affecting Protective Function: *Infections*

## Vaginitis—Inflammation of Vagina

I. **Pathophysiology**: local inflammatory reaction (redness, heat, irritation/tenderness, pain).

II. **Etiology/risk factors:**
   A. Common causative organisms:
      1. Bacteria—streptococci, *Escherichia coli,*gonococci, chlamydia.
      2. Viruses—herpes type II, cytomegalovirus (CMV), human papillomavirus (HPV).
      3. Protozoa—*Trichomonas vaginalis.*
      4. Fungi—*Candida albicans.*
   B. Atrophic changes—due to declining hormone level (postmenopausal women).

III. **Assessment**—differentiate among common vaginal infections:
   A. Vulvovaginal erythema.
   B. Pruritus, dysuria, dyspareunia.
   C. Vaginal discharge.
   D. Evaluate Papanicolaou (Pap) smear results, (e.g., to aid in identifying HPV).
   E. Evaluate enzyme-linked immunosorbent assay (ELISA) test results.

IV. **Analysis/nursing diagnosis**: *pain* related to inflammation, discharge.

V. **Nursing care plan/implementation**
   A. Goal: *emotional support.*
   B. Goal: **health teaching**. *Instruct woman in self-care measures to promote comfort and healing:*
      1. Perineal care.
      2. Sitz baths.
      3. Douching (as ordered). *Not* recommended during pregnancy.

4. Exposure of vulva to air.
5. Cotton briefs.
6. Medication: dosage/administration, action, side effects, expected outcomes.
7. Proper insertion of vaginal suppository.
8. Possible sequelae: e.g., abnormal Pap smear results, cervical intraepithelial neoplasia (CIN), pelvic inflammatory disease (PID), and infertility.
   C. Goal: *prevent reinfection.*
   1. Suggest sexual partner use condom until infection is eliminated—or abstain from intercourse.
   2. Recommend sexual partner seek examination and treatment.
   D. Goal: *medical consultation/treatment.* Refer for diagnosis and treatment.

VI. **Evaluation/outcome criteria**
   A. Woman is asymptomatic; unable to recover organism from body fluids or tissue.
   B. Woman avoids reinfection.

## Gonorrhea

I. **Pathophysiology:**
   A. *Men*—early infection usually confined to: urethra, vestibular glands, anus, or pharynx. If untreated, ascending infection may involve testes, causing sterility.
   B. *Women*—early infection usually confined to: vestibular glands, endocervix, urethra, anus (vagina is resistant). May ascend to involve pelvic structures, e.g., PID: fallopian tubes, ovaries; scarring may cause sterility.
   C. Women who are *pregnant*—may result in: premature rupture of membranes (PROM), amnionitis, preterm labor, postpartum salpingitis.
   D. Sequelae (untreated):
   1. May develop carrier state (asymptomatic; organism resident in vestibular glands).
   2. Systemic spread may result in gonococcal:
      a. Arthritis.
      b. Endocarditis.
      c. Meningitis.
      d. Septicemia.
   3. Pelvic inflammatory disease (PID) and impaired fertility.
   E. Newborn—*ophthalmia neonatorum* (gonococcal conjunctivitis). If untreated, sequelae is blindness.

II. **Etiology**: gram-negative diplococcus (*Neisseria gonorrhoeae*).

III. **Epidemiology**
   A. *Portal of entry*—oral or genitourinary mucous membranes.
   B. *Mode of transmission*—usually sexual contact; or via *fomites* (nonliving material on which disease-producing organisms may be conveyed, e.g., bed linens).

C. *Incubation period*: 2–5 d; may be asymptomatic.
D. *Communicable period*—as long as organisms are present; → 4 d after antibiotic therapy begun.
E. In the United States, adolescents have the highest prevalence of gonorrhea (and of *chlamydia trachomatis*) infection.

IV. **Assessment**
   A. History of known (or suspected) contact.
   B. *Men.*
   1. Complaint of mucoid or mucopurulent discharge.
   2. *Diagnostic procedure*: Gram-stain from urethral discharge.
   C. *Women.*
   1. Often asymptomatic; acute infection: severe vulvovaginal inflammation, venereal warts, greenish-yellow vaginal discharge.
   2. *Diagnostic procedure*: endocervical culture.
   D. *Gonococcal urethritis* (men and women)—sudden severe dysuria, frequency, burning, edema.
   C. *Salpingitis/oophoritis*—severe, sudden abdominal pain, fever (with or without vaginal discharge).

V. **Analysis/nursing diagnosis**: *Tissue integrity alteration* related to tissue inflammation.

VI. **Nursing care plan/implementation**
   A. Goal: *emotional support.*
   B. Goal: **health teaching.** Prevent transmission, sequelae, reinfection.
   1. Need for accurate diagnosis and effective treatment, follow-up examination in 7–14 d, and culture.
   2. All sexual partners need examination treatment.
   3. *Avoid* spread via fomites.
   4. Possible sequelae/complications (sterility, carrier state).
   5. *Avoid* multiple sex partners.
   6. Employ "safer sex" practices.
   C. Goal: *medical consultation/treatment.*
   1. Determine allergy to *penicillin, erythromycin, probenecid.*
   2. Refer for diagnosis and treatment.
      a. Treatment:*aqueous penicillin* G, 2.4 million units in each buttock (4.8 million units total dose), and *probenecid*, 1 g PO.
      b. Follow-up culture before birth.
      c. Notification of sexual partners.

VII. **Evaluation/outcome criteria**: The woman:
   A. Verbalizes understanding of mode of transmission, prevention, importance of examination treatment of sexual contacts.
   B. Informs sexual contacts of need for examination.
   C. Returns for follow-up examinations.
   D. Successfully treated; weekly follow-up cultures: negative on two successive visits.
   E. Avoids reinfection.

## Chlamydia Trachomatis

I. **Pathophysiology:**

    A. Most common sexually transmitted disease in U.S.; highest prevalence in adolescents.

    B. Initial infection mild in women; inflammation of cervix with discharge.

    C. If untreated, may lead to urethritis, dysuria, PID, tubal occlusion, infertility.

II. **Etiology/risk factors:**

    A. *Chlamydia trachomatis* has maternal-fetal effects.

    B. Bacteria can exist only within living cells.

    C. Transmission is by *direct contact* from one person to another.

III. **Assessment—*maternal***

    A. Inflamed cervix (may be asymptomatic).

    B. Cervical congestion, edema.

    C. Mucopurulent discharge.

IV. **Assessment—*fetal-neonatal***

    A. Stillbirth (increased incidence).

    B. Preterm birth may result.

    C. Contact with infected mucus occurs during birth.

    D. Newborn may be asymptomatic.

    E. Conjunctivitis → scarring.

    F. *Respiratory* problems: tachypnea, dyspnea, apnea. Pneumonia may result.

V. **Analysis/nursing diagnosis**

    A. *Pain* related to inflamed reproductive organs.

    B. *Fatigue* related to inflammation.

    C. *Knowledge deficit* related to mode of treatment, disease transmission.

VI. **Nursing care plan/implementation**

    A. Treatment with antibiotics, generally *erythromycin, tetracycline. Ophthalmic erythromycin* instilled into newborn's conjunctival sac.

    B. Provide pain relief (e.g., sitz baths), *analgesics.*

    C. **Health teaching.** Use of condoms (even during pregnancy) and spermicidal agents (containing *nonoxynol*-9) to prevent reinfection.

VII. **Evaluation/outcome criteria**

    A. Woman understands treatment and shows compliance.

    B. Woman understands portal of entry and risk for reinfection.

## Herpes Genitalis

I. **Pathophysiology**—initial infection: varies in severity of symptoms, may be local or systemic; duration: prolonged; morbidity: severe.

II. **Etiology**—herpes virus type II.

III. **Epidemiology**

    A. *Portal of entry*—skin, mucous membranes.

    B. *Mode of transmission*—usually sexual.

    C. *Incubation*: 3–14 days.

    D. *Communicable period*—while organisms are present may shed virus for 7 wk.

IV. **Assessment**

    A. Lesions—painful, red papules; pustular vesicles that break and form wet ulcers that later crust; self-limiting (3 wk).

    B. Severe itching and/or pain.

    C. Discharge—copious; foul-smelling.

    D. Dysuria.

    E. Lymph nodes—enlarged, inflammatory, inguinal.

    F. During pregnancy—vaginal bleeding, spontaneous abortion, fetal death.

    G. *Diagnostic procedures*: multinucleated giant cells in microscopic examination of lesion exudate; culture for herpes simplex virus (HSV).

V. **Analysis/nursing diagnosis**

    A. *Pain* related to inflammation process.

    B. *Fear* related to longevity of disease, no cure for disease.

    C. *Knowledge deficit* related to transmission to future partners.

VI. **Nursing care plan/implementation**

    A. Goal: *emotional support.*

    B. Goal: **health teaching.**

        1. Virus remains in body for life (dormant, noninfectious) in 25–30% of population; small percentage have symptoms.

        2. Recurrence probable; usually shorter and milder.

        3. Annual Pap smear important—associated with later development of cervical cancer.

        4. Need for close surveillance during pregnancy; cesarean birth may be indicated if active lesions.

        5. *Avoid* multiple sex partners; practice "safer sex."

    C. Goal: *promote comfort.*

    D. Goal: *accurate definitive treatment.* Refer for diagnosis and treatment.

        1. *Diagnostic procedure*: cervical smears.

        2. Treatment—*acyclovir* given from 36 wks until delivery to suppress outbreaks.

VII. **Evaluation/outcome criteria**

    A. Woman remains asymptomatic.

    B. Pregnancy continues to term with no newborn effects.

## Syphilis

I. **Pathophysiology:**

    A. *Primary stage*: nonreactive VDRL.

        1. *Men*: 3–4 wk after contact, painless, localized penile/anal ulcer (chancre); lymph nodes—enlarged, regional.

        2. *Women*: often asymptomatic; labial, vaginal, or cervical chancre.

    B. *Secondary stage*: reactive VDRL.

        1. Six to eight wk after infection.

        2. Rash—macular, papular; on trunk, palms, soles.

3. Malaise, headache, sore throat, weight loss, low-grade temperature.

C. *Latent stage*; reactive serologic test for syphilis (STS). Asymptomatic; noninfectious.

D. *Tertiary stage.*

1. Gumma formation in skin, cardiovascular or central nervous system.

2. Psychosis.

II. **Etiology**: *Treponema pallidum* (spirochete).

III. **Epidemiology**

A. *Portal of entry*—skin, mucous membranes.

B. *Mode of transmission*—usually sexual.

C. *Incubation period*—9 d–3 mo.

D. *Communicable period*—primary and secondary stages.

IV. **Assessment**

A. *Primary stage:* chancre, when detectable. *Medical diagnosis*—procedure: dark-field examination of lesion exudate.

B. *Secondary stage:*

1. Malaise, lymphadenopathy, headache, elevated temperature.

2. Macular, papular rash on palms and soles; may be disseminated.

3. *Medical diagnosis*—see **D.** below.

C. *Tertiary stage:*

1. Subcutaneous nodules (gumma).

2. NOTE: Gumma formation may affect any body system; symptoms associated with area of involvement.

D. *Diagnostic procedures*: (other than *primary stage*)—STS: **VDRL**, rapid plasma reagin (**RPR**), *Tr. pallidum* immobilization (**TPI**), fluorescent treponemal antibody absorption (**FTA**). *False-positive* STS in: collagen diseases, infectious mononucleosis, malaria, systemic tuberculosis.

V. **Analysis/nursing diagnosis**

A. *Pain* related to inflammation process.

B. *Knowledge deficit* related to treatment and transmission of the disease.

VI. **Nursing care plan/implementation**

A. Goal: *emotional support.*

1. Nonjudgmental.

2. Caring, supportive manner.

B. Goal: **health teaching.**

1. Need for accurate diagnosis and treatment, follow-up examinations.

2. All sexual partners need examination and treatment.

3. *Avoid* multiple sex partners; practice "safer sex."

C. Goal: *medical consultation/treatment.*

1. Refer for diagnosis and treatment. NOTE: In pregnancy—treatment by 18th gestational week prevents congenital syphilis in neonate; however, treat at time of diagnosis.

2. Treatment

a. *Primary, secondary stages—benzathine penicillin G,* 2.4 million units.

b. Other stages—7.2 million units over 3 wk period.

c. *Erythromycin* for clients who are allergic to penicillin.

VII. **Evaluation/outcome criteria**

A. If treated by 18th week of pregnancy, congenital syphilis is prevented.

B. Appropriate treatment after 18th week cures both mother and fetus; however, any fetal damage occurring before treatment is irreversible.

C. Follow-up *VDRL*: nonreactive at 1, 3, 6, 9, and 12 mo.

D. *Tertiary stage*—cerebrospinal fluid examination negative at 6 mo and 1 yr following treatment.

E. Woman verbalizes understanding of mode of transmission, potential sequelae without treatment, importance of examination/treatment of sexual contacts, preventive techniques.

F. Woman informs contacts of need for examination.

G. Woman returns for follow-up visit.

H. Woman avoids reinfection.

## Pelvic Inflammatory Disease (PID)

I. **Pathophysiology**: ascending pelvic infection; may involve fallopian tubes (*salpingitis*), ovaries (*oophoritis*); may develop pelvic *abscess* (most common complication), pelvic *cellulitis*, pelvic *thrombophlebitis, peritonitis.*

II. **Etiology**

A. *Chlamydia trachomatis.*

B. Gonococci.

C. Streptococci.

D. Staphylococci.

III. **Assessment**

A. Pain: acute, abdominal.

B. Vaginal discharge: foul-smelling.

C. Fever, chills, malaise.

D. Elevated white blood cell count.

E. Number of sex partners.

F. Sex practices (e.g., consistent use of "safer sex" practices).

IV. **Analysis/nursing diagnosis**

A. *Pain* related to occluded tubules.

B. *Infertility risk* related to permanent block of tubes.

C. *Knowledge deficit* related to transmission of disease.

D. *Urinary elimination alteration* related to dysuria.

V. **Nursing care plan/implementation**—for hospitalized woman:

A. Goal: *emotional support.*

B. Goal: *limit extension of infection.*

1. Bedrest—*position*: semi-Fowler's, to promote drainage.
2. *Force fluids* to 3000 mL/d.
3. Administer antibiotics, as ordered.

C. Goal: *prevent autoinoculation/transmission*.
1. Strict aseptic technique (handwashing, perineal care).
2. Contact-item isolation.
3. **Health teaching.** If untreated, high risk of: tubal scarring, sterility, or ectopic pregnancy, pelvic adhesions, transmission of disease.

D. Goal: *promote comfort*.
1. *Analgesics*, as ordered.
2. External heat, as ordered.

VI. **Evaluation/outcome criteria**
A. Woman responds to therapy; uneventful recovery.
B. Woman avoids reinfection.

## HIV-Positive Status and AIDS

I. **General aspects**: AIDS is a serious condition affecting the immune system. It is the fourth leading cause of death among women of reproductive age in the U.S. Heterosexual women are considered at risk if they or their sexual partners:
A. Are HIV positive.
B. Are IV drug users (50%).
C. Received blood between 1977 and 1985 (9%).
D. Are homosexual or bisexual men (39%).
E. Have hemophilia.

II. **Assessment**—general symptoms:
A. Malaise.
B. Chronic cough; possible tuberculosis.
C. Chronic diarrhea.
D. HIV positive.
E. Weight loss: 10 pounds in 2 mo.
F. Night sweats; lymphadenopathy.
G. Skin lesions; thrush.
H. PID; STDs; vulvovaginitis—usually yeast (*candidiasis*), often refractory and severe.
I. Cervical cytologic abnormalities; often infected with HPV.

III. **Analysis/nursing diagnosis**
A. *Nutritional deficit* related to general malaise.
B. *Fatigue* related to altered health status, weight loss.
C. *Fear* related to progressively debilitating disease.
D. *Knowledge deficit* related to disease progression, treatment, life expectancy.
E. *Individual coping impairment* related to disease progression.

IV. **Nursing care plan/implementation**
A. Identify women at risk.
B. Protect confidentiality.
C. Implement standard precautions:
1. Use proper gloves, gown, handwashing.
2. Use protective eyewear and mask in labor, birth.

V. **Evaluation/outcome criteria**
A. Further transmission of virus is avoided.
B. Woman's confidentiality maintained.
C. Standard precautions implemented.
D. Emotional support implemented.
E. Supportive groups contacted.

## Woman Who is HIV-Positive

I. *Antepartum*
A. **Epidemiology:**
1. Increased incidence of other STDs (gonorrhea, syphilis, herpes, HPV, candidiasis).
2. Increased incidence of CMV.
B. **Assessment:** differential diagnosis for all pregnancy-induced complaints.
C. **Health teaching.**
1. Counsel regarding nutrition.
2. Advise about risk to infant.
3. Counsel regarding safer sex (e.g., using condoms even during pregnancy).

II. *Intrapartum*
A. **Assessment**
1. External electronic fetal monitoring (EFM) preferred.
a. *Avoid* use of fetal scalp electrodes or sampling.
B. **Nursing care plan/implementation**
1. Goal: **health teaching.**
a. Focus on prevention of transmission (use standard precautions).
b. Mode of birth is not based on the disease.

III. *Postpartum*
A. **Pathophysiology**: no remarkable alteration in disease progression.
B. **Nursing care plan/implementation**
1. Breastfeeding **contraindicated**.
2. Implement standard precautions for mother and infant.
3. Refer to specialists in AIDS care and treatment.

IV. *Nurse with needle-stick injury should receive zidovudine (ZDV) STAT.*

V. **Health teaching.** Use an effective disinfectant against HIV, e.g. household bleach 1:10 (*sodium hypochlorite*).

## Newborn or Neonate with AIDS

I. **General aspects**: neonatal AIDS—exact mode of transmission unknown, but possibly transplacental, contact with maternal blood at birth, and/or postnatal exposure to a parent who is infected (i.e., breastfeeding).

II. **Assessment**
A. Classic signs evident in adult often not present.
B. *Common signs*: lymphadenopathy, hepatosplenomegaly, oral candidiasis, bacterial infections, failure to thrive.

C. If a new mother is HIV positive, newborn has an *ELISA test* for presence of HIV antibodies at 6 mo of age. (About 30–50% of infants of HIV+ mothers are HIV+.) A positive test indicates only that antibodies from the mother have passed to the fetus.

**III. Nursing care plan/implementation**

A. *Zidovudine* (ZDV) is the first-line therapy for HIV; it can reduce the rate of transmission during pregnancy from over 25% to just over 8%. Women can be offered the option of this medication starting at 14 wk gestation if they have not had it before and if their CD4 count is less than 200 mcg/L.

B. **Goal:** *provide supportive nursing care* (thermoregulation, respiratory).
   1. Monitor intake and weight gain.
   2. Observe for signs of infection.
   3. Bathe immediately after delivery in Palmolive liquid soap to decrease infant's contact with mother's blood.

C. **Goal:** *encourage parent-infant contact.*
   1. Provide opportunities for sensory stimuli and touch.

D. **Goal:** *referral.*
   1. Initiate social service consultation.

## Other Infections

I. *TORCH* infections (see **Table 3.2**).

II. Other infections of concern: Coxsackie virus B, *varicella* (*chickenpox*), influenza, listeriosis, Lyme disease, mumps (parotitis), parvovirus B-19, rubeola, *tuberculosis, human papillomavirus* (genital warts). Brief comments follow regarding selected infections.

A. *Chickenpox (varicella-zoster virus). Maternal consequences*: pneumonia, which could be life-threatening, and encephalitis with long-term neurologic sequelae. Therefore, exposed women who are not immune can receive *varicella-zoster immune globulin* (VZIG), which is considered safe to administer during pregnancy. The woman with varicella-zoster pneumonia is given *acyclovir*. Women with chickenpox at the time of birth should **not** have contact with their newborns until all vesicles have crusted. *Newborns* with varicella lesions should be *strictly isolated* from other hospitalized infants. The nurse must remember that transmission of this virus occurs through aerosol spray (sneezes) or through contact with vesicular fluid and cells from fresh skin lesions.

B. *Tuberculosis*. Pregnancy is not jeopardized by pulmonary tuberculosis, but spontaneous abortion does occur in one of five infected women. A woman who has had tuberculosis needs to wait 1 ½–2 yr after she is declared free of the disease before attempting pregnancy.

C. *Human papillomavirus* (HPV), responsible for venereal or genital warts, can have serious consequences for the woman and for her fetus/

newborn. It is the *most* common viral sexually transmitted infection—3 times greater than genital herpes. Having multiple sex partners increases the likelihood of HPV infection; other *risk factors* include smoking and use of oral contraceptives. Smoking and substance abuse impair the immune system.
   1. *Women*: Several strains are associated with cervical neoplasia, cervical intraepithelial neoplasia (CIN). Women who are at-risk need frequent *Pap* smears for early identification. Coexistence of herpes and chlamydia infection may play a role in development of CIN or invasive cervical cancer. In women under 18 yr of age, the metaplastic condition of the adolescent cervix, plus the other risk factors, may also increase the risk of cervical cancer.
   2. *Children*: congenitally-derived respiratory papillomatosis.

# Age-Related Risk Factors

## The Adolescent Who is Pregnant

I. *General aspects*
   A. Pregnancy in women ≤ 17 yr old have been declining each year since 1990.
   B. Incidence increasing dramatically; nationally approximately 15% of all births are to adolescents.

II. **Risk factors:** early menarche, early experimentation with sex (vaginal and cervical mucosa is not mature before age 18 yr)
   A. *Associated health problems*: pre-eclampsia/eclampsia, preterm labor, SGA infants, anemia, bleeding disorders, infections, cephalopelvic disproportion (CPD).
   B. *Social problems*: mothers who are poorly educated, child abuse, single-parent families, mothers who are unemployed or working at minimum wage, or who lack support system; poor family relationships, low socioeconomic status, late or no prenatal care.

III. **Assessment**
   A. Present physical/health status.
   B. Feelings toward pregnancy.
   C. Plans for the future.
   D. Factors influencing decisions related to self, pregnancy, baby.
   E. Signs and symptoms of complications of pregnancy (see **II. A.** above, *Associated health problems*).
   F. Potential for gestational diabetes.
   G. Need/desire for health maintenance information (family planning).
      1. Adolescents become sexually active an average of 15 mo before starting regular contraception.

## TABLE 3.2 ☼ TORCH INFECTIONS

| Infection | Maternal Effects | Fetal Effects | 🏠 Teaching/Nursing Implications |
|---|---|---|---|
| **T**oxoplasmosis | Flulike symptoms | Parasitemia | *Avoid* raw meat and litter from infected cats |
| **O**ther | | | |
| **H**epatitis A (infectious) | Abortion, fever | Anomalies, preterm birth | *Transmission*: droplet and hand contact<br>💊 Tx: gamma globulin |
| **H**epatitis B (serum) | Symptoms variable: fever, aching, etc. | Infected during birth | *Transmission*: contaminated needles, blood, etc.<br>💊 Tx: hepatitis B vaccine (series of 3) |
| **G**roup B streptococcus (GBS) | Miscarriage, preterm birth, fever, puerperal infection | Life-threatening neonatal infection | *Transmission*: from mother to infant during birth; transmission rate: 50 to 75% |
| **R**ubella | Usually mild infection | *First 2 mo*: malformations: heart, cataracts, damaged cranial VIII nerve (deafness), mental retardation | Vaccinate susceptible women after birth; woman signs informed consent to avoid pregnancy for 3 mo following vaccination |
| **C**ytomegalovirus (CMV) | Mononucleosis-like syndrome | Fetal or neonatal death; hydrocephaly, etc. | *Transmission*: transplacental infection or during birth; disease progresses through infancy/childhood |
| **H**erpes genitalis, type 2 | See **discussion, p. 60** | | |

Tx = treatment.

2. Most discontinue use within first year after starting contraception.
3. Adolescents frequently romanticize boyfriends' decisions not to use contraceptives as an affirmation of love or commitment.

◄ **IV. Analysis/nursing diagnosis**
 A. *Individual/family coping impairment* related to need to alter lifestyle, plans, expectations.
 B. *Family process alteration* related to unexpected/unwanted pregnancy.
 C. *Parenting alteration* related to intrafamily stress secondary to unexpected pregnancy, developmental tasks.
 D. *Self-esteem disturbance* related to altered self-concept, body image, role performance, personal identity.
 E. *Knowledge deficit* related to family planning, health maintenance, risk factors, pregnancy options.
 F. *Nutrition alteration* related to lifestyle.

◄ **V. Nursing care plan/implementation**
 A. Goal: *emotional support.*
  1. Assure confidentiality.
  2. Establish acceptant, supportive environment.
  3. Encourage verbalization of feelings, concerns, fears, desires, etc.

4. Maintain continuity of care—consistency of nursing approach, to establish trust, confidentiality.
 B. Goal: *facilitate informed decision making.* Discuss available options; aid in exploring implications of possible decisions.
 C. Goal: *nutritional counseling* (anemia).
  1. Needs for own growth and that of fetus.
  2. High-quality diet.
  3. Include pizza, hamburgers, milkshakes as acceptable—to minimize anger at being "different."
 D. Goal: **health teaching.**
  1. Rest, exercise, hygiene—as for other women.
  2. Prevention of infection—STD, UTI, etc.
  3. Breast self-examination; Pap smear.
  4. Future family planning options (see **Table 1.2, p. 10–12**).
 E. Goal: *assist in achievement of normal developmental tasks.* Developmental tasks of adolescence are interrupted by those of pregnancy. Encourage exploration of new role and responsibilities.
 F. Goal: *referral to appropriate resources.*
  1. Abortion.
  2. Preparation for childbirth and parenting classes that respect adolescents' needs and developmental level: use concrete examples, creativity, flexibility, humor.

3. Family counseling.

4. Social services.

G. Goal: *assist in facilitating continuing/completing basic education.*

   1. Communicate with school nurse.

   2. Explore other options available in community.

**VI. Evaluation/outcome criteria**

A. Adolescent makes informed decisions appropriate to individual and family needs, desires.

B. Adolescent actively participates in own health maintenance.

   1. Complies with medical/nursing recommendations.

   2. Minimizes potential for complications of pregnancy.

C. Adolescent copes effectively with normal physiologic and psychosocial alterations of pregnancy.

D. Both adolescent and baby's father express satisfaction with decision and management of this pregnancy. If parenthood is chosen and pregnancy is successful, accepts parenting role.

## Mothers Who are Older: Primigravida Over Age 35

**I. General aspects**: higher incidence of congenital anomalies (e.g., *Down syndrome*), increased possibility of complications of pregnancy; however, generally it is a conscious decision to have postponed childbearing. Individuals are usually used to making own decisions regarding career and health care.

**II. Assessment**

A. Same as for other women who are pregnant.

B. Reaction to reality of pregnancy.

C. Family response to pregnancy.

**III. Analysis/nursing diagnosis**

A. *Fear* related to threat to pregnancy.

B. *Knowledge deficit* related to aspects of pregnancy care.

**IV. Nursing care plan/implementation**

A. Goal: *anticipatory guidance.* Preparation for parenthood, altered lifestyle, potential change of career. Assist with realistic expectations. Refer to "over 30" parents' support group.

B. Goal: **health teaching.** Explain, discuss special diagnostic procedures. See **Amniocentesis, p. 82.**

C. Other—same as for other women who are pregnant.

**V. Evaluation/outcome criteria**

A. Woman experiences normal, uncomplicated pregnancy, labor, and birth of normal, healthy newborn.

B. Woman expresses satisfaction with decision and outcome of this pregnancy.

## Mothers Who are Older: Multipara Over Age 40

**I. General aspects**

A. Increased incidence of pre- and coexisting medical disorders (hypertension, diabetes, arthritis).

B. Increased incidence of complications of pregnancy (hypertension, hemorrhage).

C. **Major risk factor**: smoking

**II. Assessment**

A. Same as for other women who are pregnant.

B. Reaction to pregnancy (varies from pleasure at still being "young enough," to despair, if facing decision to abort).

C. History, signs and symptoms of coexisting disorders.

D. Indications of reduced physical ability to cope with normal physiologic alterations of pregnancy.

E. Family constellation: stage of family developmental cycle, responses to this pregnancy (especially adolescents' reaction to mother's pregnancy).

**III. Analysis/nursing diagnosis**: same as for over 35 age group.

**IV. Nursing care plan/implementation**

A. Goal: *emotional support.* Encourage verbalization of feelings, fears, concerns.

B. Goal: *referral to appropriate resource.*

   1. Genetic counseling.

   2. Abortion/support groups.

   3. Preparation for childbirth and parenthood classes.

C. Goal: *facilitate/support effective family process.* Involve family in preparation for birth and integration of newborn into family unit.

D. Other—same as for other women who are pregnant.

**V. Evaluation/outcome criteria**

A. Woman makes informed decisions related to pregnancy.

B. Woman expresses satisfaction with decision and outcome of this pregnancy.

C. Woman experiences uncomplicated pregnancy, labor, and birth of normal, healthy newborn.

# Other Medical-Surgical Conditions Placing Pregnancy at Risk

## Asthma: Medical Management

**I.** Effect on pregnancy is unpredictable.

**II.** Woman with preexisting asthma has an increased possibility of: hyperemesis, hemorrhage, pre-eclampsia, and complicated labor. Other dangers are: prematurity, low birth weight, and neonatal hypoxia.

III. Asthma status can be monitored by a *pulmonary flow test* using a portable peak-flow meter to assess the greatest flow velocity during forced expiration from fully inflated lungs.

IV. Most asthma medications are safe to take during pregnancy—for up to 4 doses/d; inhaled medications are preferable.

A. *Theophylline* is one of the mainstays of asthma therapy during pregnancy; may exacerbate gastroesophageal reflux (severe heartburn).

B. Inhaled *glucocorticoids*.

C. Inhaled ß₂ agonists (e.g., *terbutaline, [Brethaire, Brethine, Bricanyl]*) are useful in managing acute asthma during pregnancy.

D. Inhaled *Altrovent* (ipratropium bromide) may be beneficial in presence of mucus-producing cough.

E. Acute episodes may require *steroids, aminophylline, oxygen*, and correction of fluid-electrolyte imbalance.

F. *Labor.*

1. Meperidine (*Demerol*) relieves bronchospasm; *morphine is not* used in labor because it may cause bronchospasm.

2. Vaginal birth with local or regional anesthesia is method of choice.

G. Breastfeeding is possible if medications are inhaled, because of their low systemic bioavailability.

H. *Hemabate* is not used to control postpartum hemorrhage due to bronchospasm.

V. Teratogenic effects, if they occur, do so during the first trimester, the period of organogenesis.

## Sickle Cell Disease (Hemoglobin Type SS): Management

I. *Heart failure* is a potential problem: Assess vital signs, auscultate for rales (crackles) frequently, place in *semirecumbent* position, prevent bearing down (pushing) with second-stage labor.

II. *Control asthma*, because it can promote **sickling crises** by shifting the oxygen-hemoglobin dissociation curve to the right.

III. *Prevent infection*—pneumococcal pneumonia (but also salmonella osteomyelitis, and urinary tract infections) can promote **sickling crises** by shifting the oxygen-hemoglobin dissociation curve to the right.

IV. Ensure adequate *hydration* to prevent/treat infection.

*Crisis is caused by*: hypoxia, hypotension, acidosis, dehydration, exertion, sudden cooling, and low-grade fever. Thrombophlebitis may occur from increased blood viscosity.

V. For *crises*: *analgesia* is administered, prn.

VI. Blood transfusions given to maintain hemoglobin at ≥ 8 mg/dL, hemoglobin A at over 40%, and hematocrit at ≥ 30%.

VII. Prepare for birth with forceps assistance or vacuum assistance under local or regional anesthesia.

VIII. Assess for pseudo pre-eclampsia (hypertension and proteinuria, but with *no* weight gain) that often accompanies bone pain crisis.

## Systemic Lupus Erythematosus (SLE): Health Teaching

I. Maternal complications correlate with degree of cardiac or renal involvement.

II. SLE should be in remission at least 6 mo *before* pregnancy is attempted.

III. If SLE has been controlled well on low doses of corticosteroids for 2 yr, pregnancy may be considered. *Prednisone* and *azathioprine* can be continued during pregnancy; they do not appear to be teratogenic. Many other medications used in treating SLE are not recommended during pregnancy.

IV. **Health teaching.** While planning for pregnancy, the woman with SLE needs to know:

A. Risk of miscarriage is higher than in normal pregnancy.

B. She is twice as likely to suffer a flare-up during pregnancy.

C. Hypertension is a major problem.

D. Contraception.

1. Oral contraceptives are **contraindicated**.

2. Condoms and diaphragms are the preferred methods if pregnancy is desired in the future.

## Women Who Have Had Phenylketonuria (PKU): Health Teaching

I. Strict adherence to a *phenylalanine-restricted diet before* and *during* pregnancy is essential; phenylalanine is teratogenic.

II. Fetal damage (microcephaly, mental retardation, cardiac defects) and intrauterine growth restriction (IUGR) *can* be largely prevented, but even careful management of phenylalanine levels does *not ensure* the birth of a normal infant.

## Cystic Fibrosis: Woman With Both Recessive Genes

I. **Pathophysiology:**

A. Most women are infertile, but pregnancy is not uncommon.

B. *Pulmonary* function: unable to maintain vital capacity, so that there is *decreased* oxygen to the myocardium, *decreased* cardiac output, and an *increase* in hypoxemia. Severe pulmonary infection is associated with increased maternal and perinatal mortality.

C. Amount of *sodium* lost through sweat can be significant; *hypovolemia* can occur.

II. *Medical management.*

A. In the presence of any degree of *cor pulmonale*, she must be guarded against *fluid overload*.

B. Oxygen is given freely during labor; epidural or local *anesthesia* is given for birth.

**III. Health teaching.**

A. Genetics:

1. Child will carry at least one gene for cystic fibrosis, since this is an *autosomal-recessive* disorder.

2. If the father of the child also carries the gene and passes it on, this child *will* exhibit the disease; if the father contributes a normal gene, the child will carry one gene for cystic fibrosis.

B. Breastfeeding is *deferred* until after the sodium content of the woman's breast milk has been estimated; it may be as high as 280 mmole/liter. Breastfeeding is encouraged *if* levels of sodium are acceptable.

C. Formula feeding is encouraged if this is the woman's choice, even if her breast milk has an acceptable amount of sodium.

## Hyperthyroidism: Medical Management

I. Affects approximately 1 to 2/1000 pregnancies.

II. May be responsible for *anovulation* and amenorrhea; not a recognized cause of spontaneous abortion or fetal malformation.

III. Surgical treatment of hyperthyroidism (subtotal thyroidectomy) may be performed during the *second* and *third trimesters*.

IV. Controlled with *propylthiouracil* (PTU).

A. Readily crosses the placenta.

B. May induce fetal hypothyroidism and goiter; at birth, a *free $T_4$ index determination* on cord blood is needed to assess newborn status.

## Epilepsy

I. Risk of congenital anomalies: 3% overall chance of having a baby with an anomaly.

II. *Valproic acid* associated with 1–2% incidence of neural tube defects; *not* recommended during pregnancy.

III. Phenytoin (*Dilantin*): anticonvulsant.

A. Can cause *fetal hydantoin syndrome*: microcephaly, mental retardation, developmental delay, intrauterine growth restriction, facial clefts, and nail hypoplasia.

B. Interferes with normal *folate* absorption from GI tract; 1 mg/d ordered.

C. Interferes with normal *vitamin D* production; supplementation recommended.

## Spinal Cord Injury (SCI): Management

I. Although individuals with SCI are physiologically the same as other women, some normal *adaptations* do require *special consideration*: urinary frequency, urinary tract infection, constipation, and need to relieve pressure on ischial spines and gluteal muscles and to straighten body, since pregnancy precludes lying prone.

II. *Oxytocin*, if needed, is used cautiously and only when personnel are versed in the recognition and treatment of autonomic dysreflexia. The headache and hypertension must not be confused with pre-eclampsia.

III. Although women with SCI do *not* experience labor as other women do, they are in tune with their bodies and know when something is happening.

IV. The woman with SCI experiences no trouble with a vaginal birth even though she has no ability to push. Uterine contractions, plus a relaxed perineum, facilitate a vaginal birth.

## Life-Threatening Situations: Nursing Management

I. *Cardiopulmonary resuscitation* (CPR).

A. Done with woman *supine with lateral uterine tilt*.

B. Maintain 30:2 ratio; pause at end of every fifth compression. Total: 6 breaths/min.

C. If mother is resuscitated, the fetus will be too.

II. *Foreign body airway obstruction (FBAO) maneuver (Heimlich).*

A. If *conscious*: encircle her chest and provide chest thrusts.

B. If *unconscious*: give chest compressions same as for women without a pulse.

III. *Anaphylaxis* (an immediate hypersensitivity reaction)

A. **Assessment**

1. *Local* reactions: angioedema (redness and swelling).

2. *Systemic* reactions: cardiovascular collapse; nausea, vomiting, diarrhea; asthma-like symptoms.

B. *Medical management*

1. *Epinephrine* by injection is the drug of choice. It dilates the bronchi, constricts blood vessels, increases blood pressure, and increases rate/strength of heartbeat (and, therefore, the circulation of oxygen throughout body).

## Surgical Emergencies

I. **Acute suppurative appendicitis**—*medical aspects*

A. The appendix is carried high and to the right, away from McBurney's point, by the enlarged uterus, complicating diagnosis. Increased *sedimentation rate* is normal during pregnancy, and therefore *cannot* be used in diagnosis.

B. Therapeutic abortion is **never** indicated.

C. Maternal mortality: increases to about 10% in the third trimester; 15% if it occurs during labor.

D. Perinatal mortality: approximately 10% with unruptured appendicitis; 35% if complicated with peritonitis.

E. Rupture and peritonitis: 2–3 times more often than in women who are not pregnant.

II. **Intestinal obstruction** (adynamic ileus)—*management*

A. Not common during pregnancy.

⋈ B. **Assess** *signs/symptoms*

    1. Persistent cramplike abdominal pain.

    2. Auscultatory rushes within the abdomen and "laddering" of the intestinal shadows on x-ray films aid in diagnosis.

C. Immediate surgical intervention to release the intestinal obstruction (adynamic ileus) rarely adversely affects pregnancy.

### III. Nonobstetric surgery: Preoperative Care

A. *Antacids* are given *before* surgery because the hydrochloric acid in the stomach (if aspirated) may cause an asthmalike syndrome with necrotizing bronchitis.

    1. *Cimetidine*: a histamine blocker; decreases production of gastric acid.

    2. Metoclopramide (*Reglan*) increases gastric emptying.

B. Prolonged NPO can lead to *ketosis* and *hypoglycemia*; IV fluids with dextrose are given to prevent them.

C. Greater risk of *postoperative atelectasis* and pulmonary complications because of the decreased respiratory excursion associated with the enlarged uterus.

D. Stress of surgery may stimulate the onset of labor.

☞ E. Fetal monitoring before and after surgery to ensure fetal well-being, if fetus is viable. If previable, FHT with doppler before and after surgical procedure.

## Cancer and Pregnancy

I. For each 1800 pregnant women, 1 will also have cancer. In order of frequency, the types are: breast cancer, leukemia and lymphomas as a group; melanomas, gynecologic (cervical and ovarian) tumors, and bone tumors.

II. With diagnosis, many complex issues and reactions arise:

A. Decision to continue or terminate pregnancy.

B. Selection of therapies: surgery, chemotherapy, radiation.

C. Moral and philosophic dilemmas.

III. Key points: cancer therapy and pregnancy.

A. Chemotherapy and radiation are specific against rapidly growing cells. Therefore, the embryo/ fetus is *most at risk* during the first trimester, the period of organogenesis and tissue growth.

B. After the first trimester, live births with few congenital abnormalities occur following judicious use of chemotherapy. *Alkylating agents, 5-fluorouracil* and *vincristine*, are relatively safe for the fetus.

C. Radiation can cause damage at any stage of embryonic/fetal development.

D. Surgery may be performed safely in many cases.

### Breast Cancer

I. Approximately 1–2% of women are pregnant when breast cancer is diagnosed. The nurse needs to counsel women that breastfeeding is **contraindicated** because lactation increases vascularity and possible metastasis.

### Malignant Melanoma

(Rare in women who are pregnant)

I. Effect on *woman*: although the effect of pregnancy on melanoma is unknown, women with melanoma are *cautioned* about getting pregnant because there is a natural increase in melanocyte-stimulating hormone (MSH) during pregnancy. Adrenocorticotropic hormone (ACTH) production also increases during pregnancy, which heightens MSH activity. Stage for stage, there is no significant difference in the survival of women who are pregnant and not pregnant with malignant melanoma.

II. Effect on *fetus*: 50% of placental metastases and almost 90% of fetal metastases occur from maternal melanoma.

## Violence

### Rape: Sexual Assault

I. *Rape trauma syndrome*—characteristics:

A. *Acute phase*: fear, humiliation, anger, and self-blame; feels unclean and wants to bathe and douche despite fact she would be destroying evidence.

B. Desire to forget the incident is characteristic of the *first* reorganization phase (*adjustment*).

C. Urgency to change residence or phone number is characteristic of the *first* reorganization phase (*adjustment*).

D. Nightmares and eating disorders are very common in the *second* reorganization phase (*integration*) and the *third* reorganization phase (*recovery*).

II. *Medical management.*

☞ A. Specimens are obtained from orifices, e.g., vaginal vault.

B. Physical injuries are treated.

C. Prophylaxis for infection is given.

D. Prophylaxis for pregnancy is provided.

### Assault and Battery

I. **General comments**

A. Violence against women respects no social, economic, racial or ethnic categories.

B. Prevalence of abuse toward women who are pregnant ranges from 8-17%; violence often starts and/or becomes worse during pregnancy.

C. Cycle of violence occurs in *three phases: building, battering, calm.*

D. Alcohol has not been causally related to battering, but batterers do have a high rate of alcohol abuse.

**!** E. Women who are abused are 1 ½ times more likely to have low-birth-weight (LBW) infants and more likely to have associated risk factors for LBW, such as poor obstetric history, infections, and alcohol or drug use.

F. A woman in a battering situation is *more likely* to seek help early *if* she has not experienced violence in her family of origin; that is, she has not been taught "learned helplessness." Others who seek help early are those beaten frequently and severely and those who see an alternative to life in their marriages—specifically, those with jobs.

G. Women *less likely* to seek help are those who: have just learned they are pregnant, have one or more preschool children, or are afraid that the batterer will punish them.

**II. Assessment**: Nursing interview technique must be skillful, help the woman focus on the situation, avoid implication that she is somehow responsible, and be unthreatening. Example: "Have you had any relationships in which you have been abused emotionally, physically, or sexually?" does not place blame on the woman or accuse the partner.

**III. Nursing intervention**: Most therapeutic action is to assist the woman in identifying her options, which may include remaining in the relationship. *Avoid* taking sides against the batterer or suggesting that the woman leave the batterer.

**IV. Evaluation/outcome criteria of nursing intervention**: Goals have been met when the woman can use phrases such as "*I am . . . ,*" which indicate a developing self-esteem, feelings of worth and personal adequacy, and independence. NOTE: following the "advice" of counselors is a submissive, passive, and dependent act—a continuation of "learned helplessness."

### Trauma—Nursing Management

**I.** *First* intervention: *tilt* uterus off the major vessels to facilitate venous return and prevent supine hypotension and placental congestion. If on backboard, *tilt* entire board. If CPR needed, perform while keeping uterus tilted off vessels (see p. 67).

**II.** Do **not** place in Trendelenburg's position, which could severely impair maternal respirations when the heavy enlarged uterus presses up against the diaphragm.

**III.** Establish an *intravenous line* for fluid and electrolyte replacement.

**IV.** Place a *central venous or pulmonary artery catheter* to monitor fluid therapy. The woman may sustain a *significant blood loss* of approximately 30% without the usual signs and symptoms of hypovolemia. A rapid pulse may reflect only the usual increase of 10–15 beats/min during pregnancy, or it may be a sign of hypovolemia.

**V.** Insert a *retention urinary catheter*. Although not the priority action, the catheter is inserted to: measure hourly urine output during fluid therapy, assess for shock, and assess for bladder injury secondary to the trauma. (During pregnancy, the bladder is pulled up above the symphysis pubis and is more vulnerable to **!** *injury*.)

**VI.** Auscultate fetal heart rate (FHR) after the woman's condition is assessed and therapy is instituted. When her condition has been stabilized, attention is given to the FHR and to the possibility of *preterm labor* and **!** *abruptio placentae.*

**VII.** Observe the maternal-fetal unit for 48 hr to rule out **!** complications such as *preterm labor* and *abruptio placentae.*

# Common Complications: First Trimester

## Complications Affecting Fluid–Gas Transport: *Hemorrhagic Disorders*

### General Aspects

See **Emergency Conditions, Table 3.3.**

**I. Assessment**
   A. Vital signs, output, general status.
   B. Evidence of internal/external bleeding.
   C. Pain.
   D. Emotional response.
   E. Perineal pads saturated and number.
   F. Speculum examination.

**II. Analysis/nursing diagnosis**
   A. *Knowledge deficit* related to diagnosis, prognosis, treatment, sequelae.
   B. *Anxiety/fear* related to loss of pregnancy, surgery.
   C. *Fluid volume deficit, potential/actual*, related to excessive blood loss.
   D. *Pain.*
   E. *Individual/family coping impairment*, related to knowledge deficit and fear.
   F. *Anticipatory/dysfunctional grieving*, related to loss of pregnancy.
   G. *Disturbance in self-esteem, body image, role performance*, related to threat to self-image as woman and childbearer.

**III. Nursing care plan/implementation**
   A. Goal: *minimize blood loss, stabilize physiologic status.*
      1. Facilitate prompt medical management.
      2. Administer IV fluids, blood, as ordered.
      3. Administer *analgesics*, as needed.
   **B.** Goal: *prevent infection.* Strict aseptic technique.

C. Goal: *emotional support.*
   1. Encourage verbalization of anxiety, fears, concerns.
   2. Supportive care for grief reaction (see **Loss of Pregnancy, Table 3.6**).

▶ IV. **Evaluation/outcome criteria**
   A. Woman's blood loss is minimized; physiologic status stable.
   B. Woman (family) copes effectively with loss of pregnancy.

## Spontaneous Abortion: Before Viable Age of 20–22 wk

I. **Etiology/risk factors:**
   A. Defective products of conception.
   B. Insufficient production of progesterone.
   C. Acute infections.
   D. Reproductive system abnormalities, e.g., incompetent cervical os.
   E. Trauma (physical or emotional).
   F. Rh incompatibility.

▶ II. **Assessment: types**
   A. *Threatened*—mild bleeding, spotting, cramping; cervix closed.
   B. *Inevitable*—moderate bleeding, painful cramping; cervix dilated, positive *Nitrazine test* (membranes ruptured).
   C. *Imminent*—profuse bleeding, severe cramping, urge to bear down.
   D. *Incomplete*—fetal parts or fetus expelled; placenta and membranes retained.
   E. *Complete*—all products of conception expelled; minimal vaginal bleeding.
   F. *Habitual/recurrent*—history of spontaneous loss of three or more successive pregnancies.
   G. *Missed*—fetal death with no spontaneous expulsion within 4 wk.
      1. Anorexia, malaise, headache.
      2. Fundal height—inconsistent with gestational estimate.
      3. Laboratory tests—*prolonged* clotting time, due to resultant concurrent *hypofibrinogenemia* (disseminated intravascular coagulation [DIC], a major threat to mother).
   H. Elective abortions (intentionally introduced loss of pregnancy).

▶ III. **Analysis/nursing diagnosis**
   A. *Family processes alteration* related to pregnancy, circumstances surrounding abortion.
   B. *Sexual dysfunction* related to compromised self-image, altered interpersonal relationship, guilt feelings.

▶ IV. **Nursing care plan/implementation**
   A. *Threatened*—goal: **health teaching.** Suggest: *avoid coitus and orgasm,* especially around normal time for menstrual period.
   B. *Incomplete, inevitable, imminent*

1. Goal: *safeguard status.*
   a. Save all perineal pads, clots, tissue for expert diagnosis.
   b. Report **immediately** any change in status, excessive bleeding, signs of infection, shock.
   c. Prepare for surgery.
2. Goal: *comfort measures.*
   a. Administer *analgesics*, as necessary.
   b. *Bedrest*, quiet diversional activities.
3. Goal: *emotional support.*
   a. Encourage verbalization of fear, concerns.
   b. Reduce anxiety, as possible.
   c. If pregnancy terminates, facilitate grieving process; assist in working through guilt feelings (see **Table 3.6**).
   d. Supportive care for grief reaction (see **Table 3.6**).
4. Goal: *prevent isoimmunization.* See **Rh incompatibility, p. 52-53.**
5. *Medical management*
   a. Laboratory tests–blood type and Rh factor, indirect Coombs', platelets, serum fibrinogen, clotting time.
   b. Replace blood loss; maintain fluid levels with IV.
   c. Dilatation and curettage.
C. *Habitual*—determine etiology.

▶ V. **Evaluation/outcome criteria**
   A. *Threatened abortion*—woman responds to medical/nursing regimen; abortion avoided, successfully carries pregnancy to term.
   B. *Spontaneous abortion*—after uterus emptied:
      1. Woman's bleeding is controlled.
      2. Woman's vital signs are stable.
      3. Woman (family) copes effectively with loss of pregnancy.
      4. Woman (family) expresses satisfaction with care.
   C. *Habitual abortion*—cause identified and corrected; woman carries subsequent pregnancy to successful termination.

## Hydatidiform Mole (Complete)

I. **Pathophysiology**: gestational trophoblastic disease (GTD), in which chorionic villi degenerate into grapelike cluster of vesicles (**Figures 3.1** and **3.2**); may be antecedent to **choriocarcinoma.**

II. **Etiology**: genetic base of complete mole (sperm enters empty egg and its chromosomes replicate; 23 pairs of chromosomes are all of paternal origin); rare complication; more common in women *over 45 yr* of age and Asian women.

▶ III. **Assessment** (see **Table 3.3**).
   A. Uterus—rapid enlargement; fundal height inconsistent with gestational estimate.

**TABLE 3.3** ⚕ **EMERGENCY CONDITIONS**

## FIRST TRIMESTER

| ► Assessment/Observations | Possible Problem | ► Nursing Care Plan/Implementation |
|---|---|---|
| **Fluid-Gas Transport** | | |
| a. *Cramping*—with or without bleeding or passage of tissue | Abortion (before 24 wk) Threatened Imminent Incomplete Septic | • Bedrest, sedation, *avoid* coitus—if threatened; start IV fluids and draw blood for *laboratory* work: CBC, type/ cross-match, electrolytes, platelets, hCG levels |
| b. *Passage of tissue* (products of conception; grapelike vesicles) or *brown spotting*; absent FHT; fundus too high for gestational age; *blood pressure elevated*; often associated with *hyperemesis gravidarum* and pre-eclampsia | Hydatidiform mole (gestational trophoblastic disease) | • Vital signs q 5–15 min, prn<br>• Maintain hydration; assess for dehydration<br>• Refer to MD |
| c. Severe *pain, shock* out of proportion to amount of overt blood; shoulder-strap pain (*Kehr's sign*), a "referred pain" that indicates intraabdominal bleeding (or rupture of ovarian cyst); amenorrhea of 6–12 wk | Ectopic pregnancy | • Save all pads or tissue passed through vagina for physician evaluation<br>• **No** rectal or vaginal examination until physician is present |
| d. Malodorous *discharge; hyperthermia and chills;* tender abdomen | Septic abortion (self-induced or "criminal") | • Take complete history, if possible<br>**!** • Convulsion precautions if hypertensive |
| e. *Ecchymosis or bleeding*—with a history that includes any or all of the following: had symptoms of pregnancy, but they subsided; pregnancy test *negative*; uterine size diminishing; no FHT | Missed abortion with possible DIC (*retained dead fetus syndrome*) | • Emotional support for loss of pregnancy (through nurse's: manner, tone of voice, touch, use of woman's name) keep her informed of what is happening<br>☞ • Oxygen, prn |

**TABLE 3.4** ⚕ **EMERGENCY CONDITIONS**

## SECOND TRIMESTER

| ► Assessment/Observations | Possible Problem | ► Nursing Care Plan/Implementation |
|---|---|---|
| **Fluid-Gas Transport** | | |
| a. Cramping; passage of products of conception | Late abortion | • Same as for first trimester |
| b. Labor—cervical changes, "show" | Incompetent cervical os | • See MD immediately for possible cerclage |
| c. Preterm labor (see **Chapter 5**) | | |

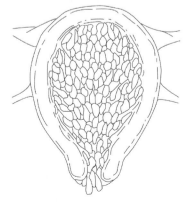

**FIGURE 3.1  HYDATIDIFORM MOLE IN UTERUS**

B. Brownish discharge—beginning about *week 12*; may contain vesicles.

C. Signs and symptoms of pre-eclampsia/eclampsia (*before* third trimester), increased incidence of
**!** hyperemesis gravidarum (see **p. 74-75**).

〰 D. *Medical evaluation—diagnostic tests/procedures:*

1. Sonography, amniography—no fetal parts present; "snow storm." See **Figure 3.2**.

2. *Laboratory test*—for *elevated* human chorionic gonadotropin (hCG) levels.

3. Follow-up surveillance of hCG levels for at least one year; *persistent hCG* level is consistent with choriocarcinoma.

**TABLE 3.5** ⊕ **EMERGENCY CONDITIONS** *(continued)*

## THIRD TRIMESTER

| ▶ *Assessment/Observations* | *Possible Problem* | ▶ *Nursing Care Plan/Implementation* |
|---|---|---|
| **Sensory-Perceptual** | | |
| a. *Pre-eclampsia/eclampsia* (also see **p. 75-77**) *Assessment*: hypertension first noted after 24 wk; followed by increased proteinuria *Symptoms*: blurred or double vision; pain: headache, epigastric (late sign)<br><br>*Signs*: BP 160/110; 3⁺ proteinuria; edema: facial, digital, pulmonary; oliguria; hyperreflexia | With increased severity: renal failure circulatory collapse stroke coagulation defects (DIC) abruptio placentae | • Pharmacologic management of woman with hypertension (**p. 79**)<br>☞ *Convulsion (seizure) precautions* (**p. 77**)<br>  1. Emergency tray at bedside<br>  2. Oxygen/suction<br>  3. Start IV<br>  4. Padded siderails<br>  5. Indwelling urinary catheter<br>  6. Constant observation<br>  7. Deep tendon reflexes<br>  8. Daily weight<br>  9. I&O<br>  10. Note any complaints and changes<br>〰 11. Prepare for *lab work* (type and cross-match, CBC, platelets, BUN, liver function tests, uric acid and creatinine) |
| b. *Convulsions* in absence of hypertension, proteinuria, or facial edema | Stroke Epilepsy Drug toxicity Intracranial injury Diabetic complications Encephalopathy | ☞ *Convulsion (seizure) care*: see **p. 77**<br>  1. Oxygen/mask; drugs (*Valium* to control seizures)<br>  2. Observe:<br>    a. Uterine tone, FHRs, fetal activity<br>    b. Signs of labor<br>  3. Emotional support for woman and family |
| **Fluid-Gas Transport** | | |
| a. *Bleeding*: painless, bright red, vaginal; Contractions and/or uterine tone normal | **Placenta previa** | • **No vaginal examination**<br>☞ • Apply fetal monitor; assess for labor<br>☞ • *Position*: semi- to high-Fowler's |
| b. *Pain*: abdomen rigid and tender to touch increased uterine tone; signs of shock disproportionate to visible blood loss; may have loss of FHTs; associated with: pre-eclampsia, multiparity, precipitous labor, oxytocin induction, trauma, cocaine use | **Abruptio placentae** | • Same as for placenta previa; *position*: Sims' |

FHR = fetal heart rate; DIC = disseminated intravascular coagulation; CBC = complete blood count; hCG = human chorionic gonadotropin
*Source*: Lagerquist, S. *Davis's NCLEX-RN® Success*, Philadelphia.

▶ **IV. Analysis/nursing diagnosis**
  A. *Anxiety/fear* related to treatment, possible sequelae of hydatidiform mole (choriocarcinoma).
  B. *Potential for injury* related to hemorrhage, perforation of uterine wall, pre-eclampsia/eclampsia.
  C. *Fluid volume deficit* related to injury.

▶ **V. Nursing care plan/implementation**
  A. *Medical management*.
  ! 1. Monitor for pre-eclampsia/eclampsia.
    2. Evacuate the uterus—hysterectomy may be necessary.
    3. *Strict* contraception for at least 1 yr to enable accurate assessment of status.
  ⊂⊃ 4. Choriocarcinoma—chemotherapy (*methotrexate* plus *dactinomycin*) and/or radiation therapy.

B. **Nursing management.**
  1. Goal: *safeguard status*. Observe for hemorrhage, passage of retained vesicles and abdominal pain, or signs of infection (because woman is at-risk for perforation of
  ! uterine wall).
  ◻ 2. Goal: **health teaching.**
    a. Explain, discuss diagnostic tests; prepare for tests.
    b. Discuss contraceptive options.
    c. Discuss importance of follow-up.
  3. Goal: *preoperative and postoperative care*.
  4. Goal: *emotional support*. Facilitate grieving (see **Table 3.6**).

## TABLE 3.6 LOSS OF PREGNANCY

| Stage of Grief | Possible Maternal Response | ▶ Nursing Care Plan/Implementation |
|---|---|---|
| Shock, disbelief | Pulls back, withdraws: not interested in events around her; may stay in bed, staring at wall, with shades drawn | Since client cannot communicate effectively now, nurse demonstrates caring behaviors by: *staying* with her, touching or *massaging* her; providing *physical* care; giving her opportunity to talk if she wants to; do *not* make light of her situation |
| Anger, fear | Verbal fault-finding and possible physical aggression, irritability, insomnia | State that it is normal to be angry; help her identify her questions and concerns (guilt); be available to her (and her family) |
| Helplessness, despair, guilt | Dependent behaviors—may become demanding, may cry, may exhibit regressive behaviors; may see no purpose to anything; may feel very guilty, worthless | Help her *verbalize* her actual and implied feelings: "It is hard to understand," "You probably feel you are to blame . . ."; "The way you feel may seem strange or even 'crazy' to you." Do provide *physical* care, give massage, keep her physically comfortable |
| Reorganization (after discharge) | Begins to be interested in events around her, to have increased amounts of energy; inquires again about events leading to the situation, the etiology, the medical and nursing management, as she tries to integrate the experience. | Community health or clinic nurse listens, clarifies, fills in gaps. Reexplain the grieving process—that her (their) behaviors were normal; that acute grief lasts 6 wk, while the entire process lasts about 1 yr or more. Talk about what older siblings or other family members may be feeling—a young child's return to bed-wetting may be a response to the parents' tension, etc.; older siblings may show regressive behavior: fear of the dark, fear of school, or behavioral difficulties |

▶ **VI. Evaluation/outcome criteria**

    A. Woman verbalizes understanding of diagnosis, tests, and treatment.

    B. Woman complies with medical/nursing recommendations.

    C. Woman tolerates surgical procedure well.

       1. Bleeding controlled.

       2. Vital signs stable.

       3. Urinary output adequate.

    D. Woman copes effectively with loss of pregnancy.

    E. Woman returns for follow-up care/surveillance.

    F. Woman selects and effectively implements method of contraception; *avoids* pregnancy for 1 yr or more.

    G. Tests for hCG remain negative for 1 yr; no evidence of malignancy.

    H. Woman achieves a pregnancy when desired.

    I. Woman successfully carries pregnancy to term; normal, uncomplicated birth of viable infant.

**FIGURE 3.2 HYDATIDIFORM MOLE PREGNANCY**

### Ectopic Pregnancy

    I. **Pathophysiology**: implantation outside of uterine cavity.

    II. **Types (see Figure 3.3):**

       A. Tubal (most common).

       B. Cervical.

       C. Abdominal.

       D. Ovarian.

    III. **Etiology/risk factors:**

       A. Pelvic inflammatory disease (PID)—pelvic salpingitis and endometritis.

       B. 43% caused by sexually transmitted disease (STD); related factors: 25%, chlamydial; 20%, previous STD.

       C. Tubal or uterine anomalies, tubal spasm.

       D. Adhesions from PID or past surgeries.

       E. Presence of intrauterine device (IUD).

**IV. Assessment** (dependent on implantation site)

A. *Early signs*—abnormal menstrual period (usually following a missed menstrual period), spotting, some symptoms of pregnancy; possible dull pain on affected side.

B. *Impending or posttubal rupture*—sudden, acute, lower abdominal pain; nausea and vomiting; signs of shock; referred shoulder pain (*Kehr's sign*) or neck pain—due to blood in peritoneal cavity; blood in cul-de-sac may → rectal pressure.

C. *Cullen's sign*: ecchymotic blueness of umbilicus, indicative of *hematoperitoneum*. Sharp, localized pain when cervix is touched during vaginal examination; shock and circulatory collapse in some, usually *following* vaginal examination.

D. Positive pregnancy test in most women.

**V. Analysis/nursing diagnosis**

A. *Fear* related to abdominal pain and pregnancy status.

B. *Grief* related to pregnancy loss.

**VI. Nursing care plan/implementation**

A. *Medical management*: surgical removal/repair.

B. **Nursing management.**
1. Goal: **health teaching.** *Preoperative and postoperative care.*
2. Goal: *supportive care for grief reaction*; encourage verbalization of anxiety and concerns of further pregnancies.

**VII. Evaluation/outcome criteria**

A. Woman experiences uncomplicated postoperative course.

B. Woman copes effectively with loss of pregnancy.

## Complications Affecting Nutrition/Elimination

### Hyperemesis Gravidarum

I. **Definition:** pernicious vomiting during first 14–16 wk (peak incidence around 10 wk gestation); excessive vomiting at any time during pregnancy.

II. **Pathophysiology:** secretion of hCG, *decrease* in free gastric HCl, *decreased* gastrointestinal motility.

! Increased incidence in hydatidiform mole and multifetal pregnancy (due to high levels of hCG).

Potential hazards include:

A. *Dehydration* with fluid and electrolyte imbalance.

B. *Starvation*, with loss of 5% or more of body weight; protein and vitamin *deficiencies*.

C. *Metabolic acidosis* due to breakdown of fat stores to meet metabolic needs.

D. *Metabolic alkalosis* which can be caused by vomiting all gastric acids.

E. Hypovolemia and hemoconcentration; *increased* blood urea nitrogen (BUN); *decreased* urinary output.

III. **Risk factor/causes:** (other than **Pathophysiology;** see II. above)

A. *Psychological*—thought to be related to rejection of pregnancy and/or sexual relations.

**IV. Assessment**

A. Intractable vomiting.

B. Abdominal pain.

C. Hiccups.

D. Marked weight loss.

E. Dehydration—thirst, tachycardia, skin turgor.

F. Increased respiratory rate (*metabolic acidosis*).

G. Laboratory—*elevated* BUN.

H. *Medical evaluation*: rule out other causes (infection, tumors).

Abdominal implantation (intestine)

Tubal implantation

Ovarian implantation

Cervical implantation

**FIGURE 3.3 ECTOPTIC PREGNANCY SITES**

### V. Analysis/nursing diagnosis

A. *Nutritional deficit* related to inability to retain oral feedings.

B. *Fluid volume deficit* related to dehydration.

C. *Individual coping impairment* related to symptoms, insecurity in role, psychological stress of unwanted pregnancy.

D. *Personal identity disturbance* related to symptoms and/or perception of self as inadequate in role, sick, socially unpresentable.

### VI. Nursing care plan/implementation

A. Goal: *physiologic stability.*

1. Rest GI tract (keep NPO), e.g., maintain IV fluids, parenteral nutrition.

2. Progress *diet*, as ordered; present small feedings attractively. *Avoid* citrus fruit, juice.

3. Weigh daily, assess hydration; note weight gain.

B. Goal: *minimize environmental stimuli.*

1. Limit visitors and phone calls.

2. *Bedrest* with bathroom privileges.

C. Goal: *emotional support.*

1. Establish accepting, supportive environment.

2. Encourage verbalization of anxiety, fears, concerns.

3. Support positive self-image.

### VII. Evaluation/outcome criteria

A. Woman's signs and symptoms subside; she takes oral nourishment and gains weight.

B. Woman's pregnancy continues to term without recurrence of hyperemesis.

# Common Complications: Second Trimester

See **Table 3.4** for **Emergency Conditions.**

## Complications Affecting Comfort, Rest, Mobility

### Incompetent Cervix

I. **Pathophysiology**: inability of cervix to support growing weight of pregnancy; associated with repeated spontaneous second trimester abortion.

II. **Etiology/risk factors:**

A. Unknown.

B. Congenital defect in cervical musculature.

C. Cervical trauma during previous birth, abortion; aggressive, deep, or repeated dilatation and curettage.

III. **Assessment**

A. History of habitual, second trimester abortions.

B. Painless, progressive cervical effacement and dilatation during second trimester.

C. Signs of threatened abortion or (early third trimester) preterm labor.

### IV. Analysis/nursing diagnosis

A. *Pain* related to early dilatation.

B. *Fear* related to possible pregnancy loss.

### V. Nursing care plan/implementation

A. *Medical management.*

1. Cerclage surgical procedure (*Shirodkar, McDonald*).

B. *Preoperative* **nursing management.**

1. Goal: r*educe physical stress on incompetent cervix. Bedrest*, supportive care.

2. Goal: *emotional support.* Encourage verbalization of anxiety, fear, concerns.

3. Goal: **health** (*preoperative*) **teaching.** Explain procedure—purse-string suture encircles cervix and reinforces musculature.

4. Goal: *preparation for surgery.*

C. *Postoperative* **nursing management.**

1. Goal: *maximize surgical result with bedrest*, supportive care.

2. Goal: **health teaching.**

a. *Avoid*: strenuous physical activity; straining.

b. Report promptly: signs of labor (vaginal bleeding, cramping).

c. Need for continued, close health surveillance.

### VI. **Evaluation/outcome criterion**: Woman carries pregnancy to successful termination.

## Complications Affecting Protective Functions

### Preterm Labor

Preterm birth is that which occurs *after week 20* but *before* the *end of week 37* of gestation. Preterm birth is responsible for almost two-thirds of infant deaths. Because of the high incidence, all women who are pregnant need to learn the signs and symptoms of preterm labor. See **Chapter 5, p. 128-131** for discussion.

# Common Complications: Third Trimester

See **Table 3.5** for Emergency Conditions.

## Complications Affecting Sensory/Perceptual Functions

### Pre-eclampsia/Eclampsia

I. **Pathophysiology:**

A. Generalized arteriospasm → increased peripheral resistance, decreased tissue perfusion, and hypertension.

B. *Kidney:*
1. Reduced renal perfusion and vasospasm → glomerular lesions.
2. Damage to membrane → loss of serum protein (*albuminuria*). NOTE: *Reduced* serum albumin-globulin (A/G) ratio alters blood osmolarity → edema.
3. Increased tubular reabsorption of sodium → increased water retention (edema).
4. Release of angiotensin contributes to vasospasm and hypertension.

C. *Brain*: decreased oxygenation, cerebral edema, and vasospasm → visual disturbances and hyperirritability, convulsions, and coma.

D. *Uterus*: decreased placental perfusion → increased risk of a baby who is SGA, abruptio placentae.

II. **Etiology**: unknown. **Risk factors**:

A. Pregnancy—occurs only when a functioning trophoblast is present; more common in *first* pregnancies; develops after week 24 of gestation.

B. Age related—*under* 17 and *over* 35 yr of age.

C. Coexisting conditions—diabetes, multifetal gestation, polyhydramnios.

III. **Assessment**—types:

A. **Pre-eclampsia**—"*mild*":
1. Hypertension—systolic increase of 30 mm Hg or more over baseline; diastolic rise of 15 mm Hg or more over baseline.
2. Proteinuria—1 g/d.
3. Edema—digital and periorbital; weight gain over 0.45 kg (1 pound)/wk.

B. **Pre-eclampsia**—*severe*:
1. *Increasing hypertension*—systolic at or above 160 mm Hg or more than 50 mm Hg over baseline; diastolic, 110 mm Hg or more.
2. Urine: proteinuria (5 g or more in 24 hr); oliguria (400 mL or less in 24 hr).
3. Hemoconcentration, hypoproteinemia, hypernatremia, hypovolemic condition.
4. Persistent vomiting.
5. Epigastric pain—due to edema of liver capsule.
6. Cerebral or visual disturbances (*before* convulsive state):
   a. Disorientation and somnolence.
   b. Severe frontal headache.
   c. Increased irritability; hyperreflexia.
   d. Blurred vision, halo vision, dimness, blind spots.

C. **Eclampsia**
1. Tonic and clonic convulsions; coma.
2. Renal shutdown—oliguria, anuria.

IV. **Assessment**—*hospitalized woman*

A. Vital signs (blood pressure, pulse, respirations)—q 2–4 hr, while awake (if mild to moderate preeclampsia) and/or as necessary. NOTE: record, report persistent hypertension.

B. Fetal heart rate (FHR) at time of vital signs.

C. Deep tendon reflexes (DTR) and clonus—to identify/monitor CNS hyperirritability.

D. I&O—to identify diuresis. (NOTE: oliguria indicates pathologic progression.)

E. Urinalysis (clean catch) for protein, daily or after each voiding, as necessary.

F. Signs of pathologic progression (see **III. Assessment**—types, **p.76**).

G. Signs of labor, abruptio placentae (NOTE: High blood pressure, or a rapid drop, may initiate abruptio), DIC.

H. Emotional status.

I. Daily weight, amount/distribution of edema (pitting; pedal, digital, periorbital)—to identify signs of mobilization of tissue fluid, diuresis.

V. **Analysis/nursing diagnosis**

A. *Fluid volume deficit*: hemoconcentration, edema related to altered blood osmolarity (due to loss of protein from vascular compartment) and sodium/water retention. Hypovolemia results.

B. *Nutritional deficit*: protein deficiency related to dietary lack and/or loss through damaged renal membrane.

C. *Tissue perfusion alteration* related to increased peripheral resistance and vasospasm in renal, cardiovascular system.

D. *Urinary elimination alteration* oliguria, anuria related to hypovolemia.

E. *Sensory/perceptual alterations*: visual disturbances, hyperirritability related to cerebral edema, decreased oxygenation to brain.

F. *Anxiety* related to symptoms, implications of pathophysiology.

G. *Diversional activity deficit* related to need for reduced environmental stimuli, bedrest.

H. *Injury risk* related to seizure.

VI. **Prognosis**

A. *Good*—symptoms mild, respond to treatment.

B. *Poor*—convulsions (number and duration); persistent coma; hyperthermia, tachycardia (120 beats/min); cyanosis.

C. *Terminal*—pulmonary edema, heart failure, acute renal failure, cerebral hemorrhage. The earlier the symptoms appear, the poorer the outcome for the pregnancy.

VII. **Nursing care plan/implementation**

A. Goal: **health teaching.** Home care and health maintenance.
1. Education—learning about the condition.
2. Education—self-care:
   a. Taking own blood pressure.
   b. Checking for proteinuria.
   c. Monitoring weight gain and **STAT** reporting of gain of more than 1 pound/wk.
3. Fetal well-being—daily fetal movement count (DFMC).

4. Rest—frequent naps in *lateral Sims' position*, or bedrest.
   a. Coping with bedrest.
      (1) Increasing fluid intake.
      (2) Using diversional activities.
      (3) Exercising gently—hands, feet, alternately tensing and relaxing muscles.
      (4) Using relaxation techniques.
5. Involve family.
6. Nutrition.
   a. Diet should be well balanced.
   b. Do *not* eliminate sodium; do *avoid* foods with *high* salt (potato chips, pickles, etc.).
   c. *Avoid* alcohol and smoking.
   d. *Fluids*—8–10 8 oz. glasses/d.
   e. Foods with *roughage*.
7. Importance of regular prenatal visits.
8. Immediate recognition and reporting of **warning signs** indicating increasing severity:
   1. Digital and periorbital edema.
   2. Severe headache, irritability.
   3. Visual disturbances.
   4. Epigastric pain.

**VIII. Nursing care plan/implementation**—*hospital care*

A. Goal: *reduce environmental stimuli.* Minimize stimulation of hyperirritable CNS. Limit visitors and phone calls.
B. Goal: *emotional support.*
   1. Encourage verbalization of anxiety, fears, concerns.
   2. Explain all procedures, seizure precautions.
C. Goal: *supportive care.*
   1. Encourage bedrest in *lateral Sims' position* to increase tissue perfusion, promote diuresis, and reduce risk of supine hypotensive syndrome.
   2. Suggest diversional activities, teach relaxation techniques to reduce stress.
D. Goal: *administer medications as ordered and monitor effects.*
   1. See **Pharmacology box 3.1, p. 79.**
   2. **Emergency: magnesium sulfate toxicity**
      *Assess for signs/symptoms:*
      Respirations ≤ 12/min
      DTRs: hyporeflexia, or absence (patella)
      Urinary output ≤ 30 mL/hr
      Toxic *serum levels* ≥ 9.6 mg/dL
      Fetal distress: drop in FHRs, no fetal movement
      Significant drop in maternal pulse or BP
      *Collaborative management:*
      **STAT**: discontinue MgSO₄; open maintenance IV line
      Call for assistance **STAT**; notify attending physician

Administer *calcium gluconate or calcium chloride* as ordered (e.g., 1 g by IV injection **given over 3 min. period**)
Monitor frequently: DTRs, respirations, urinary output, MgSO₄ serum levels
Notify nursery nurses about possible neonatal effects

E. Goal: **seizure precautions**, to safeguard maternal-fetal health and well-being (see **Table 3.5, p. 72**).
   1. *Environment*: nonstimulating, quiet, subdued lighting.
   2. *Safety*: padded siderails; equipment for suctioning and oxygen administration, tested and ready for use; call button easily reached.
   3. Emergency fluids and medication tray easily accessible
      a. *Magnesium sulfate and hydralazine.*
      b. *Calcium gluconate* available in a well-labeled syringe.
   4. Emergency birth pack readily available.
   5. **Observe for warning signs and symptoms of impending seizure:**
      a. Frontal headache.
      b. Epigastric pain.
      c. Sharp cry.
      d. Eyes fixed; unresponsive.
      e. Facial twitching.
   6. Continue close observation for 48 hr postpartum.
F. Goal: **seizure care** (client with eclampsia):
   1. Maintain patent *airway*—prop in *lateral position*; after seizure, suction and administer oxygen by face mask.
   2. Administer medications/fluids as ordered.
   3. Assess uterine activity for labor and/or abruptio placentae.
   4. Check perineum for impending birth.
   5. Check FHR.
   6. Observe, report, and record:
      a. Onset and progression of convulsion.
      b. If followed by coma and/or incontinence.

**IX. Evaluation/outcome criteria**
   1. Woman complies with medical/nursing plan of care.
   2. Woman's symptoms respond to treatment; progression halted.
   3. Woman carries uneventful pregnancy to successful termination.

## HELLP Syndrome

**I. Definition**: a critical complication of severe pre-eclampsia.

**II. Assessment**

A. Signs and symptoms of severe pre-eclampsia (see **III. B, p. 76**), plus **Table 3.5, p. 72.**
B. **H**emolysis, **E**levated **L**iver enzymes, and **L**ow **P**latelets.

III. **Analysis/nursing diagnosis**
   A. *Injury risk* (**mother**) related to CNS irritability secondary to cerebral edema, vasospasm, decreased renal perfusion; seizures.
   B. *Injury risk* (**fetus**) related to altered tissue perfusion (uteroplacental insufficiency, abruptio placentae) and/or preterm birth.

IV. **Nursing care plan/implementation**
   A. Assist at birth, the only definitive treatment.
      1. *Vaginal*, if cervix is favorable and fetal presentation and position are favorable.
      2. *Cesarean*, if induction for an extended period of time would be needed or for other indications such as fetal intolerance of labor or CPD.
   B. Administer prescribed medications:
      1. Magnesium sulfate—seizure prophylaxis.
      2. *Antihypertensive* agent for diastolic ≥ 110 mm Hg.
   C. Prevent/treat hypoglycemia (a major factor in maternal mortality in this disorder): ≤ 40 mg/dL.
   D. To permit seepage of edematous fluid, the cesarean incisional wound may be left open from the fascial layer; scrupulous *wound care* is imperative.
   E. Monitor breath sounds and woman's symptoms to identify and promptly treat *adult respiratory distress syndrome* (ARDS), which is one risk factor for women with the **HELLP** syndrome.
   F. Alert nursery nurse to observe newborn for *thrombocytopenia*, a common sequel to **HELLP** syndrome.

V. **Evaluation/outcome criteria**
   A. Woman/fetus does not suffer adverse sequelae to HELLP syndrome or its management.
   B. Family is able to cope effectively with this complication, its management, and outcomes.

# Complications Affecting Fluid-Gas Transport

(see **Table 3.5, p. 72**)

## Placenta Previa

**Definition**: abnormal implantation; near or over internal os. Increased incidence with smokers, and women > 40 yrs of age.

See **Figure 3.4 Placental Locations** and **Figure 3.5 Comparison of Normal Placental Implantation and Placenta Previa.**

I. **Assessment**
   A. Painless vaginal bleeding (may be intermittent); absence of contractions, abdomen soft.
   B. If in labor, contractions usually normal.
   C. Boggy lower uterine segment—palpated on vaginal examination. (NOTE: If placenta previa is suspected, internal examinations are **contraindicated**.)

D. *Medical diagnosis—procedure*: sonography to determine placental site.

II. **Analysis/nursing diagnosis**
   A. *Anxiety* related to bleeding, outcome.
   B. *Fluid volume deficit* related to excessive blood loss.
   C. *Tissue perfusion alteration* related to blood loss.
   D. *Urinary elimination alteration* related to hypovolemia.
   E. *Fear* related to fetal injury or loss.

III. **Nursing care plan/implementation**
   A. *Medical management.*
      1. *Ultrasound* is used to locate placental site; if unavailable, a sterile vaginal examination is conducted in a surgical suite under *double setup* (i.e., physicians and client are ready for an immediate vaginal or cesarean birth).
      2. Vaginal birth possible if: bleeding is *minimal*; placental implantation is *marginal*; and *fetal vertex* is presenting so that presenting part acts as tamponade.
      3. Cesarean birth for complete previa.
   B. **Nursing management.** Goal: *safeguard status.*

IV. **Evaluation/outcome criteria**: see Abruptio Placentae, **p. 72** and **79**, and **Tables 3.5** and **3.7**.

## Abruptio Placentae

**Definition**: premature separation of normally implanted placenta

I. **Assessment**
   A. *Sudden* onset, *severe* abdominal pain.
   B. Increased uterine tone—may contract unevenly, fails to relax between contractions; very tender.
   C. Shock usually more profound than expected on basis of external bleeding or internal bleeding.
   D. *Medical evaluation—procedures*: DIC screening (bleeding time, platelet count, prothrombin time, activated partial thromboplastin time, fibrinogen).

II. **Analysis/nursing diagnosis**
   A. *Fluid volume deficit* related to bleeding.
   B. *Fetal injury risk* related to uteroplacental insufficiency.
   C. *Fear* related to unknown outcome.

III. **Potential complications:**
   A. Afibrinogenemia and DIC.
   B. *Couvelaire* uterus—bleeding into uterine muscle.
   C. Amniotic fluid (pulmonary) embolus.
   D. Hypovolemic shock.
   E. Renal failure.
   F. Uterine atony, hemorrhage, infection in postpartum.

IV. **Nursing care plan/implementation**
   A. *Medical management*
      1. Control: hemorrhage, hypovolemic shock, replace blood loss.
      2. Cesarean birth.

## 🔵 PHARMACOLOGY BOX 3.1   HYPERTENSION IN PREGNANCY AND LABOR

| Drug/Dosage | Indication/Action | ◄ Assessment: Side Effects | ◄ Nursing Management |
|---|---|---|---|
| **Anticonvulsant** | | | |
| Magnesium sulfate (injection) *IM*: 1–5 g, prn *IV*: 1–4 g 1 h *Infusion*: 4 g in 250 mL 5% dextrose at ≤ 3 mL/m (loading dose) through infusion pump | Anticonvulsant activity due to inhibition of peripheral neuromuscular transmission Severe pre-eclampsia, eclampsia, HELLP syndrome | See box: **magnesium sulfate toxicity, p. 77** | Education: explain procedure, rationale to woman, family Take safety precautions Provide comfort measures 🔲 *Warning*—do *not* give to women on digoxin (arrhythmias may occur); emergency artificial ventilation may be necessary |
| **Antihypertensives** | | | |
| Hydralazine (*Apresoline, Neopresol*) (arteriolar vasodilators), 50–200 mg (0)/d | Peripheral arterioles: decreases muscle tone, thereby decreasing peripheral resistance | **Mother:** Headache Flushing Palpitation Tachycardia **Fetus:** Tachycardia: late decelerations and bradycardia if maternal diastolic pressure < 90 mm Hg | Monitor effects of medications Alert mother (family) to expected effects of medications ☞ Monitor BP (precipitous drop can lead to shock and perhaps to abruptio placentae); monitor ☞ urinary output Maintain bedrest in *lateral position* with siderails for safety |
| Labetalol hydrochloride (*Normodyne*) | Beta-blocking agent causing vasodilatation in peripheral arterioles, without significant change in cardiac output | Dizziness, drowsiness Bradycardia, postural hypotension Nausea/vomiting/diarrhea | See *Hydralazine* |
| Methyldopa (*Aldomet*) (used if maintenance therapy is needed): 250–500 mg orally q8h ( $\alpha_2$ -receptor agonist) | Reduces peripheral vascular resistance CNS: sedation | **Mother:** Sleepiness Postural hypotension Constipation 〰 Positive Coombs' | See *Hydralazine* NOTE: 10%-20% of women receiving medication over 1 yr will have *direct* and *indirect* Coombs'-positive hemolytic anemia |
| *Nitroglycerin* | Potent vasodilator of venous system Decreases BP by decreasing cardiac output | If maternal BP drops, FHR variability may decrease | Monitor: BP electronically, FHRs Need special IV setup See *Hydralazine* |

NOTE: Diuretics such as *thiazides* and *furosemide* (*Lasix*) are used only in severe situations: pulmonary edema. If used, the physician must be ready to justify the action.

🔵 3.  *IV heparin*—by infusion pump—to reduce coagulation and fibrinolysis.

B. **Nursing management.** Goal: *safeguard status*. Implement or assist with medical management.

◄ **V.   Evaluation/outcome criteria**

A. Woman experiences successful termination of pregnancy
1. Gives birth to viable newborn (via vaginal or cesarean method).
2. Has minimal blood loss.
3. Maintains assessment findings within normal limits.
4. Retains capacity for further childbearing.

B. Woman has no evidence of complications (anemia, hypotonia, DIC) during postpartal period.

## Complications Affecting Comfort, Rest, Mobility

### Polyhydramnios

**Definition**: amniotic fluid in excess of 2000 mL (normal volume: 500–1200 mL).

I.   **Etiology**: unknown. **Risk factors**:
A. Maternal diabetes.
B. Multifetal gestation.
C. Erythroblastosis fetalis.
D. Pre-eclampsia/eclampsia.
E. Congenital anomalies (e.g., anencephaly, upper GI anomalies, such as esophageal atresia).

◄ II.   **Assessment**
A. Fundal height: *excessive* for gestational estimate.
B. Fetal parts: *difficult* to palpate, *small* in proportion to uterine size.

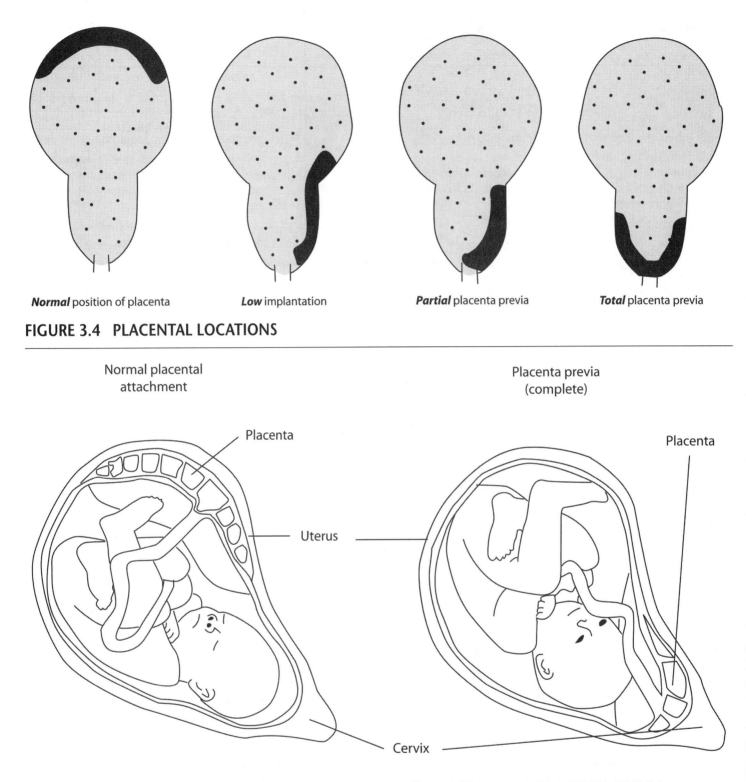

*Normal* position of placenta

*Low* implantation

*Partial* placenta previa

*Total* placenta previa

**FIGURE 3.4 PLACENTAL LOCATIONS**

Normal placental attachment

Placenta previa (complete)

Placenta

Placenta

Uterus

Cervix

**FIGURE 3.5 COMPARISON OF NORMAL PLACENTAL IMPLANTATION AND PLACENTA PREVIA.**

C. Increased discomfort—due to large, heavy uterus.

D. Increased edema in vulva and legs.

E. Shortness of breath.

F. GI discomfort—heartburn, constipation.

G. Susceptibility to *supine hypotensive syndrome*—due to compression of inferior vena cava and descending aorta while in supine position.

H. *Medical diagnosis—procedures*:

1. *Sonography*—to diagnose multifetal pregnancy, gross fetal anomaly, locate placental site.

2. *Amniocentesis*—to diagnose anomalies, erythroblastosis.

**III. Potential complications:**

A. Maternal respiratory compromise.

B. Premature rupture of membranes (PROM) with prolapsed cord and/or amnionitis.

C. Preterm labor.

D. Postpartum hemorrhage—due to overdistention and uterine atony.

## TABLE 3.7 COMPARISON OF PLACENTA PREVIA AND ABRUPTIO PLACENTAE

| Pathology | Etiology/Risk Factors | ▶ Assessment | ▶ Nursing Care Plan/ Implementation |
|---|---|---|---|
| **Placenta Previa** | | | |
| Types: *Marginal*—low lying *Partial*—partly covers internal os *Complete*—covers internal os | Unknown More common with multiparity, advanced maternal age Fibroid tumors Endometriosis Old scars Smoking | Painless vaginal bleeding Usually manifests in 8th mo **Postpartum**: signs of: hemorrhage, infection | • No vaginal or rectal exams or enemas • Bedrest (*high-Fowler's* if marginal previa) ☞ • Continuous fetal monitor • Maternal vital signs q 4 h, or as needed • Note character and amount of bleeding • Emotional support |
| **Abruptio Placentae** | | | |
| Types: *Partial*—small part separates *Complete*—total placenta separates *Retroplacental*—bleeding (concealed) *Marginal*—occurs at edges; ⬭ external bleeding | Pre-eclampsia/eclampsia Before birth of second twin Traction on cord Rupture of membranes High parity Chronic renal hypertension ⬭ Oxytocin induction/ augmentation of labor Cocaine addiction Trauma | Pain: sudden, severe Abdomen: rigid Uterus: very tender to touch Fetal hyperactivity; ⚡ bradycardia, death Shock: rapid, profound Port-wine amniotic fluid Signs of DIC **Postpartum**: signs of: atony, infection, pulmonary emboli | • *Position*: *supine*; *elevate* (R) hip ☞ • Monitor: vital signs, blood loss, fetus 〰 • I&O (anuria, oliguria; hematuria) • Prepare for surgery • Emotional support |

*Source*: ©Lagerquist, S. *Davis's NCLEX-RN® Success*, Philadelphia.

▶ **IV. Analysis/nursing diagnosis**

    A. *Pain* related to excessive size of uterus impinging on diaphragm, stomach, bladder.

    B. *Physical mobility impairment* related to increased lordotic curvature of back, increased weight on legs.

    C. *Tissue perfusion alteration* related to decreased venous return from lower extremities, compression of body structures by overdistended uterus.

    D. *Fluid volume deficit* related to potential uterine atony in immediate postpartum, secondary to loss of contractility due to overdistention.

    E. *Sleep pattern disturbance* related to respiratory compromise and discomfort in side-lying position.

    F. *Anxiety* related to discomfort, potential for complications, associated with congenital anomalies.

    G. *Urinary elimination alteration* (frequency) related to pressure of overdistended uterus on bladder.

▶ **V. Nursing care plan/implementation**

    A. *Medical management*.

      〰 1. *Amniocentesis*—remove excess fluid very slowly, to prevent abruptio placentae.

      2. Termination of pregnancy—if fetal abnormality present *and* woman desires.

    B. **Nursing management.**

      🏠 1. Goal: **health teaching.**

        a. Need for lateral *Sims' position* during resting; *semi-Fowler's* may alleviate respiratory compromise.

        b. Explain diagnostic and/or treatment procedures.

      ! c. Signs and symptoms to be *reported* **immediately**: bleeding, loss of fluid through vagina, cramping.

      2. Goal: *prepare for diagnostic and/or treatment procedures*.

        a. *Force* fluids—for sonography.

        b. Ensure that informed consent for amniocentesis is signed and in woman's chart.

      3. Goal: *emotional support for loss of pregnancy* (if applicable).

        a. Encourage verbalization of feelings.

        b. Facilitate grieving. Permit parents to see, hold infant; if desired, take photograph, footprints for them.

**◄ VI. Evaluation/outcome criteria**

    A. Woman complies with medical/nursing management.

    B. Woman's symptoms of respiratory compromise, etc. reduced; comfort promoted.

    C. Woman experiences normal, uncomplicated pregnancy, labor, birth, and postpartum.

# Diagnostic Tests to Evaluate Fetal Growth and Well-Being

## Daily Fetal Movement Count (DFMC)

    I. Noninvasive test done by a woman who is pregnant.

    II. Assesses *fetal activity*.

        A. Ten movements/hr = normal activity.

        B. Nine movements or less/hr may indicate fetal jeopardy.

    III. Assess for fetal sleep patterns; best time: just after a meal.

## Nonstress Test (NST)

    I. Correlates fetal movement with FHR. Requires electronic monitoring at least 20 minutes.

    II. *Reactive test*—acceleration of FHR 15 beats/min above baseline FHR, lasting for 15 sec or more, 3 times in 20 minutes.

    III. *Nonreactive* test—acceleration less than 15 beats/min above baseline FHR, lasting less than 3 times in 20 minutes; may indicate *fetal jeopardy*.

## Contraction Stress Test (CST); Oxytocin Challenge Test (OCT)

    I. Correlates fetal heart rate response to induced uterine contractions.

    II. Requires electronic monitoring.

    III. Indicator of *uteroplacental sufficiency*.

    IV. Identifies pregnancies at risk for fetal compromise from uteroplacental insufficiency.

    V. Increasing doses of oxytocin are administered to stimulate uterine contractions; requires 3 contractions lasting 40 sec in 10 minutes.

    VI. Interpretation: *negative* results indicate *absence* of abnormal deceleration with all contractions.

    VII. *Positive* results when 2 out of 3 contractions have late decelerations.

    VIII. Nipple stimulation (*breast self-stimulation test*) may also release enough systemic oxytocin to contract uterus to obtain indicators of fetal well-being or fetal jeopardy.

## Biophysical Profile (BPP)

    I. Observation by ultrasound of five variables for 30 min:

        A. Fetal body movements.

        B. Fetal tone.

        C. Amniotic fluid volume > 5.

        D. Reactive nonstress test.

        E. Fetal breathing movements.

    II. Variables are scored at 2 if present; score of *less than 6* is associated with perinatal *mortality*.

## Ultrasound

    I. Noninvasive procedure involving passage of high-frequency sound waves through uterus to obtain data regarding fetal growth, placental positioning, and the uterine cavity.

    II. Purpose may include:

        A. Pregnancy confirmation.

        B. Fetal viability.

        C. Estimation of fetal age.

        D. Biparietal diameter measurement (BPD).

        E. Placenta location.

        F. Detect fetal abnormalities.

        G. Confirm fetal death.

        H. Identify multifetal gestations.

        I. Estimated fetal weight.

    III. No risk to mother with infrequent use. Fetal risk not determined on long-term basis.

## Amniocentesis

    I. *Invasive* procedure for amniotic fluid analysis to assess fetal growth and maturity; done after 14 wk gestation.

    II. *Procedure*—needle placed through abdominal-uterine wall; designated amount of fluid is withdrawn for examination.

    III. Empty bladder if gestation greater than 20 wk.

    IV. Risk of complications less than 1%. Ultrasound *always* precedes this procedure.

    V. *Possible complications*: onset of contractions; infections (probably amnionitis); placental, cord puncture; bladder puncture.

    VI. Advise women to observe and *report* to physician: fetal hypo- or hyperactivity, vaginal bleeding, vaginal discharge (clear or colored), signs of labor.

## Analysis of Amniotic Fluid

    I. Chromosomal studies to detect *genetic* aberrations.

    II. Biochemical analysis of fetal cells to detect inborn errors of *metabolism*.

    III. Determination of fetal *lung maturity* by assessing L/S ratios.

IV. Evaluation of *phospholipids* (PG and PI); aids in determining lung *maturity*; new and accurate.

V. Determination of *creatinine* levels, aids in determining *fetal age*. (Greater than 1.8 mg/dL indicates fetal maturity and the fetal age.)

VI. Assessment of isoimmune disease.

VII. Assessment of *alpha-fetoprotein* (AFP) levels for determination of *neural tube* defects.

! VIII. Presence of meconium may indicate *fetal hypoxia*.

## Chorionic Villous Sampling (CVS)

I. Cervically *invasive* procedure.

II. *Advantage*—results can be obtained after 10 wk gestation due to fast-growing fetal cells.

III. *Procedure*—removal of small piece of tissue (chorionic villi) from fetal portion of placenta. Tissue reflects genetic makeup of fetus.

IV. Determines some genetic aberrations and allows for earlier decision for induced abortion (if desired) from abnormal results. Does *not* diagnose neural tube defects; Further diagnoses needed with ultrasound and serum AFP levels.

V. Protects "pregnancy privacy" because results can be obtained before the pregnancy is apparent and decisions can be made regarding abortion or continuation of gestation.

VI. *Risks* involve: spontaneous abortion, infection, hematoma, intrauterine death.

# Summary

Assessment for risk factors helps to identify the population that would benefit from timely intervention. Early identification is essential in order to plan and implement management of care throughout the childbearing cycle.

This chapter focuses on diseases that may *predate the pregnancy*: cardiac disease, Rh incompatibility, diabetes, substance abuse, STDs, age-related factors, cancer, violence, and other medical-surgical conditions.

In addition, *pregnancy-related conditions* are discussed: hemorrhagic disorders; metabolic disorders; pre-eclampsia, eclampsia, and HELLP syndrome; and hydramnios.

*Diagnostic tests* to evaluate fetal growth and well-being are outlined.

## Study and Memory Aids

### Insulin Requirements in Pregnancy

Trimester *one*: ↓
Trimester *two*: ↑
Trimester *three*: ↑
Postpartum: ↓

### Gestational Diabetes—Assessment: "3 P's"

**P**olydipsia
**P**olyphagia
**P**olyuria

### Heart Failure—Assessment

Heart rate is the most sensitive and reliable indicator of impending heart failure.

### RHoGAM

RhoGam is given to **Rh-negative** *woman only*!

### Indications for RHoGAM—Give RhoGAM to:

1. Rh- mother who gives birth to Rh+ neonate.
2. Rh- mother after spontaneous or induced abortion (> 8 wk).
3. Rh- mother after amniocentesis or chorionic villous sampling (CVS).
4. Rh- mother between 28 and 32 wk gestation.

### RhoGAM and Rubella Titer

Since RhoGAM is an immune globulin, rubella vaccination, given at about the same time, may *not* ! "take"; rubella titer needs to be redone at 3 mo.

### Fetal Maturity— Assessment

*Phosphatidyl glycerol* is more accurate indicator of fetal lung maturity in women who are diabetic.

### Infections

- *Vaginitis: avoid* douching during pregnancy.
- *STDs* in the U.S.: highest prevalence among teens.
- *AIDS* in the U.S.: fourth leading cause of death among women of reproductive age.

### TORCH Infections

**T**oxoplasmosis
**O**ther (hepatitis A virus [HAV], hepatitis B virus [HBV], group B streptococcus [GBS])
**R**ubella
**C**ytomegalovirus (CMV)
**H**erpes type 2

### Asthma

*Avoid* morphine for woman with asthma who is in labor.

## Cancer

**Malignant melanoma:** the *only* cancer that crosses the placenta to the fetus.

## Cycle of Violence

**Phase 1**—*building*: increased tension, anger, blaming, and arguing

**Phase 2**—*battering*: hitting, slapping, kicking, choking, use of objects or weapons; sexual abuse; verbal threats and abuse

**Phase 3**—*calm* state (may decrease over time): batterer may deny violence, state he was drunk, say he's sorry, and "promise it will never happen again," **returns to phase 1.**

Modified from A Helton. *A Protocol of Care for the Battered Woman.* White Plains, NY: March of Dimes Birth Defects Foundation.

## Hydatidiform Mole

**Complete H. mole:** *only* condition that can lead to maternal cancer.

## Pre-eclampsia

- *Proteinuria* differentiates pre-eclampsia from other pregnancy-induced hypertension (PIH) states.
- Pre-eclampsia is a disorder of *hypovolemia*.
- Home care may eliminate the need for hospitalization for "mild" pre-eclampsia.

## 🍎 Pre-eclampsia—Diet

Do *not eliminate* sodium from the diet.

## Hypertension—Standard American College of Obstetricians and Gynecologists (ACOG) Definition

Systolic: 30+ mm Hg above baseline
Diastolic: 15+ mm Hg above baseline

## HELLP Syndrome—Assessment

**H**emolysis
**E**levated **L**iver (enzymes)
**L**ow **P**latelets

## HELLP Syndrome—Complication

Hypoglycemia: ≤ 40 mg/dL
Hypoglycemia can lead to maternal mortality..

## Placenta Previa

Vaginal examinations **contraindicated** with undiagnosed vaginal bleeding.

# Questions

1. The nurse is planning to lead a seminar for young adults on violence against women, concentrating on abuse of women who are pregnant. Which statement is accurate and would be part of the nurse's discussion?
   1. Most of these women live below poverty level.
   2. Alcohol has been causally related to battering.
   3. The prevalence of violence lessens during pregnancy, dropping to a range of 2–4%.
   4. Women who are abused are more likely to have infants who are low-birth-weight (LBW) infants than women who are not abused during pregnancy.

2. The mode of birth of children with mothers who are HIV+ follows obstetric indications. Which is an unnecessary precaution for this client?
   1. Avoid scalp electrodes for electronic fetal monitoring.
   2. Avoid scalp pH determinations.
   3. Remove newborn to special care nursery immediately after birth.
   4. Delay amniotomy to reduce possibility of vertical transmission of HIV.

3. A nurse is discussing sexually transmitted diseases with a class of high school seniors. The students submitted a list of what they knew. The nurse evaluated the list. The only accurate statement is that gonorrhea:
   1. Is often spread through fomites.
   2. Is only spread through promiscuous sex.
   3. Is easily cured with penicillin.
   4. Can be prevented if condoms are used for sexual encounters.

4. The nurse considers a blood pressure of 120/80 in a woman who is pregnant as indicative of pre-eclampsia if:
   1. The woman has gained 2 pounds for each of the previous 2 wks.
   2. The woman is carrying a hydatidiform mole.
   3. The woman has had ankle edema each evening for the previous 2 wks.
   4. The woman's systolic pressure has increased by 30 mm Hg; the diastolic by 15 mm Hg.

5. A nurse case manager is developing a plan of care for a woman who is 4 wk pregnant with a Class I functional classification of organic heart disease. The nurse knows to plan for what normal adaptation to pregnancy that can place a client with cardiac disease at risk?
   1. Physiologic anemia.
   2. Increase in cardiac output after the 34th week.
   3. Gradual increase in size and weight of the uterus.
   4. Increased heart rate during the last half of pregnancy.

6. The nurse must teach the woman with cardiac disease and who is pregnant the symptoms specific to cardiac decompensation, which include:
   1. Fatigue.
   2. Periodic shortness of breath even when at rest.
   3. Transient palpitations.
   4. Coughing or feeling of smothering with coughing attacks.

7. The nursing plan of care for a woman in sickle cell crisis who is pregnant needs to be reevaluated if it includes:
   1. Adequate hydration with intravenous fluids.
   2. Blood transfusion to maintain hemoglobin at more than 10 mg/dL.
   3. Analgesia, as necessary.
   4. Control of asthma symptoms.

8. A nursing plan of care for home management of "mild" pre-eclampsia would include a diet consisting of:
   1. High protein, high calories, no added salt.
   2. High protein, high fiber, restrict salt.
   3. Low protein, fiber, and fat; no more than four (8 oz.) glasses of water/d.
   4. Low protein, high fiber, low salt; water to eight (8 oz.) glasses/d.

9. A woman with pre-eclampsia is admitted to the labor unit. Magnesium sulfate therapy is ordered. The nurse reviews the woman's chart and decides to confer with the physician before giving the medication when the following data are noted in her record:
   1. Mean arterial pressure = 107.
   2. Deep tendon reflexes are +2.
   3. Diabetic condition is controlled with insulin.
   4. Cardiac condition is controlled with digitoxin.

10. A woman who is attending a clinic for asthma sufferers tells the nurse she is pregnant. The nurse knows that, during pregnancy, preexisting asthma:
    1. Can be safely medicated with up to six doses of asthma medication per day.
    2. Increases the possibility of hyperemesis gravidarum.
    3. Is best treated with oral or parenteral formulations.
    4. Cannot be treated with sympathomimetic therapy (beta-agonist medications such as terbutaline sulfate [*Brethaire, Brethine, Bricanyl*]).

11. A woman at 32 wk gestation has been severely beaten and pushed down a flight of stairs. Although no external bleeding is noted, internal bleeding is a possibility. When clinical signs of shock appear due to loss of blood, the nurse knows the woman who is pregnant and injured has lost at least what percentage of her blood volume?
    1. 30%.
    2. 40%.
    3. 50%.
    4. 60%.

12. Preconception counseling should include information about the importance of vaccinations to bolster a woman's immune system. The nurse must teach potential parents that although varicella-zoster virus (VZV) infections are infrequent during pregnancy, they can cause serious consequences for the mother/fetus/newborn, which include:
    1. Mother: pneumonia, encephalitis.
    2. Placenta: abruption.
    3. Fetus: spontaneous abortion.
    4. Newborn: conjunctivitis.

13. A woman who is pregnant is Rh negative; her husband is Rh positive. Which statement by the woman demonstrates to the nurse that the woman understands Rh isoimmunization?
    1. "A small amount of my red blood cells crosses the placenta; the baby then becomes allergic to them."
    2. "If my baby is Rh positive, I could develop antibodies against my baby's red blood cells."
    3. "The first pregnancy is most at risk; subsequent pregnancies are not nearly as dangerous."
    4. "Coombs' positive means that my baby and I are protected against Rh isoimmunization."

14. During a preconception class, the discussion turns to questions about drug dependence and pregnancy. The nurse's response is based on knowledge that maternal withdrawal from cocaine dependence puts the fetus/newborn at risk for:
    1. Intrauterine asphyxia.
    2. Facial dysmorphia.
    3. Disseminated intravascular coagulation (DIC).
    4. Bronchopulmonary dysplasia (BPD).

15. A woman who is pregnant becomes frightened when she overhears a physician say she had a reactive nonstress test (NST). The nurse clarifies the physician's comment and states that a reactive NST suggests:
    1. Intrauterine asphyxia.
    2. Fetal well-being.
    3. Need for immediate cesarean birth.
    4. Need for confirmation with a contraction stress test (CST).

16. Digitalis preparations may be ordered to maximize ventricular contractions. The nurse can expect to administer higher doses (or more frequent doses) of digitalis for a woman who is pregnant because:
    1. Maternal hormones increase the effect of digitalis.
    2. Maternal hormones decrease the effect of digitalis.
    3. During pregnancy, drugs are metabolized more rapidly.
    4. Increased plasma volume may lower circulating levels of the drug.

17. To meet the standard of care for risk management of the woman who is pregnant and diabetic, the nurse must develop a plan of care to maintain (during pregnancy) the target range for postprandial (2 hr after meals) blood glucose levels between:
    1. 60–90 mg/dL.
    2. 60–105 mg/dL.
    3. 60–120 mg/dL.
    4. 90–140 mg/dL.

18. During preconception counseling, the nurse's teaching plan must include information that acidosis in a woman who is pregnant and has a type 1 diabetes may be precipitated if she:
    1. Limits salt in her diet.
    2. Decreases activity.
    3. Experiences nausea, vomiting, and loss of appetite.
    4. Increases intake of simple sugars.

19. A nurse case manager's plan of care for a woman who is pregnant and has diabetes recognizes that labor may be induced several weeks before term in the client with poorly controlled diabetes, because early birth:
    1. Prevents the baby from getting too large.
    2. Improves chances for a live-born baby.
    3. Prevents diabetes from developing in the baby.
    4. Decreases the infant's chances of developing respiratory distress syndrome (RDS).

20. To meet the standard of care for risk management, *all* nurses must be aware of how maternal adaptations to pregnancy alter assessment techniques and findings, so that timely intervention is possible. Acute suppurative appendicitis complicates about 1/1000 pregnancies. What statement is accurate about this condition during pregnancy?
    1. Appendiceal rupture and peritonitis rarely occur during pregnancy.
    2. Maternal and perinatal morbidity and mortality are greatly increased when appendicitis occurs during pregnancy.
    3. Therapeutic abortion is indicated in appendicitis.
    4. Appendicitis is easier to diagnose during pregnancy than in the woman who is not pregnant.

21. The ability to achieve pregnancy is not affected by spinal cord injury (SCI). The nurse should plan care for a woman who is pregnant and has a SCI that is based on knowledge that:
    1. Physiologically, the woman with SCI encounters many of the same problems that women who are pregnant also generally experience.
    2. She will be assessed frequently during the last weeks of pregnancy, since she is unable to know when she is having labor contractions.
    3. Since she cannot push to give birth, she will have a forceps-assisted birth.

    4. Oxytocin induction of labor is warranted if she is prone to autonomic dysreflexia (sweating, flushing, pounding headache, severe hypertension).

22. A woman who is pregnant slipped on her front porch steps and sustained a deep cut in her leg. Her husband has picked her up, wrapped her in a blanket, and placed her in Trendelenburg's position, and is applying direct pressure over the wound with some clean linen while waiting for the ambulance. A home health nurse, going to visit a client in the neighborhood, stops and evaluates the care her husband is providing. The nurse should:
    1. Reposition her out of Trendelenburg.
    2. Compliment her husband for using Trendelenburg.
    3. Apply a tourniquet above the wound on her leg.
    4. Go to visit the home health client; the husband has everything under control.

23. All nurses must know that rectal or vaginal examinations are contraindicated for women with undiagnosed third trimester vaginal bleeding because:
    1. It is undesirable to stimulate labor.
    2. A low-lying placenta may be dislodged, and bleeding will follow.
    3. There is danger of rupturing the membranes.
    4. Cervical dilatation is of little importance in this situation.

24. The nurse develops a plan of care to incorporate physician-ordered treatment for the woman who is pregnant with mild pre-eclampsia, which would most likely include:
    1. Bedrest.
    2. Analgesics.
    3. Thiazide diuretics.
    4. Magnesium sulfate.

25. A woman in labor is experiencing increasingly severe symptoms of pre-eclampsia. When she complains of epigastric pain, the nurse realizes that this complaint suggests:
    1. Impending convulsions.
    2. Impending digestive disorder.
    3. Impending birth.
    4. No clinical significance.

26. When providing care for a woman in labor who has severe pre-eclampsia (or eclampsia), the nurse must be constantly alert for increasing severity of symptoms and for a possible associated complication—HELLP syndrome. Which finding needs to be present for a woman to be diagnosed with HELLP syndrome?
    1. Hyperglycemia.
    2. Platelet count of 100,000 or more.
    3. Disseminated intravascular coagulopathy (DIC).
    4. Elevated liver enzymes.

27. Following a woman's eclamptic seizure, and after ensuring a patent airway, the nurse will do all of the following. Which should the nurse do *first*?
    1. Assess fetal status: FHR, movement.
    2. Assess labor status: contractions, cervical dilatation/effacement, membranes, station.
    3. Assess maternal vital signs, deep tendon reflexes, and I&O.
    4. Document seizure event.

28. Magnesium sulfate IV is ordered for the client with severe pre-eclampsia. Which sign would lead the nurse to suspect magnesium sulfate toxicity?
    1. Increased urine output.
    2. Decreased deep tendon reflexes (DTRs).
    3. Increased respiratory rate.
    4. Cold, clammy skin.

29. Which assessment finding would prompt the nurse to stop the intravenous infusion of $MgSO_4$ for treatment of severe pre-eclampsia?
    1. Respirations at 16/min.
    2. Patellar and brachial reflexes at +1.
    3. Urine output at 90 mL/4 hr.
    4. Pulse pressure at 30 mm Hg.

30. The clinic nurse would suggest that a woman be brought to the emergency department if she has signs/symptoms of acute rupture of a tubal pregnancy, such as:
    1. Profuse vaginal bleeding.
    2. Referred shoulder pain.
    3. Irregular fetal heart rate.
    4. Elevation of temperature.

31. A woman is admitted to the labor unit with a diagnosis of partial placenta abruptio. The nurse would question the diagnosis if assessment reveals:
    1. A history of multiparity or hypertension.
    2. Appearance of port-wine-stained amniotic fluid.
    3. Normal uterine contractions.
    4. Mild uterine hypertonicity.

32. The nursing plan of care for a woman with cardiac disease who is in labor is modified to meet her special needs. Which intervention is specific for this woman?
    1. Auscultate for crackles (rales) q30 min
    2. Turn from side to side qh.
    3. Monitor blood pressure qh.
    4. Assess bladder filling and encourage voiding as necessary.

33. A woman in active labor has a positive culture for *herpes genitalis*. Her membranes are intact; the cervix is 5 cm dilated. The nurse should be prepared for what type of birth?
    1. Cesarean.
    2. Vacuum-assisted.
    3. Low forceps-assisted.
    4. Spontaneous-vaginal.

34. A woman in active labor is HIV positive. Which fetal monitoring method should the nurse choose?
    1. Leff scope or DeHillis scope.
    2. Penard's stethoscope.
    3. External electronic fetal monitor.
    4. Internal electronic fetal monitor.

35. Asthma is not uncommon in pregnancy and the nurse must know about the disorder since the effect of pregnancy on asthma is unpredictable. The nurse's plan of care must recognize that acute episodes may require steroids, aminophylline, oxygen, and correction of fluid-electrolyte imbalance. Regarding the management of labor for a woman with bronchial asthma, the nurse anticipates that:
    1. Vaginal birth with local or regional anesthesia is the method of choice.
    2. Morphine is used in labor because it usually relieves bronchospasm.
    3. Ephedrine and corticotropin (pressor drugs) are used if pre-eclampsia develops.
    4. Asthma does not affect the incidence of abortion or preterm labor, or produce adverse effects on the fetus.

36. The nurse who gives anticipatory guidance related to labor anticipates the following variation(s) from the normal routine for a woman with heart disease:
    1. The woman will probably lie flat in bed, but only on her side.
    2. Assessment of pulse and respirations will be more frequent than usual.
    3. The woman will have an unmedicated second stage of labor.
    4. Low forceps-assisted birth is contraindicated.

37. The woman with a known cardiac condition must be watched carefully during labor. To prevent cardiac decompensation, she should be:
    1. Maintained with oxytocin to increase contractions.
    2. Monitored more frequently.
    3. Maintained with an IV infusion.
    4. Positioned on her side with her shoulders elevated.

38. The nurse monitoring a woman who is pregnant and on digitalis must be on the alert for:
    1. Delay in the onset of labor.
    2. Shortening of the length of labor.
    3. Prolonged length of labor.
    4. Secondary uterine inertia during labor.

39. If a woman in labor vomits during a convulsion, the nurse's first action is to:
    1. Quickly obtain the necessary equipment and suction her.
    2. Position the woman on her side with her head lower than her shoulders.
    3. Insert a padded tongue blade.
    4. Start oxygen by face mask.

40. The nurse knows that the sign which distinguishes pre-eclampsia from gestational hypertension is:
    1. A rise in systolic pressure of at least 30 mm Hg.
    2. Edema in the ankles.
    3. A diastolic pressure of 90 mm Hg or more.
    4. Proteinuria.

41. A common condition in individuals with rheumatic heart disease (RHD) is mitral stenosis. Ventricular failure, pulmonary edema, and atrial fibrillation can occur. The nurse needs to counsel the woman who is pregnant and has RHD that she may expect the following interventions:
    1. Warfarin sodium (*Coumadin*).
    2. Unmedicated labor and birth.
    3. Bearing down in semi-Fowler's position with legs in stirrups.
    4. Digoxin and anticoagulants.

42. A clinic client with systemic lupus erythematosus (SLE) tells the nurse that she is anticipating having a child. She asks the nurse how SLE could affect pregnancy. The nurse's response is based on the knowledge that:
    1. The risk of miscarriage is high with SLE.
    2. Hypotension is a major problem during pregnancy with SLE.
    3. Many medications used in treating SLE can be used during pregnancy.
    4. The incidence of flare-ups of SLE is decreased during pregnancy.

43. A preconception conference is particularly important for women with a history of medical complications. Before collaborating with a physician to develop a teaching plan for these women, the nurse reviews a list of medical conditions in which pregnancy with a favorable outcome is possible. This list would include:
    1. A woman who is a transplant recipient.
    2. Women with Marfan's syndrome.
    3. Women with pulmonary hypertension.
    4. A woman with diabetes and proliferative retinopathy.

44. A nurse case manager is developing a plan of care for women who are pregnant and considered to be at high risk. The plan for a woman who is pregnant and has sickle cell disease must include close monitoring, especially for infection with:
    1. Pneumococcus.
    2. Streptococcus.
    3. Staphylococcus.
    4. Enterococcus.

45. The nurse analyzes the following assessment data about a woman who is receiving magnesium sulfate intravenously for severe pre-eclampsia: some bleeding from her gums and a small amount of blood oozing from her IV infusion site. The nurse's *first* action should be to:
    1. Restart the IV at another site.
    2. Provide good mouth care.

3. Obtain an order for a stat platelet determination.
4. Continue with routine monitoring.

46. A woman who is pregnant asks her home health care nurse what she needs to know about her drug therapy for asthma during pregnancy. The nurse's best response is that:
    1. Most asthma medications are safe to take.
    2. Asthma medications make it impossible for her to breastfeed.
    3. Teratogenic effects of these medications can occur well into the second trimester.
    4. Beta-agonists cannot be used during pregnancy.

47. A woman at 32 wk gestation has been severely beaten and pushed down a flight of stairs; spinal cord injury is a possibility. The nurse plans to continuously monitor the maternal-fetal unit for at least:
    1. 4 hr.
    2. 12 hr.
    3. 24 hr.
    4. 24–48 hr.

48. The nurse analyzes the following data: on admission, the hematocrit (Hct) of a woman with pre-eclampsia was 34%; 3 d later, it is 38%. The nurse determines that this is probably the result of:
    1. Improved diet resulting in increased hematopoiesis.
    2. Improved perfusion of the spleen, causing depressed hemolysis of red blood cells (RBCs).
    3. A shift of fluid out of the vascular compartment.
    4. Normal physiologic polycythemia of pregnancy.

49. Which assessment finding would prompt the nurse to stop IV infusion of $MgSO_4$ for treatment of severe pre-eclampsia?
    1. Respirations: 14/min.
    2. Patellar and brachial reflexes: 0.
    3. Urinary output: 150 mL/4 h.
    4. Blood pressure: 142/94.

50. The home health nurse advice is that, in addition to hospital disinfectants, another substance that is effective against HIV for washable surfaces is:
    1. Normal saline solution.
    2. Household cleanser.
    3. Household bleach (sodium hypochlorite) 1:10 solution.
    4. Detergent (¼ c) and hot water (1 gallon).

51. The nurse should be alert to the fact that, among leading causes of death among women of reproductive-age in the United States, acquired immunodeficiency syndrome (AIDS) ranks:
    1. Third.
    2. Fourth.
    3. Fifth.
    4. Sixth.

52. A 17-year-old woman comes to the woman's clinic with the chief complaint of dysuria and painful blisters on the outside of her vagina for 2 days. Her history reveals feeling feverish and achy 1 wk ago, and having sex with a new partner 3 wk ago. The clinic nurse suspects:
    1. Syphilis.
    2. Venereal warts.
    3. Primary herpes.
    4. Recurrent herpes.

53. To relieve periurethral discomfort caused by vaginal infection with *Chlamydia trachomatis*, the nurse recommends:
    1. Douching.
    2. A perineal heat lamp.
    3. Sitz baths.
    4. Ambulation.

54. A woman's menstrual cycles are regular, lasting 31 days. Her LMP started on March 15. When can she expect to ovulate next?
    1. March 25.
    2. March 29.
    3. April 2.
    4. April 15.

55. The nurse tells the woman that a symptom to watch for that is indicative of a chlamydial infection is:
    1. +1 Protein in urine.
    2. Burning on urination.
    3. Purulent vaginal discharge.
    4. Dependent edema.

56. In about 3% of cases of complete hydatidiform moles, a progression toward choriocarcinoma occurs. The nurse counsels strict adherence to the follow-up management, which continues for one year and includes:
    1. Regularly scheduled suction curettage.
    2. Frequent measurement of serum hCG levels.
    3. Contraception with diaphragm, spermicide, and condoms.
    4. Treatment with methotrexate and dactinomycin.

# Answers/Rationale

1. **(4)** Women who are abused are 1 ½ times more likely to have infants who are LBW than women not abused during pregnancy, and they are more likely to have associated risk factors for LBW, such as poor obstetric history, infections, and alcohol or drug usage. Violence against women respects no social, economic, or racial categories (**1**). Alcohol (**2**) has not been causally related to battering, but batterers have a high rate of alcohol abuse. The prevalence of abuse toward women who are pregnant ranges from 8–17%; violence may become *worse* during pregnancy, rather than improving (**3**). **AN, RE/KN, 7, PsI, Psychosocial integrity**

2. **(3)** Newborns do *not* need to be separated from their mothers on the basis of the mother's HIV status. Options 1, 2, and 4 are all *appropriate* precautions to take when caring for mothers and newborns who are HIV +. **IMP, APP, 1,SECE, Safety and infection control**

3. **(1)** Gonorrhea can be spread through fomites, which are nonliving material, e.g., linens, on which disease-producing organisms may be conveyed. Option **2** is incorrect because even sex with *one* partner who has gonorrhea can cause infection. Option **3** is incorrect because gonorrhea is *more difficult* to cure, since some bacterial *Neisseria gonorrhoeae* have developed resistance to penicillin, which used to cure the disease with comparative speed, especially in the early stages, and some women are allergic to penicillin. (Ceftriaxone in a single dose is recommended for treatment of women who are pregnant and not pregnant; spectinomycin is the preferred alternative therapy.) Option **4** is incorrect because condoms only *protect* against (*not prevent*) transmission during penile-vaginal contact; gonorrhea can be transmitted into the rectum or the oropharynx, or through fomites. **EV, RE/KN, 1, SECE, Safety and infection control**

4. **(4)** An increase in systolic pressure by ≥ 30 mmHg and in diastolic pressure by ≥ 15 mmHg is the accepted definition of pre-eclampsia. A weight gain of 2 pounds in 2 wk does not fit the definition of pre-eclampsia (**1**). While pre-eclampsia *can* occur before the twentieth week in the presence of a hydatidiform mole, the presence of an H. mole does *not* indicate the presence of pre-eclampsia (**2**). Ankle edema can occur in women who are *healthy* and experiencing normal pregnancy (e.g., after a long period of standing or in the evening of a hot day), not just in pre-eclampsia (**3**). **EV, ANL, 6, PhI, Physiological adaptation**

5. **(4)** The increased blood volume and cardiac output and the increase in heart rate during the last half of pregnancy can stress the heart beyond its ability to compensate. Physiologic anemia alone (**1**) does not stress the heart beyond its ability to compensate (although *true* anemia can lead to cardiac failure).

---

**Key to Codes**

**Nursing process: AS,** assessment; **AN,** analysis; **PL,** planning; **IMP,** implementation; **EV,** evaluation. (See **Appendix J** for explanation of nursing process steps.)

**Cognitive level: RE/KN,** recall/knowledge; **COM,** comprehension; **APP,** application; **ANL,** analysis; **EVL,** evaluation; **SYN,** synthesis. (See **Appendix J** for explanation.)

**Category of human function: 1,** protective; **2,** sensory-perceptual; **3,** comfort, rest, activity, and mobility; **4,** nutrition; **5,** growth and development; **6,** fluid-gas transport; **7,** psychosocial-cultural; **8,** elimination. (See **Appendix L** for explanation.)

**Client need: SECE,** safe, effective care environment; **HPM,** health promotion and maintenance; **PsI,** psychosocial integrity; **PhI,** physiological integrity. (See **Appendix M** for explanation.)

**Client subneed:** See **Appendix M** for explanation.

The cardiac output does not continue to increase after the 34th week (2); it declines to about a 20% increase at 40 weeks. Although the size and weight of the uterus (3) can impede venous return to the heart when the woman is supine, proper positioning (side-lying with shoulders elevated) supports cardiac functioning. **PL, ANL, 6, PhI, Physiological adaptation**

6. (4) Congestion develops as the heart is increasingly unable to maintain adequate circulation. The symptoms in options 1, 2, and 3 *may be* symptoms of cardiac decompensation, but they are *also normal* findings during pregnancy. **IMP, COM, 6, PhI, Physiological adaptation**

7. (2) Blood transfusion is given to maintain hemoglobin at more than *8 mg/dL* and hemoglobin A at over 40%. The other options do not require reevaluation: adequate hydration (1) *is* essential; analgesia (3) *should* be administered as necessary; asthma *must* be controlled (4), since it is a condition that can promote sickling crises by shifting the oxygen-hemoglobin dissociation curve to the right. **EV, ANL, 6, PhI, Reduction of risk potiental**

Test-taking tip: Look at what is being asked; options that do *not* require reevaluation are *true*.

8. (1) Women who are pre-eclamptic especially need high protein to replace that lost in the urine. The high caloric intake is needed to meet the extra demands of stress as well as the needs of maternal/fetal growth. All protein of high biologic value has salt; however, the woman should not add extra to her food. The other diets would not be therapeutic. Option 2: Salt should not be *restricted*, and she needs extra calories. (The high fiber is generally advisable, although it is not specific to this condition.) Options 3 and 4: She needs high, *not* low, protein, and she *should* have plenty of water to quench her thirst (8 glasses/d is acceptable, but does not need to be stated as a limit). **PL, APP, 4, PhI, Basic care and comfort**

9. (4) Magnesium sulfate should *not* be given to women who are pre-eclamptic with cardiac disease and who are taking digitoxin. Arrhythmias may occur; emergency artificial ventilation may be necessary. A MAP of 107 (1) is indicative of mild pre-eclampsia; the client may be a candidate for magnesium sulfate therapy. DTRs of +2 (2) are within *normal* range. Magnesium sulfate is not contraindicated for clients with diabetes controlled with insulin (3). **EV, ANL, 2, PhI, Physiological adaptation**

10. (2) The woman with preexisting asthma has an increased possibility of hyperemesis, hemorrhage, pre-eclampsia, and complicated labor. Other dangers are prematurity, low birth weight, and neonatal hypoxia. She can be safely medicated with up to four doses per day; dosing in excess of 4 times/d (1)

is a warning sign for the woman to seek medical attention immediately. *Inhaled* medications are preferable to oral or parenteral medications (3). She *can* be treated with sympathomimetic therapy (4). **AN, APP, 6, HPM, Health promotion and maintenance**

11. (1) During pregnancy, the woman may sustain a significant blood loss, approximately 30%, without the usual signs and symptoms of hypovolemia. The blood loss in options 2, 3, and 4 is over 30%; while signs and symptoms of hypovolemia would already have appeared, these percentages do not represent the *minimum* amount lost before they appear. **NOTE:** A rapid pulse may reflect only the usual increase of 10-15 beats/min during pregnancy, or it may be a sign of hypovolemia. **AS, ANL, 6, PhI, Physiological adaptation**

12. (1) Consequences for VZV infection for the mother are pneumonia (mortality of severe varicella pneumonia is about 3%, but can be as high as 15–40% if specific antiviral therapy is not administered) and encephalitis (mortality is between 5 and 20%; long-term neurologic manifestations may occur in as many as 15% of survivors). Abruptio placentae (2) is *not* a consequence. Spontaneous abortion rate (3) is *not* higher (however, these women are more likely to give birth at or before 37 wk gestation; congenital anomalies can occur). Conjunctivitis (4) is *not* one of the consequences; however, newborns may develop pneumonia, disseminated intravascular coagulation (DIC), and infection (mortality 30%). **IMP, APP, 1, SECE, Safety and infection control**

13. (2) If the fetus is Rh positive, the woman could develop antibodies against the fetal red blood cells. It is the entry of Rh positive blood into the blood stream of Rh negative *woman*, not into the fetus' circulation (1) that stimulates the formation of antibodies against the Rh factor. The first pregnancy (3) is at *least* risk (risk arises only if the woman had previously developed antibodies against the Rh factor due to an erroneous blood transfusion). "Coombs' positive" (4) refers to the titer of Rh antibodies present in the woman's blood stream; the Rh positive fetus is at great risk of hemolysis with subsequent anemia, edema formation, and cardiac decompensation. **EV, EVL, 6, PhI, Physiological adaptation**

14. (1) Maternal withdrawal from cocaine puts the fetus at risk for intrauterine asphyxia. Its significant and agonizing withdrawal is felt as violent movements in utero. Maternal episodes of vasospastic hypertension during cocaine use cause numerous small strokes; withdrawal may cause sudden maternal hypotension, which can be a cause of fetal asphyxia. Facial dysmorphia (2) is characteristic of *fetal alcohol syndrome* (FAS). DIC (3) has not been documented as being associated with maternal dependence on cocaine and withdrawal symptoms. BPD (4) is characteristic of *lung dysplasia* that

develops in preterm infants dependent on long-term oxygen and ventilator support. **AN, RE/KN, 6, PhI, Physiological adaptation**

15. **(2)** A reactive NST suggests fetal well-being. The criteria for a reactive test: two or more accelerations of 15 beats/min lasting for 15 sec over a 20 min period; normal baseline rate; long-term variability amplitude of 10 or more beats/min. Because fetal *well-being* is assured by a reactive NST, there is no indication of a problem such as asphyxia (1), and there is no need for immediate cesarean birth (3). If the test were *non*reactive, a CST should be performed (4). **IMP, APP, 5, PhI, Reduction of risk potential**

16. **(4)** 30–50% is added to the circulating plasma volume during pregnancy, which lowers the circulating levels of the drug. Options 1, 2, and 3 are not relevant to the need to increase the dose of digitalis preparations for the woman who is pregnant and has cardiac disease. NOTE: Other medications that may be ordered for this woman with cardiac disease are heparin (vs. warfarin [*Coumadin*]) and antibiotics. **PL, COM, 6, PhI, Pharmacological and parenteral Therapies**

17. **(3)** 60–120 mg/dL is the target range. The range in option 1 is the target range for *fasting* blood sugar (before breakfast), and the range in option 2 is the target range *before* lunch, dinner, and bedtime. The range in option 4 is too high. NOTE: Good diabetic control is associated with good pregnancy outcome, e.g., absence of sequelae of poor control: congenital anomalies, hydramnios, macrosomia, respiratory distress syndrome (even if born at term). **PL, APP, 4, PhI, Reduction of risk potenial**

18. **(3)** When a person does not eat, the body begins to break down its own tissues; metabolic acidosis results. None of the actions in options 1, 2, and 4 would precipitate acidosis in a woman who is pregnant and diabetic. **PL, APP, 4, PhI, Physiological adaptation**

19. **(2)** The incidence of intrauterine fetal death rises dramatically starting with week 37; reasons are not known. An infant who is macrosomal (1) could still be born at term, vaginally or abdominally; however, in this case early birth increases the chances for the infant's *survival*. Early birth is not related to developing diabetes (3); diabetes is familial (possibly inherited) but may also be viral-related. The baby of a poorly controlled woman with diabetes is at risk for RDS (4) whether preterm or term, because high insulin levels in the fetus delay the production of surfactant in the lungs. **PL, APP, 6, PhI, Reduction of risk potential**

20. **(2)** Maternal mortality increases to about 10% in the third trimester; 15% of it occurs during labor. Perinatal mortality is approximately 10% with unruptured appendicitis; 35%, with peritonitis. Rupture and peritonitis (1) occur 2–3 times *more often* than in women who are not pregnant. Therapeutic abortion (3) is *never* indicated in appendicitis. The appendix is carried high and to the right away from McBurney's point by the enlarged uterus, making diagnosis more *difficult*, not easier (4). Also, increased sedimentation rate cannot be used as an indicator of infection during pregnancy. **AS, RE/KN, 1, HPM, Health promotion and maintenance**

21. **(1)** The woman with SCI is physiologically the same as other women. Some of the normal adaptations, however, do require special consideration: urinary frequency, urinary tract infection, constipation, the need to relieve pressure on ischial spines and gluteal muscles, and to straighten (as pregnancy precludes lying prone). Although women with SCI do not experience labor as other women do (2), they are in tune with their bodies and know when something is happening. The woman with SCI experiences *no* trouble with a vaginal birth (3) even though she has no ability to push. Uterine contractions, plus a relaxed perineum, facilitate a vaginal birth. Oxytocin (4), if needed, is used cautiously and only when personnel are versed in the recognition and treatment of autonomic dysreflexia (the headache and hypertension must not be confused with pre-eclampsia). **PL, RE/KN, 5, HPM, Health promotion and maintenance**

22. **(1)** Trendelenburg's position could severely impair maternal respirations since the heavy enlarged uterus will press against her diaphragm. She must *not* remain in Trendelenburg (2); she should be repositioned on her side. Tourniquets (3) must be used with care; direct pressure is appropriate in this case. The nurse *cannot* leave (4) until the client's safety is assured. **EV, ANL, 1, PhI, Reduction of risk potential**

23. **(2)** Third trimester bleeding suggests a low-lying placenta, which may be dislodged during examination causing further bleeding. Stimulating the cervix or actually touching the placenta during the examination can result in further separation of the placenta and life-threatening hemorrhage. Options 1 and 3 are *not* relevant to precautions for third trimester vaginal bleeding. Although the statement in option 4 is true, it is not the *reason* that rectal or vaginal examination is contraindicated. **IMP, RE/KN, 6, PhI, Reduction of risk potential**

24. **(1)** Bedrest in the side-lying position increases perfusion of the uterus and kidneys and often reduces stress. (Increased perfusion of the kidneys decreases their production of angiotensin-II.) Although some authors have postulated that aspirin can have a preventive/curative effect on pre-eclampsia (2), no definitive evidence is available. Diuretics (3) are *contraindicated* during pregnancy, except in the case of cardiopulmonary decompensation; they can cause electrolyte imbalance. Magnesium sulfate (4) is an anticonvulsant and CNS depressant; it does *not* prevent pre-eclampsia. **PL, APP, 3, PhI, Basic care and comfort**

25. (1) "Epigastric" pain is the subjective description of pain from the edematous liver capsule and liver infarcts; it often heralds impending convulsions. The epigastric discomfort is *not* related to a gastrointestinal tract problem (2), and it is *not* a sign of impending birth (3). It *does* have clinical significance (4), as it should alert the nurse to possible convulsive seizures. **EV, ANL, 2, PhI, Physiological adaptation**

26. (4) H = hemolysis; EL = *elevated liver enzymes*; LP = low platelets. None of the findings in options 1, 2, and 3 is part of the definition of the **HELLP** syndrome. **AN, APP, 6, PhI, Physiological adaptation**

27. (1) This activity takes very little time, and while doing it, the nurse can also begin assessment of uterine irritability. This provides data about fetal oxygen needs so that oxygen by face mask would be in place while continuing with assessments. Labor status (2) is assessed *after* fetal status (birth may be IMMINENT!), *then* maternal status (3). Documentation (4) is essential (characteristics of seizure and aftermath; assessment findings and woman's response to interventions), but would *follow* the other steps listed. **AN, ANL, 2, PhI, Reduction of risk potential**

28. (2) Magnesium sulfate acts on the myoneural junction; reflexes must be at least at 1+ so that paralysis of muscles does not occur. Increased urine output (1), or diuresis, is a *good* prognostic sign—the magnesium sulfate therapy is effective. Respirations are *depressed* with toxicity, *not increased* (3). Cold, clammy skin (4) is a sign of *shock, not* magnesium sulfate toxicity. **AS, ANL, 2, PhI, Pharmacological and parenteral therapies**

29. (3) Urinary output should be at least 120 mL/4 hr, as renal ischemia from hypertension can cause dangerous concentrations of $MgSO_4$. Respirations must be 12/min or more to continue therapy, so a rate of 16/min (1) *is* within limits. Reflexes must be at least +1 to continue therapy, so a value of +1 (2) *is* within limits. Pulse pressure (4) is unaffected by $MgSO_4$. **EV, ANL, 8, PhI, Physiological adaptation**

30. (2) Referred shoulder pain (Kehr's sign) is a common finding with acute rupture of a tubal pregnancy. Referred pain probably occurs because pain signals from the viscera travel along the same neural pathways used by pain signals from the shoulder; the woman perceives the pain but interprets it as having originated in the shoulder, rather than in the deep-seated viscera—the fallopian tube. Bleeding (1) occurs into the *peritoneal* cavity instead of into the intrauterine cavity. FHTs (3) are *never* heard; the tube cannot sustain a pregnancy long enough for the fetus to develop enough to have audible FHTs. Elevation of temperature (4) is *not* one of the usual findings of acute rupture of a tubal pregnancy. **EV, ANL, 1, PhI, Physiological adaptation**

31. (3) Premature separation of the placenta (placenta abruptio) is usually accompanied by *mild to severe* uterine hypertonicity; the uterus may contract unevenly, and fail to relax between contractions. Options 1, 2, and 4 *are* all associated with placental abruption. NOTE: The following may also be seen with placenta abruptio: history of abdominal trauma or cocaine use; pain, mild to severe, localized over one region of the uterus, or diffuse over the uterus with a boardlike abdomen. Maternal hypertension has been identified in approximately half of the cases. **EV, ANL, 5, HPM, Health promotion and maintenance**

32. (1) Since these women are at risk for heart failure during labor, the nurse auscultates for crackles (rales) every 30 min. Side-lying position facilitates venous return; it is *not* necessary for her to turn from side to side (2). Blood pressure (3) and bladder filling (4) are monitored for *all* women in labor; for *this* woman, assessment for heart failure is a priority. **IMP, ANL, 6, PhI, Physiological adaptation**

33. (1) The route of *herpes simplex* virus (HSV) transmission from mother to newborn is via an infected birth canal during birth. Although cesarean birth is no longer recommended for all mothers with HSV, transplacental infection can occur; mothers with clinical evidence of active lesions will likely give birth abdominally. Vaginal birth, whether assisted (2 and 3) or spontaneous (4), is likely to be *contraindicated*. **PL, COM, 1, SECE, Safety and infection control**

34. (3) This woman should be monitored with an external electronic fetal monitor. Leff and DeHillis stethoscopes (1) are used for intermittent assessment of the fetal heart rate (FHR), and are *not* the method of choice during a *high-risk* labor. Penard's stethoscope (2), a small tubelike instrument, is used for *low*-risk labors (it is not commonly used in the U.S., but may be used by some midwives). The risk of transmission of HIV is increased with any intrusive procedure, such as an internal monitor (4). **IMP, RE/KN, 1, PhI, Reduction of risk potential**

35. (1) Vaginal birth with local or regional anesthesia is the method of choice since respiratory reflexes remain intact and it decreases the stress of labor and birth on the respiratory tract, liver, kidney, and metabolic system. Morphine (2) is *not* used in labor because it may cause bronchospasm in the woman. Meperidine (*Demerol*) will usually relieve bronchospasm. Use of ephedrine and corticotropin, pressor drugs (3), is *avoided* or limited in the treatment of eclampsia. Asthma (4) *increases* the incidence of abortion and preterm labor, but the fetus itself is unaffected. **IMP, RE/KN, 6, PhI, Reduction of risk potential**

36. (2) She is at risk for cardiac decompensation and will need frequent assessment of vital signs. The woman will be positioned with her head and shoulders *up*, not flat in bed (1) and her arms at the level of her heart. This position gives the heart more room

within the cavity, and also avoids compression of the vena cava, allowing for easier and better cardiac functioning. She *will* need medication (3). Pain causes stress, which compromises cardiac function, and she must not bear down. She will need to be medicated (epidural), must not bear down, and *will* need assistance to give birth (4). **PL, ANL, 6, PhI, Reduction of risk potential**

37. **(4)** This position places the least stress on cardiac function, and therefore serves to *prevent* decompensation. Maintaining contractions with oxytocin (1) does *not* prevent decompensation. Monitoring (2) does *not* prevent decompensation. Maintaining an IV infusion (3) does *not* prevent decompensation. **PL, APP, 3, PhI, Reduction of risk potential**

☀ When all options are correct, look for *key word*. In this case, the most important word in the stem is "prevent."

38. **(2)** Shortening of the length of labor is a side effect of digitalis preparations taken by woman who are pregnant. Options 1, 3, and 4 do *not* describe effects of digitalis preparations on labor. **AS, COM, 5, PhI, Pharmacological and parenteral therapies**

39. **(2)** This position utilizes gravity drainage to keep her from aspirating. Suction equipment (1) should be readily available *at the bedside*; suctioning will need to be done *after* the convulsion, but the priority during the convulsion is a side-lying position. Insertion of a padded tongue blade (3) is almost always difficult, if not impossible, and can itself lead to injury. Oxygen (4) is started only *after* the airway is clear. NOTE: The FHR is assessed only *after* the woman is out of immediate danger. **IMP, ANL, 1, PhI, Reduction of risk potential**

40. **(4)** Proteinuria is characteristic *only* of pre-eclampsia, *not* of gestational hypertension. A rise in systolic pressure of 30 mm Hg or more over baseline (1), without a rise in diastolic pressure of 15 mm Hg or more over baseline, is *not* indicative of pre-eclampsia; also, in pre-eclampsia, the rise is accompanied by proteinuria. Edema in the ankles (2) occurs in many women who are pregnant, especially late in pregnancy, during hot humid weather, or after standing for long periods; physiologic edema is a *normal* finding in women who are pregnant. A diastolic pressure of 90 mm Hg or more (3) is *not specific* for pre-eclampsia. Diastolic pressure characteristic of pre-eclampsia represents a rise of 15 mm Hg over baseline, and is accompanied by a rise in systolic pressure of 30 mm Hg or more over baseline; in addition, proteinuria must be present before pre-eclampsia is diagnosed. **AS, ANL, 6, PhI, Physiological adaptation**

41. **(4)** Digoxin and anticoagulants are given prophylactically to improve the function of the heart and to prevent emboli secondary to atrial

fibrillation. If the woman needs an anticoagulant, *heparin* is the drug of choice; heparin's larger molecules are less likely to cross the placenta than are the small molecules of *Coumadin* (1). Options 2 and 3 are incorrect because these women must be spared any stress during labor, and their hearts *cannot* tolerate the stress of pushing; stress leads to cardiac decompensation. **IMP, APP, 6, PhI, Reduction of risk potential**

42. **(1)** The risk of miscarriage is higher with SLE than in a normal pregnancy. *Hyper*tension, *not* hypotension (2), is a major problem during pregnancy. Many medications used in treating SLE (3) are *not* recommended during pregnancy. Clients with SLE are *twice* as likely to suffer a flare-up during pregnancy, *not* less likely (4). **AN, RE/KN, 5, HPM, Health promotion and maintenance**

43. **(1)** Transplant recipients *can* become pregnant, but they must postpone conception for 1–2 yr so that graft function stabilizes and immunosuppressive agents can be given at maintenance levels. Women with Marfan's syndrome (2) must be evaluated for aortic root involvement, complicated coarctation of the aorta, and dilated cardiomyopathy—conditions associated with a marked increase in maternal *mortality*. Pulmonary hypertension (3) is associated with a 50% maternal *mortality*. Proliferative retinopathy (4) often *worsens* despite advances in diagnosis and treatment. **AN, COM, 1, HPM, Health promotion and maintenance**

44. **(1)** Infections—especially pneumococcal pneumonia, but also salmonella, osteomyelitis, and urinary tract infections—can promote sickling crises by shifting the oxygen-hemoglobin dissociation curve to the right. It is *not* streptococcus (2), staphylococcus (3), or enterococcus (4) that places the woman most at risk. **AS, COM, 1, SECE, Safety and infection control**

45. **(3)** Those signs indicate that disseminated intravascular coagulation (DIC) may be present (secondary to severe hypertension). The index of presence of DIC is the platelet count. Restarting the IV at another site (1) will not address the problem of possible DIC. Good mouth care (2) and monitoring (4) are warranted only *after* diagnosis and initiation of treatment for DIC, if it is the problem; the cause of the signs must be investigated and treated at this time. **IMP, ANL, 6, PhI, Pharmacological and parenteral therapies**

46. **(1)** Most asthma medications are safe to take during pregnancy. Breastfeeding (2) *is* possible if medications are inhaled; inhaled asthma medications have proved to be safe for mothers who are breastfeeding because of their low systemic bioavailability. Teratogenic effects (3) occur during the period of organogenesis, the *first* trimester. Beta-agonists (4), such as terbutaline, *are* used to manage acute asthma attacks during pregnancy. **IMP, COM, 6, PhI, Pharmacological and parenteral therapies**

47. **(4)** The complications of preterm labor or placental abruption, if they occur, usually happen within 24–48 hr. Options **1**, **2**, and **3** are all incorrect because the maternal-fetal unit must be monitored for up to *48 hr*, to rule out complications such as preterm labor and placental abruption. **IMP, RE/KN, 1, PhI, Reduction of risk potential**

48. **(3)** The hemoconcentration is due to hypovolemia, following a shift of fluid out of the vascular compartment; this woman's condition is worsening. Pre-eclampsia is a disease of hypovolemia: Protein, which retains fluid within the vascular compartment, is lost in the urine; the fluid leaves the intravascular space and enters surrounding tissue. Options **1**, **2**, and **4** are all incorrect because, again, hemoconcentration due to hypovolemia is responsible for the increase in hematocrit. **AN, COM, 6, PhI, Physiological adaptation**

49. **(2)** These reflexes must be *at least at +1* to continue therapy ($MgSO_4$ suppresses reflexes by preventing nerve impulses from crossing the myoneural junction to the muscles). The first sign of $MgSO_4$ *toxicity* is the *disappearance* of the knee-jerk (patellar) reflex. Respirations of 14/min **(1)** *is an acceptable* value; respirations must be 12/min or more to continue therapy ($MgSO_4$ suppresses respiratory activity). Urinary output of 150 mL/4 hr **(3)** *is acceptable*; the minimum limit is 120 mL/4 hr. (the level of urinary output must be monitored since renal ischemia from hypertension can cause dangerous concentrations of $MgSO_4$ if output is not maintained.) A blood pressure of 142/94 **(4)** is still elevated, and further treatment *is needed*. **EV, ANL, 2, PhI, Pharmacological and parenteral therapies**

50. **(3)** An effective disinfectant (for washable surfaces) against HIV is household bleach (sodium hypochlorite) 1:10 solution. The substances in options **1**, **2**, and **4** are not effective disinfectants against HIV. **IMP, RE/KN, 1, SECE, Safety and infection control**

51. **(2)** AIDS is the fourth leading cause of death among women who are of reproductive-age in the U.S. (In many major *metropolitan* areas, it is the *leading* cause of death for that age group.) Options **1**, **3**, and **4** are all incorrect because AIDS ranks fourth. **AN, RE/KN, 1, HPM, Health promotion and maintenance**

52. **(3)** Dysuria, painful blisters, and her history support the diagnosis of primary herpes. Other symptoms include malaise, anorexia, painful lymphadenopathy, and dyspareunia; incubation time: 2–4 wk. Syphilis **(1)** is characterized by chancres at the entry site; they have a red base with firm, rolled edges and are painless. Early infection is asymptomatic. Venereal warts **(2)** are caused by human papillomavirus; incubation period is 2–3 mo. Recurrent herpes **(4)** may be preceded by itching, a burning sensation in the genital area, tingling in the legs, or a slight increase in vaginal discharge. **AS, APP, 1, SECE, Safety and infection control**

53. **(3)** Sitz baths would be the best method to promote the client's comfort. The actions in options **1**, **2**, and **4** would *not* be the best measures to promote periurethral comfort. **IMP, APP, 1, SECE, Safety and infection control**

54. **(3)** Ovulation occurs 14 days *before* the next menstrual period; 31 – 14 = day 17, her ovulation day; add 17 to March 15 to arrive at the answer, April 2. Options **1**, **2**, and **4** do not reflect accurate calculations of her expected date of ovulation based on her LMP. **IMP, APP, 5, HPM, Health promotion and maintenance**

55. **(3)** The most obvious sign of an active chlamydial infection is a cervical vaginal discharge; the woman may be otherwise asymptomatic. Generally, there is no renal involvement **(1)**. Burning **(2)** is indicative of a urinary tract infection. Edema **(4)** is not related to vaginal infections. **IMP, RE/KN, 1, SECE, Safety and infection control**

56. **(2)** Initially, serum hCG levels are monitored every 1 to 2 weeks until there are two normal determinations; then every 3 months for a year. Suction curettage **(1)** offers a safe, rapid, and effective method of evacuation of the mole in almost all women; however, it is done *only* at the time of diagnosis. Oral hormonal contraceptives are recommended instead of barrier methods **(3)**, because contraception is essential; the hCG of trophoblastic cells (mole) cannot be differentiated from that of pregnancy. Methotrexate and dactinomycin **(4)** are given *only* in the presence of rising titers of hCG and an enlarging uterus; the tumor is extremely sensitive to these agents. **IMP, APP, 5, PhI, Reduction of risk potential**

# The Intrapartal Experience

4

## Chapter Outline

## 🔑 Key Points

- The nurse assumes much of the responsibility of monitoring labor and keeping the physician/nurse midwife informed of normal findings and possible deviations from normal findings.

- Coaching, support, and comfort measures assist the woman (and her family) in using her energy constructively to relax and work with her contractions.

- During the *second stage of labor*, each woman must have someone in constant attendance to provide continuous monitoring, support, and coaching.

- The *fourth stage* of labor (the first 1-2 hr postbirth) is a critical period for mother and newborn; the primary concern is *hemorrhage*. Other important concerns are: *bladder distention*, *safety*, *comfort*, and *nutrition* (including fluids).

## Key Words

Apgar scoring system
Cardinal movements of labor
Dilatation
Effacement

Fetal
    Attitude
    Lie
    Presentation
    Position
Hyperventilation
Leopold's maneuvers
Lightening
Pain
    Somatic
    Visceral
Pelvis
    False
    True
Presentation
    Cephalic-vertex
    Breech
💡 REEDA
Trial of labor after cesarean (TOLAC)
Vaginal birth after cesarean (VBAC)
Valsalva maneuver
Warm water immersion/hydrotherapy

# Biophysical Foundations of Labor

**General overview:** This review of the anatomic and physiologic determinants of successful labor provides baseline data against which the nurse compares findings of an ongoing assessment of the woman in labor. Nursing actions are planned and implemented to meet the present and emerging needs of the woman (and her family) in labor.

I. **Premonitory signs**
  A. *Lightening*—process in which the fetus "drops" into the pelvic inlet.
    1. *Characteristics:*
      a. Nullipara—usually occurs 2–3 wk before onset of labor.
      b. Multipara—commonly occurs with onset of labor.
    2. *Effects:*
      a. Relieves pressure on diaphragm—breathing is easier.
      b. Increases pelvic pressure
        (1) Urinary frequency returns.
        (2) Increased pressure on thighs.
        (3) Increased tendency to vulvar, vaginal, perianal, and leg varicosities.
  B. *Braxton-Hicks contractions*—may become more uncomfortable.

II. **Etiology:** unknown. *Theories* include:
  A. Uterine overdistention.
  B. Placental aging—declining estrogen/progesterone levels.
  C. Rising prostaglandin level.
  D. Fetal cortisol secretion.
  E. Maternal-fetal oxytocin secretion.

III. **Overview of labor process**—forces of labor (involuntary uterine contractions) overcome cervical resistance; cervix thins (*effacement*) and opens (0–10 cm *dilatation*) (**Table 4.1** and **Figure 4.1**). Voluntary contraction of secondary abdominal muscles during the second stage (e.g., pushing, bearing-down) forces fetal descent. Changing pelvic dimensions force fetal head to accommodate to the birth canal by *molding* (cranial bones overlap to decrease head size).

**Stages of labor:**
A. *First*—begins with establishment of regular, rhythmic contractions; ends with complete effacement and dilatation (10 cm); divided into three phases:
  1. Latent and early active.
  2. Active.
  3. Transitional.
B. *Second*—begins after complete dilatation; ends with birth of infant.
C. *Third*—begins after birth of infant; ends with expulsion of placenta.
D. *Fourth*—begins after expulsion of placenta; ends when maternal status is stable (usually 1–2 hr postpartum).

IV. **Anatomic/physiologic determinants**
  A. **Maternal**
    1. *Uterine contractions*—involuntary; birth, begin process of involution.
      a. *Characteristics:* rhythmic; increasing tone (*increment*), peak (*acme*), relaxation (*decrement*).
      b. *Effects:*
        (1) Decreases blood flow to uterus and placenta.
        (2) Dilates cervix during first stage of labor.
        (3) Raises maternal blood pressure during contractions.
        (4) With bearing-down efforts (abdominal muscles, voluntary), expels fetus (*second* stage) and placenta (*third* stage).
        (5) Begins involution.
      c. **Assessment**
        (1) *Frequency*–time from beginning of one contraction to beginning of the next. Also can be evaluated by determining number of contractions during certain period of time.
        (2) *Duration*—time from beginning of contraction to its relaxation.
        (3) *Strength* (*intensity*)—resistance to indentation on palpation or calculation of montevideo units (mmHg) using am internal intrauterine pressure catheter.
        (4) False/true labor—differentiation **Table 4.2, p. 99.**
        (5) Signs of dystocia (dysfunctional labor) See **p. 133.**
    2. *Pelvic structures and configuration.*
      a. *False pelvis*—*above* linea terminalis (line travels across top of symphysis pubis around to sacral promontory); supports gravid uterus during pregnancy.
      b. *True pelvis*—lies *below* linea terminalis; divided into:
        (1) Inlet—"brim," demarcated by linea terminalis
          (a) Widest diameter: transverse.
          (b) Narrowest diameter: anterior-posterior (true conjugate).
        (2) Midplane—pelvic cavity.
        (3) Outlet
          (a) Widest diameter: anterior-posterior (requires internal rotation of fetal head for entry).
          (b) Narrowest diameter: transverse (intertuberous); facilitates birth in occiput anterior (OA) position.

*(continued on p. 98)*

## TABLE 4.1 FIRST STAGE OF LABOR

| Phases of First Stage | ◄ Assessment: Expected Maternal Behaviors | ◄ Nursing Care Plan/Implementation |
| --- | --- | --- |
| **0–4 cm—Latent Phase and Early Active Phase** | | |
| 1. *Time*—nullipara 8–10 hr, average; multipara 5–6 hr | 1. Usually comfortable, euphoric, excited, talkative, and energetic, but may be fearful and withdrawn | 1. Provide encouragement, feedback for relaxation, companionship |
| 2. *Contractions*—regular, mild, 5–10 min apart, 20–30 sec duration | 2. Relieved or apprehensive that labor has begun | 2. *Coach* during contractions: signal beginning of contraction, mark the seconds, signal end of contraction; "Follow my breathing," "Watch my lips," etc. |
| 3. Low-back pain and abdominal discomfort with contractions | 3. Alert, usually receptive to: teaching, coaching, diversion, and anticipatory guidance | 3. *Comfort measures*: position for comfort; praise; keep aware of progress |
| 4. Cervix thins; some bloody show | | |
| 5. *Station*—nullipara 0; multipara 2 to +1 | | |
| **4–8 cm—Midactive Phase, Phase of Most Rapid Dilatation** | | |
| 1. *Average time*—nullipara 2–4 hr; multipara 1 ½–2 hr | 1. Tired, less talkative, and less energetic | 1. *Coach* during contractions; support person(s) may need some relief |
| 2. *Contractions*—2–5 min apart, 30–40 sec duration, intensity increasing | 2. More serious, malar flush between 5 and 6 cm, tendency to hyperventilate, may need analgesia, needs constant coaching | 2. *Comfort measures* (for support person(s), too—as needed): position for comfort while preventing *hypotensive syndrome*; encourage relaxation, focusing her on areas of tension; provide *counterpressure* to sacrococcygeal area, prn; praise; keep aware of progress; minimize distractions from surrounding environment (loud talking, other noises); offer *analgesics* and anesthetics, as appropriate; provide hygiene: mouth care, ice chips, clean perineum; warmth, as needed |
| 3. Membranes may rupture now | | 3. Monitor progress of labor and maternal-fetal response |
| 4. Increased bloody show | | 4. If monitors are in use, attention on mother; periodically check accuracy of monitor readouts |
| 5. *Station*: -1 to 0 | | |
| **8-10 cm—Transition, Deceleration Period of Active Phase** | | |
| 1. *Average time*; nullipara 1–2 hrs; multipara 1 hr | 1. If not under regional anesthesia, more introverted; may be amnesic between contractions | 1. Stay with woman (couple) and provide constant support |
| 2. *Contractions*—1 ½–2 min, 60–90 sec duration, strong intensity | 2. Feeling she cannot make it; increased: irritability, crying, nausea, vomiting, and belching; increased perspiration over upper lip and between breasts; leg tremors; and shaking | 2. Continue to *coach* with contractions: may need to remind, reassure, and encourage her to reestablish breathing techniques and concentration with each contraction; coach *panting* or "he-he" *respirations* to prevent pushing |

*(continued)*

**TABLE 4.1   FIRST STAGE OF LABOR** (continued)

| Phases of First Stage | ◄ Assessment: Expected Maternal Behaviors | ◄ Nursing Care Plan/Implementation |
|---|---|---|
| 3. Increased vaginal show; rectal pressure with beginning urge to bear down | 3. May have uncontrollable urge to push at this time | 3. *Comfort measures*: remind her and partner her behavior is normal and "OK"; coach breathing to quell nausea |
| 4. *Station*: +1 to +2. | | 4. Assist with *counterpressure* techniques. |
| | | ☞ 5. Monitor contractions, fetal heart rate, vaginal discharge, perineal bulging, maternal vital signs; record every 15 min. |
| | | 6. Assess for bladder filling |
| | | 7. Keep mother (couple) aware of progress |
| | | 8. Prepare for birth |

Source: ©Lagerquist, *S. Davis's NCLEX-RN® Success*, Philadelphia.

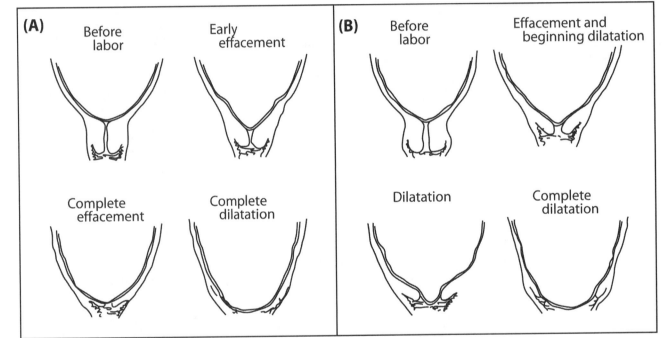

**FIGURE 4.1   COMPARISON OF (A) NULLIPARA AND (B) MULTIPARA: DILATATION AND EFFACEMENT.**

(From *Clinical Education Aid* No. 13. Columbus, OH: Ross Laboratories.)

c. *Classifications:*
 (1) Gynecoid—normal female pelvis; rounded oval.
 (2) Android—normal male pelvis; funnel-shaped.
 (3) Anthropoid—oval.
 (4) Platypelloid—flattened, transverse oval.

B. **Fetal**
 1. *Fetal head* (**Figure 4.2**):
  a. Bones—one occipital, two frontal, two parietals, two temporals.

b. Suture—line of junction or closure between bones; sagittal (longitudinal), coronal (anterior), and lambdoidal (posterior); permit molding to accommodate head to birth canal.

c. Fontanels—membranous space between cranial bones during fetal life and infancy:
 (1) *Anterior* "soft spot"—diamond-shaped; junction of coronal and sagittal sutures; closes (ossifies) in *12-18 mo.*
 (2) *Posterior*—triangular; junction of sagittal and lambdoidal sutures; closes by *2 mo* of age.

## TABLE 4.2 ◄ ASSESSMENT: DIFFERENTIATION OF FALSE/TRUE LABOR

| False Labor | True Labor |
|---|---|
| *Contractions*: *Braxton-Hicks* intensify (more noticeable at night); short, *irregular*, little change in intensity | *Contractions*: begin in *lower* back, radiate to abdomen ("girdling"); become *regular*, rhythmic; frequency, duration, intensity progressively *increase* |
| *Relieved* by change of position or activity (e.g., walking) | *Unaffected* by: change of position, activity, drinking 2 glasses of water, or moderate analgesia |
| *Cervical changes*—none; *no* progress in effacement or dilatation | *Cervical changes*—*progressive* effacement and dilatation |

2. *Fetal lie*—relationship of fetal long axis to maternal long axis (spine):
   a. Transverse—shoulder presents.
   b. Longitudinal—vertex or breech presents.
3. *Presentation*—fetal part entering inlet first: (**Figure 4.3**)
   a. *Cephalic*—vertex (most common); face, brow.
   b. *Breech*:
      (1) *Complete*—feet and legs flexed on thighs; buttocks and feet presenting.
      (2) *Frank*—legs extended on torso, feet up by shoulders; buttocks presenting. (see **Figure 4.3 (e)**)
      (3) *Footling*—single (one foot), double (both feet) presenting.
4. *Attitude*—relationship of fetal parts to one another (e.g., head flexed on chest).
5. *Position*—relationship of presenting fetal part to quadrants of maternal pelvis; vertex most common, occiput anterior on maternal left side (LOA). See **Figure 4.3 (a)**.

◄ C. **Assessment**: determine *presentation* and *position*
   ☞ 1. *Leopold's maneuvers*—abdominal palpation
      a. *First*—palms over fundus, breech feels softer, not as round as head would be.
      b. *Second*—palms on either side of abdomen, locates fetal back and small parts.
      c. *Third*—fingers just above pubic symphysis, grasp lower abdomen; if unengaged, presenting part is mobile.
      d. *Fourth*—facing mother's feet, run palms down sides of abdomen to symphysis; check for cephalic prominence (usually on right side), and if head is floating or engaged.

☞ 2. *Location of fetal heart tones* (FHTs)—heard best through fetal back or chest.
   a. *Breech* presentation—usually most audible *above* maternal umbilicus.
   b. *Vertex* presentation—usually most audible *below* maternal umbilicus.
   c. Changing location of most audible FHT—useful indicator of fetal descent.
   d. Factors affecting audibility:
      (1) Obesity.
      (2) Maternal position.
      (3) Polyhydramnios.
      (4) Maternal gastrointestinal activity.
      (5) Loud uterine souffle or bruit—origin: hissing of blood through maternal uterine arteries; synchronous with maternal pulse.
      (6) Loud funic souffle or bruit—origin: hissing of blood through umbilical arteries; synchronous with fetal heart rate (FHR).
      (7) External noise, faulty equipment.
3. *Vaginal examination*: palpable sutures, fontanels (triangular-shaped superior, diamond-shaped inferior = vertex presentation, OA position).

D. **Cardinal movements of the mechanisms of normal labor**—vertex presentation, positional changes of fetal head accommodate to changing diameters of maternal pelvis. (**Figure 4.4**)
1. *Descent*—head engages and proceeds down birth canal.
2. *Flexion*—head bent to chest; presents smallest diameter of vertex (suboccipital-bregmatic, 9.5 cm).
3. *Internal rotation*—during *second stage* of labor, transverse diameter of fetal head enters pelvis; occiput rotates 90° to bring back of neck (the nape) under symphysis (e.g., LOT to LOA to OA); presents smallest diameter (biparietal) to smallest diameter of outlet (intertuberous).
4. *Extension*—back of neck pivots under symphysis, allows head to be born by extension.
5. *Restitution*—head returns to normal alignment with shoulders (with LOA, results in head facing right thigh), presents smallest diameter of shoulders to outlet.
6. *Expulsion*—birth of neonate completed.
◄ 7. **Assessment**: relationship of fetal head to ischial spines (**degree of descent**)
   a. *Engagement*—widest diameter of presenting part has passed through pelvic inlet (e.g., biparietal diameter of fetal head).
   b. *Station*—relationship of presenting part to ischial spines (IS):
      (1) *Floating*: presenting part is above inlet, in false pelvis.

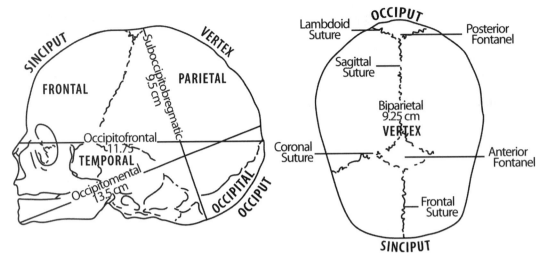

## FIGURE 4.2 THE FETAL HEAD.

**Bones**: two frontal, two temporal, two parietal, one occipital. **Sutures**: sagittal, frontal, coronal, lambdoid.
**Fontanels**: anterior, posterior.
(From *Clinical Education Aid* No. 13. Columbus, OH: Ross Laboratories.)

---

(2) Station -5: presenting part is at inlet (presenting part is well above IS).

(3) Station 0: presenting part is at IS (engaged).

(4) Station +4: presenting part is at the outlet.

V. **Warning signs during labor:**

A. *Contraction*—hypertonic, poor relaxation, or tetanic (> 90 sec long and ≤ 2 min apart).

B. *Abdominal pain*—sharp, rigid abdomen.

C. *Vaginal bleeding*—profuse.

D. *FHR*—late decelerations, prolonged variable decelerations, bradycardia, tachycardia (**Figure 4.5**).

E. *Maternal hypertension.*

F. *Meconium-stained amniotic fluid.*

G. *Prolonged rupture of membrane* (PROM).

# Pain Management During Labor and Birth

I. **Neurologic origins of pain**

A. *First stage* of labor: Pain is *visceral*, caused by dilatation of the cervix and uterine ischemia; referred to: the lower abdominal wall, the area over the lumbar region, and the sacrum.

B. *Second stage* of labor: Pain is *somatic*, caused by: hypoxia of the uterus, distention of the vagina and perineum, and pressure on adjacent tissues. Pain is felt in the lower back or suprapubic area, or referred to the flank and thighs.

C. *Third stage* of labor: Pain is similar in origin to that of the *first stage*.

II. **Psychoprophylaxis—Lamaze method** (also, see Chapter 2, p. 39.)

A. Premise—conditioned responses to stimuli occupy nerve pathways, reducing perception of pain. Emphasis is on childbirth as a natural event, with an informed woman as the active participant. The ability to relax effectively reduces the perception of pain, and the involvement of the coach fosters the family concept.

B. Childbirth partners are taught:

1. Anatomy and physiology of labor.

2. Psychology of man and woman.

3. What to expect in the hospital setting.

4. Conditioned responses to labor stimuli.

a. Concentration on focal point.

b. Breathing techniques.

c. Need for active coaching to enable woman to:

(1) Use techniques appropriate to stage of labor.

(2) *Avoid* hyperventilation.

5. Specific stage—appropriate techniques:

a. *First stage of labor—early*: slow, deep chest-breathing.

b. *Transition*(8–10 cm)—rapid, shallow breathing pattern, to prevent pushing prematurely:

(1) Panting.

(2) Pant-blow.

(3) "He-he" pattern.

c. *Second stage of labor:*

(1) Pushing (or bearing-down)—assists fetal descent through birth canal.

(2) Panting—assists relaxation between contractions; prevents explosive birth of head.

**(a) LOA**    **(b) LOP**    **(c) ROA**    **(d) ROP**

**(e) LSP**
*(Frank breech)*    **(f) Shoulder** presentation    **(g) Prolapse of umbilical cord**

## FIGURE 4.3    CATEGORIES OF FETAL PRESENTATION.

**(a) LOA**: Fetal *occiput* is in *left anterior* quadrant of maternal pelvis. **(b) LOP**: Fetal *occiput* is in *left posterior* quadrant of maternal pelvis. **(c) ROA**: Fetal *occiput* is in *right anterior* quadrant of maternal pelvis. **(d) ROP**: Fetal *occiput* is in *right posterior* quadrant of maternal pelvis. **(e) LSP** (*frank breech*): Fetal *sacrum* is in *left posterior* quadrant of maternal pelvis. **(f) Shoulder** presentation with fetus in *transverse* lie. **(g) Prolapse of umbilical cord** with fetus in **LOA** position.

(From *Clinical Education Aid* No. 18. Columbus, OH: Ross Laboratories.)

6. Effects on labor behaviors/coping:
   a. Help mother cope with and assist contractions.
   b. Prevent premature bearing-down; reduce possibility of cervical edema due to pushing on incompletely dilated cervix.
   c. When appropriate, improve efficiency of bearing-down efforts.
C. Other methods—include parent classes, classes for siblings, multiparas, and those who plan cesarean birth.

### III. Warm-water immersion/hydrotherapy
A. Proponents view labor as a normal biologic process; however, even with this type, an episiotomy may be needed.
B. Bath temperature should be maintained at 32°–37° C (89.6°–98.6° F), which is most therapeutic for both the mother and fetus.
C. **Assessment** before immersion
   1. Maternal and fetal vital signs—within normal limits.
   2. Cervical dilatation—4–5 cm; active phase of first stage.
   3. Membranes intact; or, if ruptured, fluid must be clear or only lightly stained with meconium.
   4. IV or an IV lock may be in place.
   5. Stimulation with oxytocin is a **contraindication**.

D. *Expected effects*: positive effect on labor pattern and cervical dilatation:
   1. Relief from discomfort and general body relaxation reduce a woman's anxiety, which decreases adrenalin production; → an increase in oxytocin (to stimulate labor) and endorphins (to reduce pain perception).
   2. A 30 min whirlpool bath is expected to increase cervical dilatation an additional 2–3 cm.
   3. Increases *serum level of dopamine*, which increases renal blood flow → reduces blood pressure, encourages diuresis. Blood pressure *drops* within 2 min of immersion.
E. **Nursing interventions**
   1. Continuous monitoring of labor: contractions, FHRs, BP, pulse, pain perception, signs of imminent birth, temperature.
   2. Keep woman well hydrated since dehydration may occur; can use sips of water, ice chips, IV fluids.
   3. Keep tub meticulously clean.
### IV. **Pharmacologic management of pain.** See **Table 4.3** for a discussion of categories of pain control, desired effects, nursing assessment and comments, and planning/implementation.

**FIGURE 4.4 CARDINAL MOVEMENTS IN THE MECHANISM OF LABOR** with the fetus in vertex presentation. **(a)** *Engagement*, descent, flexion. **(b)** *Internal rotation.* **(c)** *Extension beginning* (rotation complete). **(d)** *Extension complete.* **(e)** *External rotation (restitution).* **(f)** *External rotation (shoulder* rotation). **(g)** *Expulsion.*
(From *Clinical Education Aid* No. 13. Columbus, OH: Ross Laboratories.)

# Nursing Actions During First Stage of Labor

See also **Table 4.1, p. 97–98.**

▶ I. **Assessment**—careful evaluation of:
   A. *Antepartal history:*
      1. Expected date of delivery (EDD).
      2. Genetic and familial problems.
      3. Pre- and coexisting medical disorders, allergies.
      4. Pregnancy-related health problems (hyperemesis, bleeding, etc.).
      5. Infectious diseases (past and present herpes, etc.).
      6. Past obstetric history, if any.
      7. Height.
      8. Weight gain.
      9. *Laboratory test* results
         a. Blood type and Rh factor.
         b. Serology.
         c. Rubella titer.
         d. Urinalysis.
         e. Vaginal culture
      10. Prenatal care history.
      11. Use of medications.

   B. *Admission findings:*
      1. Emotional status.
      2. Vital signs.
      3. Present weight.
      4. Fundal height.
      5. Present fetal size.
      6. Edema.
      7. Urinalysis (for protein and sugar).
   ☞ C. *Fetal heart rate (FHR)*—normal, 110/min (see **Figure 4.5**).
      1. Check and record every 15–30 min—to monitor fetal response to physiologic stress of labor.
      2. *Bradycardia* < 110 BPM.
      3. *Tachycardia* > 160 BPM.
   ☞ D. *Contractions*—every 15–30 min.
      1. Place fingertips over fundus, use gentle pressure; contraction felt as hardening or tensing.
      2. *Time*: frequency and duration.
      3. *Intensity/strength* at acme:
         a. *Weak*—easily indent fundus with fingers.
         b. *Moderate*—some tension felt, fundus indents slightly with finger pressure.
         c. *Strong*—unable to indent fundus.
   E. *Maternal response to labor*—assess for effective coping, cooperation, and utilizing effective breathing techniques.
   ☞ F. *Maternal vital signs*—between contractions.
      1. Response to *pain* or use of special breathing techniques alters pulse and respirations.

*(continued on p. 108)*

| Pattern | Description | ◄ Nursing Interventions |
|---|---|---|

**A**

Head compression
**(HC)**

**Early Decelerations**

- No intervention required.
- Continue observation.

Uniform shape

180
FHR
100

Early onset  Early onset  Early onset

50
UC
0

Early deceleration (HC)

1. FHR begins to slow with the onset of the uterine contraction (UC) and returns to baseline when contraction is over.
2. *Fetal head compression* occurs.
3. Vagal nerve stimulation.
4. Transient slowing of FHR.

**B**

Placenta

Uteroplacental insufficiency
**(UPI)**

**Late Decelerations**

- Change maternal position.
- Turn off *Pitocin*; increase rate of maintenance IV.
- Begin oxygen by face mask.
- Notify MD.
- Check blood pressure and pulse rate.
- Possible candidate for *cesarean* birth.

Uniform shape

180
FHR
100

Late onset   Late onset

50
UC
0

1 Min.

Late deceleration (UP)

1. FHR begins to fall at height of the UC and returns to baseline after contractions has ceased.
2. FHR usually remains within normal range.
3. Indicates some degree of *uteroplacental insufficiency*.

**C**

Umbilical cord

Umbilical cord compression
**(CC)**

**Variable Decelerations**

- Change maternal position to alleviate cord pressure.
- Turn off *Pitocin*; increase rate of maintenance IV.
- Begin oxygen by face mask.
- Notify MD.
- Check blood pressure and pulse rate.
- Possible candidate for *cesarean* birth.
- Possible candidate for *amnio infusion*.

Variable shape

180
FHR
100

Variable onset   Variable onset

50
UC
0

Variable deceleration (CC)

1. *Slowing* of FHR either with a contraction or in between contractions. Unrelated pattern of FHR and uterine contraction.
2. Pattern may be U shaped or V shaped. Transitory acceleration precedes or follows the deceleration.
3. FHR may fall below 100 beats/min; then returns immediately to baseline.
4. Usually indicates *cord compression*.

**FIGURE 4.5  FHR DECELERATIONS AND NURSING INTERVENTIONS.**

## TABLE 4.3 ⊂⊃ PAIN MANAGEMENT DURING LABOR AND BIRTH

| Category and Desired Effect | ◄▪ Assessment and Comments | ◄▪ Planning/Implementation |
|---|---|---|
| **Systemic Medication** | | |
| *Examples*: **sedatives**<br>**Short** duration (1 hr):<br>*secobarbital (Seconal)*<br>**Intermediate** (2 hr):<br>*pentobarbital (Nembutal)*<br>**Long** duration (3 hr):<br>*phenobarbital (Luminal sodium)*<br>*Desired effect*: relieve anxiety and induce sleep only in prodromal or early latent labor:<br>*Route*: oral or IM | *Before* administration of medication note:<br>Prenatal history of allergies or medical disorders<br>Prodromal labor<br>Degree of apprehension:<br>Woman states she is anxious<br>Woman is clenching fists, restless, seems tense<br>Absence of pain<br>*After* administration of medication, note:<br>Strength and frequency of uterine contractions—should *not* decrease appreciably<br>Little change in maternal vital signs; with decreased anxiety: pulse, respirations, and blood pressure *do decrease*—but should not fall below woman's normal baseline in her prenatal record<br>Assess woman's response to medication<br>Assess FHR<br>Assess for pain | Alert physician if chart reveals history of drug allergy, other disorders<br>Administer if:<br>Woman is apprehensive, tense<br>Woman is in early latent phase of first stage of labor<br>Do *not* give sedative without an analgesic if woman has pain<br>Continue with comfort measures and general hygiene given to any woman in labor<br>If changes occur in contractions or in maternal or fetal vital signs, record and notify physician<br>If woman becomes uncomfortable, confer with physician regarding need for analgesic relief |
| *Examples*: **narcotic analgesics**<br>*Butorphanol tartrate (Stadol)*<br>*Fentanyl*<br>*Meperidine hydrochloride (Demerol)*<br>*Morphine*<br>*Nalbuphine HCl (Nubain)*<br>*Desired effect*: relief of severe, persistent, or recurrent pain, without nausea and vomiting or respiratory depression of mother or fetus<br>*Route*: IM, IV, or SC | *Before* administration of medication note:<br>Prenatal information regarding:<br>Drug allergies<br>Liver and kidney damage<br>Substance (drug) abuse<br>History of asthma<br>Stage of labor; progress in labor<br>*Nullipara*: before full dilatation<br>*Multipara*: before 7 cm dilatation<br>Degree of discomfort:<br>Mother states she is having pain; cries out with pain; clenches teeth, fists<br>Maternal and fetal vital signs<br>*After* administration of medication, note:<br>*Time* between administration of narcotic and time of baby's birth<br>*Maximum effect* (IM) in 15 min, duration of 2 hr<br>Drug may slow labor, or it may accelerate labor as woman relaxes<br>Adverse side effects assessed every 5–30 min—*respiratory depression*:<br>FHR deceleration and loss of short term variability noted by electronic fetal monitor<br>Nausea, vomiting, dizziness, sweating, dysphoria<br>Bronchospasm in women who suffer from asthma | Do *not* administer if birth is expected within 2 hr<br>Explain expected effect<br>☞ *Overdose management*: oxygen, IV fluids, and<br>⊂⊃ vasopressors<br><br><br>If baby is born when drug reaches maximum effect, baby may be depressed and require resuscitation; prepare *Narcan* (0.01/kg) to be given IM into baby's thigh |

*(continued)*

## TABLE 4.3 ⬭ PAIN MANAGEMENT DURING LABOR AND BIRTH (continued)

| *Category and Desired Effect* | ▶◀ *Assessment and Comments* | ▶◀ *Planning/Implementation* |
|---|---|---|
| **Systemic Medication—***cont'd* | | |
| *Examples*: **narcotic antagonists** Naloxone hydrochloride (*Narcan*) *Desired effect*: Reversal of narcotic depression of mother and/or baby *Route*: IV | Note which drug was given, time, amount, route; respiratory depression from any drug other than a narcotic *cannot* be reversed with these drugs | Do *not* give *Narcan* to mother addicted to narcotics because this causes instant withdrawal symptoms; *Narcan* given to mother reverses pain relief instantly, so that she must be prepared for return of pain or a second form of pain relief is given (e.g., epidural) |
| *Examples*: **analgesic-potentiating drugs** (ataractics, tranquilizers) *Hydroxyzine pamoate (Vistaril)* *Promazine hydrochloride (Sparine)* *Promethazine hydrochloride (Phenergan)* *Propiomazine hydrochloride (Largon)* *Desired effects*: increase desirable effects of analgesics *without* increasing dose of analgesics (i.e., ataractic potentiates effects of analgesic that is given with it and acts as antiemetic) *Route*: IV, IM | Same as for **narcotic analgesics** | Same as for **narcotic analgesics** |
| **General Anesthesia** | | |
| Rarely indicated for uncomplicated vaginal birth; woman is not awake; ✴ danger of *aspiration* and *respiratory depression*; safer than regional anesthesia for clients who are hypovolemic; does *not* depress neonate unless mother is anesthetized deeply *Examples*: Halothane (*Fluothane*) (inhalation)—relaxes uterus quickly, facilitates intrauterine manipulation, version, and extraction *Thiopental (Pentothal) sodium IV* produces rapid induction of anesthesia; ✴ depresses neonate; useful in controlling convulsions *Desired effect*: produces general loss of sensitivity to touch, pain, and other stimulations | Anesthetist assesses woman continuously (intubation is necessary) ☞ Monitor fetal response continuously If woman had cesarean birth, do routine postsurgery assessment—wound assessment, intake and output, etc. ☞ Provide *postanesthesia recovery care*: assess q15 min until vital signs are stable and woman is alert and reactive *Routine postpartum assessment* Assess readiness to see baby Assess her response to anesthesia and event that necessitated birth under general anesthesia (e.g., giving birth by cesarean when vaginal birth was anticipated) | If general anesthesia is being considered: Keep woman NPO ⬭ See that an IV infusion is established Premedicate with *cimetidine* to neutralize acid contents of stomach Assist with **cricoid pressure** before intubation ☞ *Recovery room care*: Maintain open airway Maintain cardiopulmonary functions Prevent postpartal hemorrhage *Routine postpartum care*: Facilitate parent-child attachment as soon as possible Answer mother's questions |

*(continued)*

**TABLE 4.3 ⬭ PAIN MANAGEMENT DURING LABOR AND BIRTH** (continued)

| *Category and Desired Effect* | ◄ *Assessment and Comments* | ◄ *Planning/Implementation* |
|---|---|---|
| **Regional (Conduction) Anesthesia** | | |
| Local anesthetics injected to block primary neuropathways that result in temporary interruption of conduction of nerve impulses, notably pain; mother remains awake<br>*Examples*: common agents in 0.5-1.0% solution<br>*Bupivacaine (Marcaine) hydrochloride*<br>*Chloroprocaine*<br>*Lidocaine (Xylocaine) hydrochloride*<br>*Mepivacaine hydrochloride (Carbocaine)*<br>*Naropin (Ropivacaine)*<br>*Tetracaine (Pontocaine) hydrochloride* | Used with epinephrine (or other vasoconstrictor drug) to delay absorption, prolong anesthetic effect, and decrease chance of hypotension | **Note any history of allergy**: note response: allergic reaction, hypotension, and lack of wearing off of anesthetic effect; **!** observe for **hypertensive crisis** if agent combined with epinephrine and oxytocin (*Pitocin*) is also being given |
| **Types of Nerve Blocks** | | |
| **Peripheral nerve block**<br>*Pudendal* (5–10 mL on each side): anesthetizes lower two-thirds of vagina and perineum; of short duration (30 min)—given for birth and repair; local anesthesia, may be done by physician or anesthetist; simple and safe, does *not* depress neonate; may *inhibit bearing-down reflex* | ☞Monitor fetal response continuously<br>Assist physician or anesthetist as necessary | See *general nursing actions*, **p. 107**<br>Provide explanation during procedure |
| **Local infiltration**: useful for perineal repairs | Assist physician or anesthetist as necessary | See *general nursing actions*, **p. 107**<br>Nurse informs physician of medication in syringe |

*(continued)*

**TABLE 4.3** 👄 PAIN MANAGEMENT DURING LABOR AND BIRTH (continued)

| Category and Desired Effect | Assessment and Comments | Planning/Implementation |
|---|---|---|

**Types of Nerve Blocks**—cont'd

**Regional nerve block:** Requires trained anesthesiologist or anesthetist; with proper administration, relieves pain completely, may prolong labor if given too early; *hypotension* from vasodilation (below anesthesia level) is likely; *fetal bradycardia* may occur as a result of maternal hypotension; *bearing-down reflex diminished or eliminated; may require forceps or vacuum assistance for delivery;* mother remains awake; absence of pain may facilitate maternal-child attachment; can be used for women with metabolic, lung, and heart diseases

*General assessment:* note degree of hydration, history of allergy, skin infection over back, previous neural or spinal injury or disease, and attitude toward anesthesia

Prebirth, monitor:
  👉 Maternal vital signs and FHR
  Return of pain
  Monitor labor if anesthesia is established during late first stage
  👉 Rate of IV fluid infusion
  Perineum to see if birth is imminent (or monitor progress by vaginal examination)

*General nursing actions:*
👄 *Hydrate by* IV infusion

Explain to woman expected feelings as anesthesia begins (warm toes) and as it wears off (tingling); help position her, offering reassurance and support; it is very frightening not to be able to see the procedure and to deal with only sensations and sounds; do *not* make promises of complete pain relief; each woman may have a differing perception of pain, or block may *not* provide complete relief

👉 Treat **hypotension**: maintain *lateral position or elevate legs;* administer oxygen by
👄 mask at 6–8 L/min; increase rate of IV maintenance fluids

**Epidural:** Useful during *first* and *second* stages; can be given as "one shot" or over a period of time; given on top of (or over) dura through third, fourth, or fifth lumbar interspace; risk of dural puncture

During labor, *analgesic* doses are given

For birth, *anesthetic* dose is given

Bearing-down reflex usually preserved

👉 Postbirth, monitor:
  Uterine tone
  Bladder tone
  Return of sensation

If contractions become *less* frequent, of *less* intensity, or of *shorter* duration, report to
❗ physician **immediately**; physician may need to augment labor; assist as necessary

Provide assistance to move; maintain good uterine tone; prevent bladder distention; prevent injury by keeping side rails up and assisting her when she ambulates

For introduction of epidural anesthesia: position woman in *modified Sims' position:* place woman on her *side,* shoulders *parallel,* legs slightly *flexed,* and back *arched*

An *alternative position* may be preferred by the anesthetist: position woman in a *sitting* position with her buttocks near edge of birth table, feet supported on a footstool; ask woman to place her arms between her knees, flex her head, and arch her back "like a rainbow"; after medication is injected, ask her to remain sitting up for 20–30 sec; then place her *supine* with a pillow under her head and a **pelvic wedge to displace uterus to left**

👉 *Postbirth:* encourage oral *fluids* (if permitted) or monitor IV fluids; ask her to report headache; keep bladder empty; maintain uterine tone

*(continued)*

**TABLE 4.3 ⊂⊃ PAIN MANAGEMENT DURING LABOR AND BIRTH** (continued)

| Category and Desired Effect | ◄ Assessment and Comments | ◄ Planning/Implementation |
|---|---|---|
| **Types of Nerve Blocks**—cont'd | | |
| **Intrathecal (spinal)** | | |
| morphine | 0.5 mg MS produces marked analgesia for 12–24 hr; onset in 20–30 min | Side effects: respiratory depression, pruritus, nausea, vomiting, sleepiness, urinary retention; keep Naloxone, 0.4 mg, at bedside and respiratory support equipment readily available |

2. BP, P, R—if *normotensive*: on admission, and then every hour and prn; *after regional anesthesia*: every 30 min (every 5 min for first 20 min).

3. *Temperature*—if within normal range: on admission, and then every 4 hr and prn. Every 2 hr after rupture of membranes.

4. *Before* and *after* analgesia/anesthesia.

5. *After* rupture of membranes (see **Amniotic fluid embolism, p. 134-135**).

G. Character and amount of *bloody show*.

H. *Bladder* status: encourage voiding every 1–2 hr, monitor output.

   1. Determine bladder distention—palpate just *above* symphysis (full bladder may impede labor progress or result in trauma to bladder).

   2. Admission urinalysis—check for protein, glucose and ketones.

I. Signs of deviations from normal patterns.

J. Status of *membranes*:

   1. Intact.

   2. Ruptured (nitrazine paper turns blue on contact with alkaline amniotic fluid). Assess, record, and report:

     a. Time—risk of infection if ruptured more than 24 hr.

     b. FHR stat and 10 min later—to check for prolapsed cord.

     c. Character and color of fluid (see below).

K. *Amniotic fluid*:

   1. *Amount*—polyhydramnios (> 2000 mL)—associated with *congenital anomalies* and *maternal diabetes*.

   2. *Character*—thick consistency and/or odor associated with *infection*.

   3. *Color*—normally clear with white specks:

     a. Yellow—indicates *fetal distress* about 35 hr previous; *Rh or ABO incompatibility*.

     b. Green or meconium stained; if fetus in vertex position, indicates recent fetal hypoxia secondary to *respiratory distress* in fetus.

     c. Port wine—may indicate *abruptio placentae*.

L. *Labor progress*:

   1. Effacement.

   2. Dilatation.

   3. Station.

   4. Bulging membranes.

   5. Molding of fetal head.

M. *Perineum*—observe for bulging.

◄ **II. Analysis/nursing diagnosis**

A. *Anxiety, fear* related to uncertain outcome, pain.

B. *Individual coping impairment* related to lack of preparation for childbirth and/or poor support from coach.

C. *Nutrition deficit (less than body requirements)* related to physiologic stress of labor.

D. *Urinary elimination alteration* related to pressure of presenting part.

E. *Thought processes alteration* related to sleep deprivation, analgesia.

F. *Fluid volume deficit* related to anemia, excessive blood loss.

G. *(Fetal) gas exchange impairment* related to impaired placental perfusion.

◄ **III. Nursing care plan/implementation**

A. Goal: *comfort measures*.

   1. Maintain hydration of oral mucosa. Encourage sucking on cool washcloth, ice chips, lollipops.

   2. Reduce dryness of lips. Apply lip balm (Chapstick, petrolatum jelly).

   3. Relieve backache. Apply sacral counter-pressure (particularly with occiput posterior presentation); change maternal position.

   4. Encourage significant other to participate.

   5. Encourage ambulation when presenting part engaged.

B. Goal: *management of physical needs*.

   1. Encourage frequent voiding—to prevent full bladder from impeding oncoming head.

   2. Encourage ambulation throughout labor; *lateral Sims' position* with head elevated to:

     a. Encourage relaxation.

     b. Allow gravity to assist in anterior rotation of fetal head.

     c. Prevent compression of inferior vena cava and descending aorta (*supine hypotensive syndrome*).

     d. Promote placental perfusion.

☞ 3. Perineal prep, if ordered—to promote cleanliness.

☞ 4. Fleet's enema, if ordered—to stimulate peristalsis, evacuate lower bowel. **NOTE:**

   ! **contraindicated** if:

   a. Cervical dilatation (4 cm or more) with unengaged head—because of possibility of *cord prolapse*.

   b. Fetal malpresentation/malposition—because of possible *fetal distress*.

   c. Preterm labor—may stimulate contractions.

   d. Painless vaginal bleeding—because of possible *placenta previa*.

🍎 5. Provide *clear fluids* (tea, apple juice) with sugar (if ordered)—to provide energy and to maintain hydration.

C. Goal: *management of psychosocial needs. Emotional support.*

   1. Encourage verbalization of feelings, fears, concerns.

   2. Explain all procedures.

   3. Reinforce self-concept ("You're doing well!").

D. Goal: *management of discomfort.*

   💊 1. *Analgesia* and/or anesthesia—may be required or desired—to facilitate safe, comfortable birth.

   2. Support/enhance/teach childbirth techniques.

   ☞ a. Reinforce appropriate *breathing techniques* for current labor status:

      (1) If **hyperventilating**, to increase PaCO$_2$, minimize fetal acidosis, and relieve symptoms of vertigo and syncope, suggest:

         (a) Breathe into paper bag.

         (b) Breathe into cupped hands.

      (2) Demonstrate appropriate breathing for several contractions—to reestablish rate and rhythm.

E. Goal: *sustain motivation.*

   1. Offer support, encouragement, and praise, as appropriate.

   2. Keep informed of status and progress.

   3. Reassure that irritability is normal.

   4. Serve as surrogate coach when necessary (if *no* partner, *before* arrival of partner, *while* partner is changing clothes, *during* needed

   ☞ breaks); assist with effleurage, breathing, focusing.

   5. Discourage bearing-down efforts by *pant-blow* until complete (10 cm) dilatation—to *avoid* cervical edema or lacerations.

   6. Facilitate informed decision-making regarding medication for relaxation or pain relief.

   7. Keep woman and family informed of her progress.

   8. Minimize distractions: quiet, relaxed environment; privacy.

⋈ IV. Evaluation/outcome criteria

   1. Woman manages own labor discomfort effectively.

   2. Woman maintains control over own behavior.

   3. Woman successfully completes first stage of labor without incident.

# Nursing Actions During Second Stage of Labor

⋈ I. Assessment

   A. Maternal (or couple's) response to labor.

   ☞ B. FHR—continuous electronic monitoring, or after each contraction with fetoscope, Doppler.

   C. Vital signs.

   D. Time elapsed—average: 2 min–1 hr; prolonged second stage increases risk of fetal distress, maternal exhaustion, psychological stress, intrauterine infection.

   E. Contraction pattern—average every 1 ½–3 min, lasting 60–90 sec.

   F. Vaginal discharge—increases.

   G. Nausea, vomiting, disorientation, tremors, amnesia between contractions, panic.

   H. Response to regional anesthesia, if administered:

      1. Signs of *hypotension*—reduces placental perfusion, increases risk of fetal hypoxia.

      2. Effect on *contractions*—note and report any slowing of labor.

   I. Efforts to bear down—increases expulsive effects of uterine contractions.

   J. Perineal bulging with contractions—fetal head distends perineum, crowns; head born by extension.

⋈ II. Analysis/nursing diagnosis

   A. *Pain* related to strong uterine contractions, pressure of fetal descent, stretching of perineum.

   B. *Injury risk*:

      1. *Infection* related to ruptured membranes, repeated vaginal examinations.

      2. *Laceration* related to pressure of fetal head exceeding perineal elasticity, and *uterine rupture* related to fundal pressure hyperstimulation.

   C. *Skin integrity impairment* related to laceration, episiotomy.

   D. *Fluid volume deficit* related to hypotension secondary to regional anesthesia.

   E. *Anxiety* related to imminent birth of fetus.

   F. *Individual coping impairment* related to prolonged sensory stimulation (contractions) and anxiety.

   G. *Urinary elimination alteration* related to anesthesia and contractions.

   H. *Sleep pattern disturbance.*

✖ III. **Nursing care plan/implementation**
   A. Goal: *emotional support.*
      1. To sustain motivation/control:
         a. **Never** leave mother and significant other alone now.
         b. Keep informed of progress.
      ☞ c. Direct bearing-down efforts (pushing) without holding breath* while pushing. Encourage pushing "out through vagina" and encourage mother to touch coming head; position mirror so woman can see perineal bulging with effective efforts; minimize distractions.
      2. To allay significant other's anxiety: reassure regarding mother's behavior if she is not anesthetized.
      3. Support family choices.
   B. Goal: *safeguard status.*
      1. Precautions when putting legs in stirrups
         a. If varicosities, **do not put legs in stirrups.**
         b. *Avoid* pressure to popliteal veins; pad stirrups.
         c. Ensure proper, even alignment by adjusting stirrups.
         d. Move legs *simultaneously* into or out of stirrups—to *avoid* nerve, ligament, and muscle strain.
         e. Provide proper support to woman not using stirrups.
      2. Support woman in whatever position selected for birth, e.g., side-lying.
      ☞ 3. Cleanse perineum, thighs, and lower abdomen, maintaining sterile technique.
   C. Goal: *maintain a comfortable environment.*
      1. Free of unnecessary noise, light, conversation.
      2. Comfortable temperature (warm).
   D. *Medical management.*
      1. Episiotomy may be performed to facilitate birth.
      2. Forceps may be applied to exert traction and expedite birth.
      3. Vacuum extraction also used to expedite birth.
   E. Use of birthing room for delivery, with alternative positions.

✖ IV. **Evaluation/outcome criteria**
   A. Woman is cooperative, actively participates in birth; maintains control over own behavior.
   B. Successful, uncomplicated birth of viable infant.
   C. All assessment findings within normal limits (vital signs, emotional status, response to birth).
   D. Presence of significant other.

* The woman must be discouraged from using the Valsalva maneuver (holding one's breath and tightening abdominal muscles) for pushing during the *second* stage. This activity increases intrathoracic pressure, reduces venous return, and increases venous pressure. The cardiac output and blood pressure increase and pulse slows temporarily. During the Valsalva maneuver, *fetal hypoxia* may occur. The process is reversed when the woman takes a breath.

# Nursing Actions During Third Stage of Labor

✖ I. **Assessment**
   A. Time elapsed—average: 5 min; prolonged third stage (> 30 min) may indicate complications.
   ! B. **Signs of placental separation:**
      1. Increase in bleeding from vagina.
      2. Cord lengthens.
      3. Uterus rises in abdomen, assumes globular shape.
   C. Assess mother's level of consciousness (LOC).
   D. Examine placenta for intactness and number of vessels in umbilical cord (*normal*: three. *NOTE*: two vessels only—associated with increased incidence of *congenital anomalies*); condition of placenta for calcification, infarcts, etc.

✖ II. **Analysis/nursing diagnosis**
   A. *Family coping: potential for growth* related to bonding, beginning achievement of developmental tasks.
   B. *Fluid volume deficit* related to blood loss during third stage.

✖ III. **Nursing care plan/implementation**
   A. Goal: *prevent uterine atony.* Administer oxytocin, as ordered (see **Pharmacology Box 6.1, p. 147**).
   B. Goal: *facilitate parent-child bonding.*
      1. While protecting neonate from cold stress, encourage parents to see, hold, touch neonate.
      2. Comment about neonate's individuality, characteristics, and behaviors.
      3. After neonate is assessed for congenital anomalies (cleft palate, esophageal atresia), encourage breastfeeding, if desired.
   C. Goal: **health teaching.**
      1. Describe, discuss common neonatal behavior in transitional period (periods of reactivity, sleep, hyperactivity).
      ☞ 2. Demonstrate removal of mucus by aspiration with bulb syringe.
      ☞ 3. Demonstrate ways of facilitating breastfeeding.

✖ IV. **Evaluation/outcome criteria**
   A. Woman has a successful, uneventful completion of labor:
      1. Minimal blood loss.
      2. Vital signs within normal limits.
      3. Fundus well contracted at level of umbilicus.
   B. Parents express satisfaction with outcome, demonstrate infant attachment.

# Nursing Actions During Fourth Stage of Labor—*1–2 hr postpartum*

▶️ I. **Assessment**—every 15 min for 4 times; then, every 30 min for 2 times—or until stable—to monitor response to physiologic stress of labor/birth.

 A. *Vital signs:*

  1. *Temperature* taken once; if elevated, requires follow-up—may indicate infection, dehydration, excessive blood loss. Note, ❗ record, report temperature of 100.4° F (38° C) or more.

  2. *Blood pressure*—every 15 min x 4.

   a. Returns to *prelabor level*—due to loss of placental circulation and increased circulating blood volume.

   b. *Elevation* may be in response to use of oxytocic drugs or pre-eclampsia (first 48 hr).

   c. *Lowered* blood pressure—may reflect significant blood loss during labor/birth, or occult bleeding.

  3. *Pulse and respirations*—every 15 min x 4.

   a. Physiologic bradycardia—due to normal vagal response.

   b. Tachycardia—may indicate excessive blood loss during labor/birth, dehydration, exhaustion, or occult bleeding.

 ☞ B. Location and tone of *fundus*—every 15 min x 4, to assure continuing contraction; prevent blood loss due to uterine relaxation.

  1. Fundus—firm; at or slightly lower than the umbilicus; in midline.

  2. May be displaced by distended bladder—due to normal diuresis; common cause of ❗ bleeding in immediate postpartum: uterine atony.

 C. Character and amount of *vaginal flow* every 15 min x 4:

  1. Moderate lochia rubra.

  2. Perineal pad saturated in 15 min, or blood pools under buttocks: may indicate excessive ❗ loss.

  3. Bright-red bleeding: may indicate cervical or ❗ vaginal laceration.

 D. *Perineum* every 15 min x 4:

  1. Edema.

  2. Bruising—due to trauma.

  3. Distention/hematoma, rectal pain.

 E. *Bladder* check for fullness every 15 min x 4—to prevent distention.

 F. Rate of IV, if present; response to added medication, if any.

 G. Intake and output—to evaluate hydration.

 H. Recovery from analgesia/anesthesia.

 I. Energy level.

 J. Verbal, nonverbal interaction between woman and significant other:

  1. Dialogue.

  2. Posture.

  3. Facial expressions.

  4. Touching.

 K. Interactions between parent(s) and newborn; signs of bonding appropriate to individual's culture:

  1. Eye contact with newborn.

  2. Calls by name.

  3. Explores with fingertips, strokes, cuddles.

➤🔖 L. Signs of **postpartal emergencies:**

  1. Uterine atony, hemorrhage.

  2. Vaginal hematoma.

▶️ II. **Analysis/nursing diagnosis**

 A. *Fluid volume deficit* related to excessive intrapartal blood loss, dehydration.

 B. *Urinary elimination alteration* related to intrapartal bladder trauma, dehydration, blood loss.

 C. *Skin integrity impairment* related to episiotomy, lacerations, cesarean birth.

 D. *Family processes alteration* related to role change.

 E. *Parenting alteration* related to interruption in bonding secondary to:

  1. Compromised maternal status.

  2. Compromised neonatal status.

 F. *Knowledge deficit* related to self-care procedures.

 G. *Fatigue* related to sleep disturbances and anxiety.

 H. *Anxiety* related to status of self and infant.

 I. *Nutrition deficit (less than body requirements)* related to decreased food and fluid intake during labor

▶️ III. **Nursing care plan/implementation**

 A. Goal: *comfort measures.*

  1. Maternal position.

  2. Pad change.

  3. Perineal care—to promote healing; to reduce possibility of infection.

  4. Ice pack to perineum, as ordered—to reduce edema, discomfort, and pain related to hemorrhoids.

 🍎 B. Goal: *nutrition/hydration.* Offer fluids, foods as tolerated.

 C. Goal: *urinary elimination.*

  1. Encourage voiding—to avoid bladder distention.

  2. Record: time, amount, character.

  3. Anticipatory guidance related to nocturnal diuresis and increased output.

 D. Goal: *promote bonding.*

  1. Provide privacy, quiet; encourage sustained contact with newborn.

  2. Encourage: touching, holding baby; breastfeeding (also promotes involution).

E. Goal: **health teaching.**
  1. Perineal care—front to back, labia closed (after *each* void/bowel movement).
  2. Handwashing—before and after each pad change; after voiding, defecating; before and after baby care.
  3. Signs to report:
     a. Uterine cramping.
     b. Increased vaginal bleeding, passage of large clots.
     c. Nausea, dizziness.

IV. **Evaluation/outcome criteria**
  A. Woman expresses comfort, satisfaction in fourth stage.
  B. Vital signs stable, fundus contracted, moderate lochia rubra, perineum undistended.
  C. Woman tolerates food and fluids well.
  D. Woman voids in adequate amount.
  E. Woman demonstrates eye contact with infant, cuddles.
  F. Woman verbalizes abnormal signs to report to physician.
  G. Woman returns demonstration of appropriate perineal care.
  H. Woman ambulates without pain, dizziness, numbness of legs.

# Nursing Management of the Newborn Immediately After Birth

I. **Assessment**
  A. Mucus in nasopharynx, oropharynx.
  B. *Apgar score*: note and record—at 1 and 5 min of age.

| Apgar Scoring System | | | |
|---|---|---|---|
| **Clinical Sign** | **Points Given According to Status** | | |
| | **0 Points** | **1 Point** | **2 Points** |
| **Appearance** (color) | Blue, pale | Body pink, extremities blue | Completely pink |
| **Pulse** (HR) | Absent | Below 100 | Over 100 |
| **Grimace** (reflex irritability to a gentle slap) | No response | Grimaces | Cries |
| **Activity** (muscle tone) | Limp | Some flexion of extremities | Active motion, general flexion |
| **Respiratory effort** | Absent | Slow, irregular | Good Strong cry |

1. *Score of 7–10*: good condition.
2. *Score of 4–6*: fair condition; assess for CNS depression; resuscitate as necessary.
3. *Score of 0–3*: poor condition; requires ongoing resuscitative measures
   **Asphyxia neonatorum**—fails to breathe spontaneously within 30-60 sec after birth.
C. Number of vessels in umbilical stump.
D. Passage of meconium stool, urine.
E. General physical appearance/status:
  1. Signs of *respiratory distress* (nasal flaring, grunting, sternal retraction, cyanosis, tachypnea).
  2. *Skin* condition (meconium-stained, cyanosis, jaundice, lesions).
  3. *Cry*—presence, pitch, quality.
  4. Signs of *birth trauma* (lacerations, dislocations, fractures).
  5. *Symmetry* (absent parts, extra digits, gross malformations, ears, palm creases, sacral dimples).
  6. *Head*: molding, caput succedaneum, cephalohematoma.
F. Identify high-risk infant.

II. **Analysis/nursing diagnosis**
  A. *Airway clearance impairment* related to excessive nasopharyngeal mucus.
  B. *Breathing pattern impairment* related to CNS depression secondary to: intrauterine hypoxia narcosis, prematurity, and lack of pulmonary surfactant.
  C. *Gas exchange impairment* related to respiratory distress.
  D. *Fluid volume deficit* related to birth trauma; hemolytic jaundice.
  E. *Skin integrity impairment* related to cord stump.
  F. *Injury risk* (biochemical, metabolic) related to impaired thermoregulation.
  G. *Thermoregulation impairment* related to environmental conditions.

III. **Nursing care plan/implementation**
  A. Goal: *ensure patent airway.*
    1. Suction *mouth first*, then nose; when stimulated, sensitive receptors around entrance to nares initiate gasp, causing aspiration of mucus present in mouth.
    2. Suction with bulb syringe.
       a. If deeper suctioning necessary, use DeLee mucus trap attached to suction.
       b. *Avoid* prolonged, vigorous suctioning:
          (1) Reduces oxygenation.
          (2) May traumatize tissue, cause edema, bleeding, laryngospasm, and cardiac arrhythmia.
    3. Assist gravity drainage of fluids; *position:head-dependent* (Trendelenburg), and *side-lying*.

B. Goal: *maintain body temperature*—to conserve energy, preserve store of brown fat, decrease oxygen needs; prevent acidosis. Prevent chilling:
   1. Minimize exposure; dry quickly.
   2. Warm; apply hat.
   3. Take temperature hourly until stable.
   4. Swaddle in warm blankets.
C. Goal: *identify infant.*
   1. Apply Identiband.
   2. Take infant's footprints and maternal fingerprints.
D. Goal: *prevent eye infection* (gonorrheal and chlamydial *ophthalmia neonatorum*). Within 1 hr of birth, apply ophthalmic *antibiotic* drops (2 drops in each eye) or ointment (1 line in each eye).
E. Goal: *facilitate prompt identification/vigilance for potential neonatal complications.*
   1. Record significant data from mother's chart:
      a. *History* of pregnancy, diabetes, hypertension, *current* drug abuse, excessive caffeine, medications, alcohol, malnutrition.
      b. Course of labor, evidence of fetal distress, medications received in labor.
      c. Birth history of anesthesia.
      d. Apgar; resuscitative efforts.
F. Goal: *facilitate prompt identification/intervention in hemolytic problems of the newborn.*
   1. Collect and send cord blood for appropriate tests:
      a. Blood type and Rh factor.
      b. Coombs' test.
   2. Give vitamin K to facilitate clotting.

**IV. Evaluation/outcome criteria:** successful transition to extrauterine life.
A. Status satisfactory; all assessment findings within normal limits.
B. Responsive in bonding process with parents.

# Nurse-Attended Emergency Birth (precipitate birth)

When woman presents without prenatal care, may represent drug abuse or ineffective coping.

## Imminent Birth

**I. Assessment:** identify signs of **imminent birth:**
A. Strong contractions.
B. Bearing-down efforts.
C. Perineal bulging; crowning.
D. Mother states, "It's coming."

**II. Analysis/nursing diagnosis**
A. *Pain* related to:
   1. Strong, sustained contractions.
   2. Descent of fetal head.
   3. Stretching of perineum.
B. *Anxiety/fear* related to imminent birth.
C. *Individual coping impairment* related to circumstances surrounding birth; anxiety, fear for self and infant.
D. *Injury* (mother) related to:
   1. Lacerations (vaginal, perineal).
   2. Infection secondary to unsterile birth.
E. *Fluid volume deficit* related to:
   1. Lacerations.
   2. Uterine atony.
   3. Retained placental fragments.
F. *Gas exchange* (infant) *impairment* related to intact membranes during birth.
G. *Injury risk* (infant) related to:
   1. Precipitate birth.
   2. Trauma.
   3. Hypoxia.

**III. Nursing care plan/implementation**
A. Goal: *reduce anxiety/fear*—reassure mother.
B. Goal: *delay birth*, if possible.
   1. Discourage bearing-down.
   2. Encourage panting.
   3. *Side-lying position* to slow descent and allow for more controlled birth.
C. Goal: *prevent infection.*
   1. Provide sterile (or clean) field for birth.
   2. *Avoid* touching birth canal without gloved hands.
   3. Support perineum (and advancing head) with sterile (or clean) towel.
D. Goal: *facilitate/assist birth* (**Figure 4.6**).

---

1. If *membranes* intact as head emerges, tear them at neck to facilitate first breath.
2. Support *head* in both hands.
3. Feel for *cord* around neck (if present, and if possible, slip cord over head; if tight, *and* sterile equipment at hand, clamp cord in 2 places, cut between clamps, unwrap cord). If *unsterile* environment, keep fetus and placenta attached—*do not* cut cord.
4. After restitution, apply gentle downward pressure to bring *anterior shoulder* under pubic symphysis.
5. Gently *lift head* to ease birth of posterior shoulder.
6. *Support infant* as body slips free of mother's body.

---

E. Goal: *facilitate drainage of mucus and fluid →* patent airway.
   1. Hold infant in *head-dependent position* (see **Figure 4.6 (e)**).
   2. Clear mucus with bulb syringe (if available), or use fingertip, wipe with towel.

*(continued on p. 115)*

**FIGURE 4.6 EMERGENCY BIRTH.** (a) **Support infant's head** as it delivers. (b) **Loosen cord** from around neck. (c) Gently guide head downward to **help upper shoulder deliver**. (d) Guide head upward to **help lower shoulder deliver**. (e) Babies are slippery! **Hold the baby firmly**, with the **head dependent**, to facilitate drainage of secretions.

☞ **F.** Goal: *prevent placental transfusion*—hold infant level with placenta until cord stops pulsating. If sterile supplies are available, cut cord (**Figure 4.7**).

☞ **G.** Goal: *prevent chilling.*
  1. Wrap infant in towel or other clean material.
  2. Place infant on *side, head-dependent*, on mother's abdomen.
  3. Dry head, cover with cap or material.

## Placental Separation

▶ **I.** **Assessment**—*third stage*: identify signs of **placental separation** (p. 110).

▶ **II.** **Nursing care plan/implementation**—*third stage*
  **A.** Goal: *avoid/minimize potential for complications* (everted uterus, tearing of placenta with fragments remaining, separation of cord from placenta).
    1. *Avoid* traction (pulling) on cord.
    2. *Avoid* vigorous fundal massage.
    3. *Discourage* maternal bearing-down efforts unless placenta visible at introitus.
    4. With fundus well contracted, and placenta visible at introitus, encourage mother to bear down to expel placenta.

☞ **B.** Goal: *stimulate respiration*. If neonate **fails to breathe spontaneously:**
    1. Maintain body temperature—dry and cover.
    2. Clear airway:
      **a.** *Position*: head *down*.
      **b.** Turn head to *side*.
    3. Stimulate:
      **a.** Rub back gently.
      **b.** Flick soles of feet.
    4. If no response to stimulation:
      **a.** Slightly extend neck to "sniffing" position (head tilt-chin lift method).
      **b.** Place mouth over newborn's nose and mouth and exhale air in cheeks, saying "ho" (prevents excessive pressure)—use bag and mask or CPR shield if available; *avoid* contact with secretions.

  **C.** Goal: begin **cardiopulmonary resuscitation (CPR) if no heart rate.**
    1. Place infant on firm, flat surface.
    2. With two-three fingers on sternum, depress ½–¾ inches 100 times/min.
    3. Assist ventilation on upstroke of every fifth compression (5:1 ratio).
    4. Go immediately to Emergency.
    5. See *Teaching parents* CPR, **Chapter 8, p. 183** and **Figure 8.7, p. 184.**

  **D.** Goal: *maintain infant's body temperature*
    1. Wrap placenta with baby, if cord intact.
    2. Place infant in mother's arms.

  **E.** Goal: *prevent maternal hemorrhage* (uterine atony).
    1. Encourage breastfeeding, or stimulate nipple.
    ☞ 2. Gently massage fundus, support lower part of uterus and express clots when uterus is contracted.
    3. Encourage voiding if bladder is full.
    4. Get to a medical facility.

  **F.** Goal: *encourage bonding/stimulate uterine contractions*. Encourage breastfeeding.

  **G.** Goal: *legal accountability* as birth attendant. Record date, time, birth events, maternal and fetal status.

▶ **III.** **Evaluation/outcome criteria**
  **A.** Woman experiences normal spontaneous birth of viable infant over intact perineum.
  **B.** Uncomplicated fourth stage—status satisfactory for both mother and infant.
  **C.** Woman expresses satisfaction with management and result.

# Alterations Affecting Protective Function

## Induction of Labor

**Definition**: deliberate initiation of uterine contraction.

▶ **I.** **Assessment**—Induction of labor. *Indications* for:
  **A.** History of rapid or silent labors, precipitate birth.
  **B.** Woman resides some distance from hospital (controversial).
  **C.** Coexisting medical disorders:
    1. Uncontrolled diabetes.
    2. Progressive pre-eclampsia.
    3. Severe renal disease.
  **D.** Premature rupture of membranes (PROM)—spontaneous rupture of membranes before onset of labor and preterm rupture of membranes less than 37 wk from last menstrual period. **Hazards:**
    1. *Maternal*—intrauterine infection (amnionitis, endometritis).
    2. *Fetal*—sepsis; prolapsed cord.
  **E.** Rh or ABO incompatibility, fetal hemolytic disease.
  **F.** Congenital anomaly (e.g., anencephaly).
  **G.** Postterm pregnancy with nonreactive (nonstress test) (NST).
  **H.** Intrauterine fetal death.

**II.** **Criteria for induction:**
  **A.** Absence of malpresentation, or malposition.
  **B.** Engaged vertex of single gestation.
  **C.** Nearing, or at, term.

**FIGURE 4.7 CUTTING THE UMBILICAL CORD.** Place clamps about 2 in. apart along the cord after it has stopped pulsating, and cut between them.

D. Fetal lung maturity.
1. Survival rate—better at 32 wk or more.
2. *Lecithin-sphingomyelin* (L/S) ratio greater than 2:1.
3. Mother who has diabetes— *phosphatidyl glycerol* is present in amniotic fluid.
E. "Ripe" cervix—softening, partially effaced, or ready for effacement/dilatation (if not already present). NOTE: Intravaginal or paracervical application of prostaglandin gel, *Cervidil* or misoprostolor may be used to prepare cervix for labor.

III. **Methods:**
A. *Amniotomy*—artificial rupture of membranes (AROM) with fetal head engaged.
B. Intravenous *oxytocin infusion*.

IV. **Potential complications:**
A. *Amniotomy*—irrevocably committed to birth
1. Prolapsed cord.
2. Infection.
B. *IV oxytocin infusion*:
1. Over-stimulation of uterus.
2. Decreased placental perfusion/fetal distress.
3. Precipitate labor and birth.
4. Cervical/perineal lacerations.
5. Uterine rupture.

6. Water intoxication—if large doses given in sterile water solution over prolonged period (antidiuretic effect increases water reabsorption).
7. Hypertensive crisis.

## Before Induction

I. **Assessment**—*before induction*
A. Estimate gestation (fundal height, EDD, cervical status, ultrasound confirmation of EDD).
B. *Bishop Score*: evaluation of cervical inducibility.
C. General health status:
1. Weight, vital signs, FHR, edema.
2. Status of membranes.
3. Vaginal bleeding.
4. Coexisting disorders.
D. History of previous labors, if any.
E. Emotional status.
F. Knowledge/understanding of anticipated procedures:
1. Amniotomy (artificial rupture of membranes).
2. IV oxytocin infusion.
3. Fetal monitoring.
G. Preparation for childbirth; coping strategies. Identify support person.

II. **Analysis/nursing diagnosis**
A. *Knowledge deficit* related to process of induction.
B. *Anxiety/fear* related to need for induction of labor.

C. *Individual coping impairment* related to psychological stress.

D. *Pain* related to uterine contractions.

**III. Nursing care plan/implementation**

A. Goal: **health teaching**.

1. Explain rationale for procedures:

    a. Amniotomy:

    (1) Induces labor.

    (2) Relieves uterine overdistention.

    (3) Increases efficiency of contractions, shortening labor.

    b. Oxytocin infusion.

    (1) Induces labor.

    (2) Stimulates uterine contractions.

    c. Internal fetal monitor.

    (1) Provides continuous assessment of uterine response to oxytocin stimulation.

    (2) Provides continuous assessment of fetal response to physiologic stress of labor.

2. *Describe procedure*—to reduce anxiety and increase cooperation.

3. *Explain advantages/disadvantages*—to ensure "informed consent."

B. Goal: *emotional support*—encourage verbalization of concerns, reassure, as possible.

**IV. Evaluation/outcome criterion:** Woman verbalizes understanding of process, rationale, procedures, and alternatives.

### During Induction

**I. Assessment**—during induction and labor

A. *Amniotomy*—same as for spontaneous rupture of membranes (SROM)

1. Observe fluid—note color, amount

2. Monitor FHR; assess for fetal distress.

3. Observe for signs of prolapsed cord.

4. Assess fetal activity:

    a. *Excessive* activity may indicate distress.

    b. *Absence* of activity may indicate distress or demise.

B. *IV oxytocin infusion:*

1. Continually assess response to oxytocin stimulation/flow rate; always given via controlled infusion.

    a. Uterine contractions.

    b. Maternal vital signs, FHR.

2. Identify signs of:

    a. *Deviation* from normal patterns:

    (1) Lack of response to increasing flow rate.

    (2) Uterine hyperstimulation (contractions— < 2 min apart).

    (3) Lack of adequate uterine relaxation between contractions.

b. *Side effects of oxytocin*: diminished output—potential water intoxication.

c. **Hazards** to mother or fetus:

(1) Sustained (> 90 sec duration) or tetanic (strong, spasmlike) contractions—potential abruptio placentae, uterine rupture, fetal hypoxia/anoxia/death.

(2) *Fetal* arrhythmias, decelerations.

(3) *Maternal* hypertension—potential for hypertensive crisis, cerebral hemorrhage.

**II. Nursing care plan/implementation**

A. Same as for other women in labor.

B. Treatment for indications of deviations from normal FHR patterns (see **Figure 4.5, p. 103**):

1. Change maternal position.

2. Stop oxytocin infusion, maintain IV with Ringer's lactate or other solution as ordered.

3. Begin oxygen per mask; up to 8–10 L/min.

4. Notify physician promptly.

5. Check maternal blood pressure and pulse rate.

C. Anticipatory guidance: may have strong contractions soon after induction starts.

**III. Evaluation/outcome criteria**

A. Woman demonstrates response to oxytocin stimulation:

1. Establishes desired contraction pattern, not hyperstimulated.

2. Progresses through labor—within normal limits:

    a. Normotensive.

    b. Voids in adequate amounts.

    c. No evidence of deviation from normal contraction patterns.

B. Fetus shows no evidence of distress.

C. Woman experiences normal vaginal birth of viable infant.

## Operative Obstetrics—*Episiotomy*

**Definition**: incision of perineum to facilitate infant's birth.

**I. Rationale*:*

A. Surgical incision reduces possibility of laceration.

B. Protects infant's head from pressure exerted by resistant perineum.

C. Shortens second stage of labor.

**II. Types:**

A. *Midline*—chance of extension into anal sphincter greater than with mediolateral.

B. *Mediolateral*—healing is more painful than midline.

## III. Assessment

A. "REEDA".
1. Color: (**r**edness).
2. Swelling: (**e**dema).
3. Bruising: (**e**cchymosis).
4. Drainage: (**d**ischarge).
5. Suture line intact, or separated (**a**pproximation).

B. Healing.

C. Hematoma.

D. Tenderness; pain. NOTE: evaluate complaints of pain carefully. If intense, and unrelieved by usual measures, report **promptly**. May indicate vulvar, paravaginal, or ischiorectal abscess or hematoma.

## V. Analysis/nursing diagnosis

A. *Pain* related to labor process.

B. *Skin integrity impairment* related to surgical incision.

C. *Fluid volume deficit* related to hematoma.

D. *Sexual dysfunction* related to discomfort.

## VI. Nursing care plan/implementation

A. Goal: *prevent/reduce edema, promote comfort and healing.*
1. Place covered ice pack during immediate postpartum.
2. Administer *analgesics*, topical sprays, ointments, witch hazel pads.
3. Encourage use of Sitz bath or rubber ring.
4. Encourage *Kegel's* exercises.
5. Do **health teaching.**
   a. Instruct in tightening gluteal muscles before sitting.
   b. Instruct to *avoid* sitting on one hip.

B. Goal: *minimize potential for infection*
1. Teach/provide perineal care during fourth stage of labor.
2. **Health teaching.** Instruct in self-perineal care after voiding, defecation, and with each pad change.

## VII. Evaluation/outcome criteria

A. Woman's incision heals by primary intention.

B. Woman demonstrates appropriate self-perineal care.

C. Woman evidences no signs of hematoma, infection, or separation of suture line.

D. Woman experiences minimal discomfort.

# Operative Obstetrics—*Forceps-Assisted* Birth

## I. Indications:

A. Fetal distress.

B. Maternal need:
1. Exhaustion.
2. Coexisting disease, such as cardiac disorder.
3. Poor progress in second stage.
4. Persistent fetal occiput transverse (OT) or occiput posterior (OP) position.

## II. Criteria for forceps application:

A. Engaged fetal head.

B. Ruptured membranes.

C. Full dilatation.

D. Absence of cephalopelvic disproportion.

E. Some anesthesia has been given; usually, episiotomy has been performed.

F. Empty bladder.

## III. *Type*: Low—outlet forceps.

## IV. Potential *complications*:

A. *Maternal*:
1. Lacerations of birth canal, rectum, bladder.
2. Uterine rupture/hemorrhage.

B. *Neonatal*:
1. Cephalohematoma.
2. Skull fracture.
3. Intracranial hemorrhage, brain damage.
4. Facial paralysis.
5. Direct tissue trauma (abrasions, ecchymosis).
6. Umbilical cord compression.

## V. Assessment

A. FHR immediately *before*—and *after*—forceps application (forceps blade may compress umbilical cord).

B. Observe mother/newborn for injury or signs of complications.

## VI. Analysis/nursing diagnosis

A. *Self-esteem disturbance* related to inability to give birth without surgical assistance.

B. *Anxiety/fear* related to infant's appearance (forceps marks) or awareness of potential complications.

## VII. Nursing care plan/implementation

A. Goal: *minimize feelings of failure due to inability to give birth "naturally".*
1. Explain, discuss reasons/indications for forceps-assisted birth.
2. Emphasize no maternal control over circumstances.

B. Goal: *reduce parental anxiety, maternal guilt over infant bruising/forceps marks.* Explain condition is temporary and has no lasting effects on child's appearance.

## VIII. Evaluation/outcome criteria

A. Woman verbalizes understanding of reasons for forceps-assisted birth.

B. Woman evidences no interruption in bonding with infant.

C. Woman experiences uncomplicated recovery.

# Operative Obstetrics—*Vacuum-Assisted Birth*

See *Forceps-Assisted Birth.*

# Operative Obstetrics—*Cesarean Birth*

**Definition**: incision through abdominal wall and uterus to give birth.

I. **Indications** for *elective* cesarean birth:

A. Known *CPD*.

B. *Previous uterine surgery* (e.g., myomectomy), repeated cesarean births (depends on type of incision done).

C. Active maternal *genital herpes II* infection.

D. *Breech* presentation (*NOTE*: to reduce infant morbidity/mortality, elective cesarean birth is recommended method of choice).

E. *Neoplasms* of cervix, uterus, or birth canal.

F. Maternal diabetes with *placental aging*; fetal macrosomia (cephalopelvic disproportion).

II. **Criteria** for elective cesarean birth: L/S ratio greater than 2:1—indicates presence of pulmonary surfactant; less risk of respiratory distress syndrome; estimated fetal weight of ≥ 4250 gms.

III. **Indications** for *emergency* cesarean birth:

A. *Fetal:*

1. *Fetal distress*: prolapsed cord.
2. *Fetal jeopardy*: Rh or ABO incompatibility.
3. *Fetal malposition*/malpresentation.

B. *Maternal:*

1. *Uterine* dysfunction.
2. *Placental* disorders:

   a. Placenta previa.
   b. Abruptio placentae, with Couvelaire uterus.

3. Severe maternal *pre-eclampsia/eclampsia*.
4. *Fetopelvic disproportion*.
5. Sudden maternal death.
6. Carcinoma.
7. Failed induction.

IV. **Types***:*

A. *Low segment*—method of choice

1. *Transverse* incision through *abdominal* wall and lower uterine segment.
2. *Transverse* incision through *abdominal* wall, with vertical incision of lower uterine segment.
3. Advantages—fewer complications:

   a. Less blood loss.
   b. More comfortable recovery.
   c. Less adhesion formation.
   d. Lower risk of uterine rupture in subsequent pregnancy/labor and birth.
   e. Cosmetically more acceptable.

B. *Classic*—*vertical* incision through abdominal wall and uterus. May be necessary for preterm due to small size of lower uterine segment.

C. *Porro's*—hysterotomy followed by hysterectomy. Necessary in presence of:

1. Hemorrhage from uterine atony.
2. Placenta previa, accreta.

3. Large uterine myomas.
4. Ruptured uterus.
5. Cancer of uterus or ovary.

V. **Assessment**

A. *Maternal* physical status:

1. Vital signs.
2. Labor status, if any.
3. Contractions (if any).
4. Membranes (intact; ruptured).
5. Signs of complications.

B. *Fetal* status:

1. FHR pattern.
2. Color and amount of amniotic fluid.
3. Biophysical profile (BPP).

C. Maternal emotional status.

D. Understanding of procedure, indications for, implications.

E. Other—as for any abdominal surgery.

VI. **Analysis/nursing diagnosis**

A. *Self-esteem disturbance* related to perceived failure to give birth vaginally.

B. *Anxiety/fear* related to impending surgery and/or reasons for cesarean birth.

C. *Individual coping impairment* related to anxiety and fear for self, infant.

D. *Fluid volume deficit* related to abdominal surgery and/or reason for cesarean birth.

E. *Pain* related to abdominal surgery.

F. *Constipation* related to decreased bowel activity.

G. *Urinary elimination alteration* related to fluid volume deficit.

VII. **Nursing care plan/implementation**

A. *Preoperative.*

1. Goal: *safeguard fetal status*.

   a. Monitor fetal heart rate continually.
   b. Notify neonatology and NICU of scheduled surgical birth.

2. Goal: **health teaching.**

   a. Describe, discuss anticipated anesthesia.
   b. Explain rationale for preoperative antacids: cimetidine, a histamine blocker, to decrease production of gastric acid; metroclopramide (*Reglan*) to hasten gastric emptying.
   c. Describe, explain anticipated procedures—abdominal shave, indwelling catheter, intravenous fluids—to woman and support person.

3. Other—as for any abdominal surgery.
4. Prepare for cesarean birth.

B. *Postoperative.*

1. Same as for other clients with abdominal surgery.
2. Same as for other women who are postpartum.

▶ VIII. **Evaluation/outcome criteria**

A. Woman verbalizes understanding of reasons for cesarean birth.

B. Successful birth of viable infant.

C. Evidence of no surgical/birth complications.

D. Woman evidences no interference with bonding.

E. Woman expresses satisfaction with procedure and result.

## Vaginal Birth After Cesarean (VBAC)—*Trial of labor after cesarean* (TOLAC)

I. **Candidates:**

A. Previous low-transverse cesarean birth.

B. Fetal head well engaged in pelvis; *no* evidence of CPD or feto-pelvic disproportion (FPD).

C. Woman in active labor, including adequate contractions, engagement and descent of presenting part, effacement and dilatation in progress; soft anterior cervix.

D. Preexisting reason for cesarean birth *not* apparent.

E. *No* history of sepsis with previous cesarean birth that may hinder new incision from healing properly.

F. *No* herpetic infection.

▶ II. **Assessment**

☞ A. Monitor FHR carefully.

☞ B. Monitor uterus for adequacy of contractions and for progress of labor.

C. Observe mother for signs of complications.

▶ III. **Analysis/nursing diagnosis**

A. *Knowledge deficit* related to trial of labor.

B. *Fear* related to outcome for fetus.

C. *Individual coping impairment* related to labor progress and outcome.

▶ IV. **Nursing care plan/implementation**

A. *Latent* phase of labor: encourage normal activities for any woman in this phase of labor.

B. *Active* phase of labor:

☞ 1. Monitor uterine activity and FHR electronically.

☞ 2. Establish IV access (e.g., IV lock).

3. Attend to woman's and family's anxiety, as well as her physical needs.

▶ V. **Evaluation/outcome criteria**

A. Woman gives birth vaginally to a healthy infant; or,

B. If a repeat cesarean birth is necessary, woman/family are supported and encouraged to verbalize feelings about outcome.

C. Whether birth is vaginal or abdominal, woman verbalizes positive feelings about herself.

# Summary

The perinatal nurse requires very special skills of assessment, analysis, planning, implementation, and evaluation to provide safe, quality nursing care during the intrapartal phase of the childbearing process. Nursing care is based on knowledge of the *biologic foundations of labor, pain management,* nursing care of the *mother-fetus/newborn and family* during the *four stages* of labor and birth, *nurse-attended emergency birth, induction of labor, operative obstetrics,* and VBAC. From admission to the hospital (or birth center) through the fourth stage of labor, the nurse considers all members of the child-bearing family, encouraging and promoting early family participation and attachment.

## 💡 Study and Memory Aids

### FHT—Assessment of Sound

**Funis:** hissing sound of blood through umbilical arteries

### Labor—Cardinal Movements

Descent
Flexion
Internal rotation
Extension
Restitution
Expulsion/birth

### Length of Labor

| Stage | Nullipara | Multipara |
|---|---|---|
| First: | 8–12 hr | 6–8 hr |
| Second: | 1–2 hr | 30 min |
| Third: | 5–60 min | 5–60 min |

### Labor—Breathing Techniques: Hyperventilation Treatment

Breathe into paper bag or cupped hands.

### ! Alert—Labor: Second Stage:

**Avoid** Valsalva maneuver when bearing down

### Placenta— Examine Cord for Blood Vessels: "AVA"

**A**rtery
**V**ein
**A**rtery

### Newborn—Assessment Components: "APGAR"

**A**ppearance
**P**ulse
**G**rimace
**A**ctivity
**R**espiratory effort

| APGAR Scores—Points for Status | |
| --- | --- |
| Good | 7–10 |
| Fair | 4–6 |
| Continue resuscitation | 0–3 |

**! Alert—Newborn Care**

Suction **mouth** first!

**Fourth Stage of Labor—Postpartum Assessments Taken: q15 min x 4; q30 min x 2**

P, R, BP
Fundus
Lochia
Perineum
Bladder
Mother's recovery

**Episiotomy—Assessment: "REEDA"**

**R**edness—color
**E**dema—swelling
**E**cchymosis—bruising
**D**ischarge—drainage
**A**pproximation—suture line

# Questions

1. The nurse informs the woman that, with lightening, the primigravida may experience:
   1. Urinary frequency, dyspnea, and leg pains.
   2. Dyspnea, constipation, and dysuria.
   3. Constipation, dysuria, and abdominal pain.
   4. Leg cramps, urinary frequency, and easier breathing.

2. The nurse knows that a woman is experiencing false labor when she reports that:
   1. She has been having bloody show.
   2. Lightening occurred 10 days ago.
   3. She is feeling her contractions beginning in the lower back.
   4. She has experienced diarrhea in the past few hours.

3. A woman in labor, sitting in a rocking chair, becomes nauseated and beads of perspiration appear over her upper lip. What is the nurse's *first* action?
   1. Notify the obstetrician because she is going into shock.
   2. Examine her to see if she is fully dilated.
   3. Quickly assess her blood pressure for hypotension.
   4. Prepare for immediate birth.

4. The nurse should discourage the use of the Valsalva maneuver during pregnancy (in exercise programs) or bearing-down during the second stage of labor because it causes:

1. A marked increase in venous return to the heart.
2. A transient hypotension followed by hypertension.
3. An increased cardiac output blood flow to the brain.
4. A decrease in fetal pH and $PO_2$ and an increase in fetal $PCO_2$.

5. A woman who is pregnant expresses concern because the doctor told her that her "spines are blunt and somewhat widely separated." The nurse's reassurance is based on knowledge that the ischial spines of the woman's pelvis are important in labor and birth because:
   1. They form the inlet of the true pelvis.
   2. The distance between them is the narrowest diameter of the pelvis.
   3. They are landmarks of the widest measurement of the pelvis.
   4. They bear the weight of the body when sitting.

6. Which statement by a nurse to a woman in labor shows understanding of the physiology of maternal positioning as related to labor progress?
   1. "When you begin pushing, you'll have your legs comfortably supported in stirrups and a pillow under your head."
   2. "Sit in the rocking chair and rest while we do a 20 min monitor strip, then we'll walk again."
   3. "You can raise the head of your bed a little and we'll support your knees with pillows."
   4. "Just stay on your left side here in bed; that will help keep your baby's heart as strong as it is now."

7. While assisting a woman to give birth, the nurse knows not to pull on the umbilical cord, because the placenta is still attached, when which finding is noted?
   1. Cord lengthens.
   2. Silver-colored tissue appears at vaginal opening.
   3. A gush of blood is seen.
   4. Uterus is discoid-shaped.

8. The labor nurse knows that maternal visceral pain is characteristic of which phase/stage of labor and birth?
   1. Latent phase of first stage.
   2. First stage.
   3. Second stage, until presenting part is on perineum.
   4. Second stage, during expulsion of baby.

9. The labor nurse knows that maternal somatic pain is characteristic of which phase/stage of labor and birth?
   1. Latent phase of first stage.
   2. First stage.
   3. Second stage.
   4. Third stage.

10. The labor nurse knows that systemic medication is best given to a nullipara when her cervix is dilated to:
    1. 3–4 cm.
    2. 5–6 cm.
    3. 8 cm.
    4. 10 cm.

11. During a vaginal examination on a woman in active labor, the nurse palpates a triangular-shaped fontanel. These data suggest:
    1. Excessive molding of fetal skull bones.
    2. The biparietal diameter is presenting.
    3. The occipitomental diameter is presenting.
    4. The suboccipitobregmatic diameter is presenting.

12. A multipara is 7–8 cm dilated. She is working, using breathing to keep in control during her frequent and strong contractions. She tells the nurse that she feels lightheaded and her fingers tingle. What is the nurse's first action?
    1. Prepare her for imminent birth.
    2. Change her position.
    3. Ask her to breathe into a paper bag.
    4. Give her oxygen by face mask.

13. During oxytocin induction of labor, the nurse must be alert for a potential complication of oxytocin, such as:
    1. Pregnancy-induced hypertension (PIH).
    2. Water intoxication.
    3. Amniotic fluid embolism.
    4. Urinary retention.

14. Assessment of a woman in labor reveals an active labor pattern and cervix dilated 4–5 cm. A 30 min whirlpool bath at this time can be expected to:
    1. Slow her labor pattern.
    2. Increase her cervical dilatation an additional 2–3 cm.
    3. Result in a precipitous birth.
    4. Have no effect on labor pattern or cervical dilatation.

15. At which time will a nullipara probably be taken to the birth room?
    1. When the vertex is seen at the introitus with contractions.
    2. When full cervical dilation occurs.
    3. At approximately 8 cm dilation.
    4. When her contractions last 50–60 sec.

16. To plan for and provide nursing care that supports a woman's self-concept and feelings of self-worth, as well as meeting her physical care needs, the nurse knows that the best description of a woman's emotional changes during labor is:
    1. She becomes increasingly dependent and needs to be handled like a child.
    2. She becomes more demanding as labor becomes more painful.
    3. She becomes more irritable as labor progresses and should be left alone.
    4. She becomes more and more introspective as labor progresses.

17. To meet the standard for care, the nurse should know that for a primigravida who is 2 cm dilated:
    1. Her blood pressure will be assessed every half hour.
    2. Vaginal examination will be done every 2 hr.
    3. The FHR will be assessed every 30 min.
    4. Her temperature will be assessed every hour.

18. The physician's examination of a woman in labor reveals the following data: cervix is 6 cm dilated and 100% effaced; the presenting part is at +1 station. Suddenly, the woman is out of emotional control, crying hysterically. The best way for the coach to assist the woman who has been prepared in childbirth education is to:
    1. Leave the room until she is composed.
    2. Suggest that she take pain medications.
    3. Tell her it will soon be over.
    4. Talk to her, using direct eye contact, and demonstrate breathing for her.

19. The nurse is confident in judging that a woman's membranes have probably ruptured if the nitrazine (pH) paper turns to the color:
    1. Dark blue.
    2. Yellow.
    3. Olive.
    4. White.

20. What nursing action should be implemented when a woman in labor in the lithotomy position experiences supine hypotension?
    1. Have the woman sit up quickly.
    2. Give oxygen by face mask.
    3. Turn the woman to her side.
    4. Have the woman stand up.

21. Immediately following the administration of epidural anesthesia, the nurse's first assessment should be the:
    1. Fetal heart rate.
    2. Maternal heart rate.
    3. Maternal blood pressure.
    4. Length of contractions.

22. The nurse's plan of care is based on knowledge that the woman who would likely be given a "trial of labor" for vaginal birth after cesarean (VBAC) is one who previously had a:
    1. Cesarean through a classic uterine incision because of severe fetal distress.
    2. Low transverse cesarean for breech presentation; in this pregnancy, the fetus is in vertex presentation.
    3. Cesarean for fetopelvic disproportion.
    4. Low transverse cesarean for active vaginal/perineal herpes infection; culture at 39 wk in this pregnancy was positive for herpes.

23. A woman is in the transition phase of labor. The fetal monitor shows a baseline FHR of 140-150 beats/min, with accelerations noted to 160 beats/min with fetal movement and occasionally with contractions. During a particularly long contraction, the nurse notes that the fetal heart slowed to 115 beats/min at the onset of the contraction and returned to baseline by the end of the contraction. What is the *priority* nursing action?
    1. Turn the woman to her side.
    2. Start an intravenous infusion of D$_5$RL.
    3. Start oxygen by face mask.
    4. Document and continue to observe.

24. If the fetal position is right occiput anterior (ROA), the nurse would locate the point of maximum impulse (PMI) of fetal heart tones (FHTs) in the mother's:
    1. Left upper quadrant (LUQ).
    2. Right upper quadrant (RUQ).
    3. Left lower quadrant (LLQ).
    4. Right lower quadrant (RLQ).

25. The nurse applies an ice pack to a new mother's episiotomy area immediately following vaginal childbirth, to reduce discomfort by:
    1. Freezing the area, thus preventing pain.
    2. Minimizing the amount of edema.
    3. Helping her focus on the cold rather than on the pain.
    4. Increasing circulation to the area for more rapid healing.

26. Which nursing assessment is appropriate during the fourth stage of labor (the 2 hr following birth)?
    1. Fundus, every 30 min x 4.
    2. Blood pressure, once at 1 hr, than per hospital protocol.
    3. Temperature, every 15 min x 4.
    4. Bladder, every 15 min x 4, then every 30 min x 2.

27. What is the nurse's *first* action immediately following rupture of the membranes of a woman in labor?
    1. Note the color and consistency of the fluid.
    2. Assess the fetal heart rate.
    3. Look for presence of the umbilical cord at the vaginal orifice.
    4. Keep her in bed until the MD is contacted

28. The labor nurse determines that the woman is experiencing false labor when:
    1. Contractions occur at regular intervals.
    2. Intensity of contractions is lessened by walking.
    3. Intervals of contractions gradually shorten.
    4. Duration of contractions increase.

29. A woman in the second stage of labor is preparing to push. The nurse must intervene *immediately* when the coach is heard to say:
    1. "Try to relax completely between contractions."
    2. "Your semirecumbent position is very good."
    3. "Push in short bursts as you feel the urge to bear down."
    4. "Push with your mouth closed and no noise!"

30. A spiral electrode and an intrauterine catheter are inserted for direct monitoring of a woman in labor. The nurse observes the following data on the monitor strip: contractions every 3 min lasting 80 sec, fetal heart rate (FHR) baseline of 135–145 beats/min, fall in FHR to 110 beats/min that begins when contraction begins and ends when contraction ends, variability 6–10 beats/min. Which nursing action is most appropriate?
    1. Implement measures for fetal distress; this is an ominous pattern.
    2. Continue monitoring per standard; this is a benign pattern.
    3. Troubleshoot the monitor; this pattern contains artifact.
    4. Notify the physician; this situation requires fetal scalp pH assessment.

31. As part of the admission procedure, the nurse performs and evaluates findings from Leopold's maneuvers as a basis for individualizing the plan of care. Leopold's maneuvers reveal the breech in the fundus and nodulations noted in the mother's left flank. This fetus is:
    1. Left sacrum posterior (LSP).
    2. Right sacrum anterior (RSA).
    3. Left occiput posterior (LOP).
    4. Right occiput anterior (ROA).

# Answers/Rationale

1. **(4)** Leg cramps, urinary frequency, and easier breathing often occur with lightening. Lightening refers to the sensation of decreased abdominal distention produced by uterine descent into the pelvic cavity, as the fetal presenting part settles into the pelvis; it occurs about 2 wk before the onset of labor in nulliparas. Lightening does *not* cause *dyspnea* (**1** and **2**) or *dysuria* (**2** and **3**), both of which would require further assessment and possible intervention (dysuria is a symptom of urinary tract infection). Lightening also does *not* result in *abdominal pain* (**3**); abdominal pain may be the result of abruptio placentae or other complications. **AS, COM, 5, HPM, Health promotion and maintenance**

2. **(4)** Although diarrhea is often a prodromal symptom of labor, it may to due to a variety of other causes. The signs/symptoms in options **1**, **2**, and **3** *are* commonly experienced by women beginning *true* labor. **AN, COM, 5, HPM, Health promotion and maintenance**

3. **(2)** The signs and symptoms described suggest that she is fully dilated (10 cm); the nurse should examine her to confirm this. These are signs/symptoms of full dilatation, not *shock* (**1**) or *hypotension* (**3**). They signify the end of the first stage and *only* the beginning of the second stage; birth (**4**) may still be *some time away*. NOTE: Other symptoms/signs include belching and shaking of the legs. **IMP, ANL, 5, HPM, Health promotion and maintenance**

4. **(4)** The Valsalva maneuver (closed glottis) does result in a decrease in fetal pH and PO$_2$, and an increase in fetal PCO$_2$. There is a marked *decrease*, not increase (**1**), in venous return to the heart. There is a transient *hypertension*, followed by a *decrease* in maternal blood pressure, rather than the reverse (**2**). There is a decrease in cardiac output blood flow to the brain, *not an increase* (**3**), that may cause orthostatic hypotension (aortocaval syndrome). **PL, COM, 6, HPM, Health promotion and maintenance**

5. **(2)** The ischial spines are the landmarks for *station* of the presenting part; the distance between them is the narrowest diameter of the pelvis. (The description given is that of an adequate, gynecoid pelvis.) The *brim* forms the inlet of the true pelvis (**1**); linea terminalis, sacral promontory, and symphysis pubis form the brim. The distance between the ischial spines is the narrowest, *not* the widest (**3**), measurement of the pelvis. The body's weight is borne by the ischial *tuberosities* when the person is sitting (**4**). **IMP, RE/KN, 5, HPM, Health promotion and maintenance**

6. **(2)** The upright position (sitting in a rocking chair, walking) is the position of preference to let gravity assist in the cervical effacement and dilatation equally around the cervix (lying in bed leads to complete effacement/dilatation "except for an anterior lip"). *Squatting* is the most efficient position for pushing with the fetus in vertex position (but not posterior); lying down (**1**) does not put the woman in best anatomic/physiologic position for pushing. Knees are *never* supported with pillows while in bed (**3**); if lying down, the woman should

be side lying. Side lying (**4**) does enhance renal and uteroplacental perfusion, but, because it does not allow gravity to work for the woman in labor, it is not the *best* choice. **EV, COM, 3, HPM, Health promotion and maintenance**

7. **(4)** Before the placenta separates, the uterus is discoid-shaped; after separation, the uterus is globular in shape. The other options are the signs that the placenta *has* separated: The cord lengthens (**1**), amniotic membranes are seen at the vaginal introitus (**2**), and a gush of blood is seen (**3**). **EV, COM, 5, HPM, Health promotion and maintenance**

8. **(2)** During the first stage of labor, pain is visceral, caused by dilatation of the cervix and uterine ischemia. This pain is referred to the lower abdominal wall, the area over the lumbar region, and the sacrum. Visceral pain characterizes the *entire* first stage, not just the latent phase (**1**). *Somatic* pain characterizes the second stage (**3** and **4**). **AN, RE/KN, 3, HPM, Health promotion and maintenance**

9. **(3)** Pain of somatic origin characterizes the second stage. It is caused by hypoxia of the uterus, distention of the vagina and perineum, and pressure on adjacent tissues. Pain may be felt in the lower back or suprapubic area, or referred to the flank and thighs. Throughout the first stage (**1** and **2**), and in the third stage (**4**), pain is *visceral* in origin. **AN, RE/KN, 3, HPM, Health promotion and maintenance**

10. **(2)** Ideally, there is less effect on the labor of the woman who is a nullipara if systemic medication is given when she is in active labor, about 5–6 cm. It is *too early* to give systemic medication to a woman who is a nullipara at cervical dilatation of 3–4 cm (**1**). It is *unnecessary to wait* until dilatation is 8 cm (**3**) before administering pain medication to the woman who is a nullipara, and 10 cm dilatation (**4**) is *too late* to give systemic medication to a woman who is a nullipara. **EV, RE/KN, 5, PhI, Pharmacological and parenteral therapies**

11. **(4)** When the suboccipitobregmatic diameter is presenting, the posterior triangular-shaped fontanel is presenting; the fetus is in an attitude of general flexion and is presenting the smallest head diameter for birth. With excessive molding (**1**), it may be difficult to feel the fontanel. (Excessive molding refers to the overlapping of cranial bones or shaping of the fetal head to accommodate and conform to the bony and soft parts of the mother's birth canal during labor.) If the fetus was presenting with the biparietal diameter (**2**), the nurse would have felt the sagittal suture. If the fetus was presenting with the largest diameter of the fetal head, the occipitomental diameter (**3**), the nurse would have felt the fetal brow or the anterior, diamond-shaped fontanel. **AN, APP, 5, HPM, Health promotion and maintenance**

---

**Key to Codes**

Nursing process: **AS**, assessment; **AN**, analysis; **PL**, planning; **IMP**, implementation; **EV**, evaluation. (See **Appendix J** for explanation of nursing process steps.)

Cognitive level: **RE/KN**, recall/knowledge; **COM**, comprehension; **APP**, application; **ANL**, analysis; **EVL**, evaluation; **SYN**, synthesis. (See **Appendix J** for explanation.)

Category of human function: 1, protective; 2, sensory-perceptual; 3, comfort, rest, activity, and mobility; 4, nutrition; 5, growth and development; 6, fluid-gas transport; 7, psychosocial-cultural; 8, elimination. (See **Appendix L** for explanation.)

Client need: **SECE**, safe, effective care environment; **HPM**, health promotion and maintenance; **PsI**, psychosocial integrity; **PhI**, physiological integrity. (See **Appendix M** for explanation.)

Client subneed: See **Appendix M** for explanation.

12. **(3)** Since these are the symptoms of hyperventilation, the nurse should ask her to breathe into a paper bag. These symptoms are not those of imminent birth (**1**). For hyperventilation, the first action is to ask her to breathe into a paper bag, *not* to change the position (**2**). She needs to rebreathe her carbon dioxide and does *not need oxygen* (**4**) at this time. **IMP, ANL, 6, PhI, Reduction of risk potential**

13. **(2)** Water intoxication is a complication associated with oxytocin induction/augmentation of labor. Neither PIH (**1**) nor urinary retention (**4**) is associated with induction. Amniotic fluid embolism (**3**) is associated with rupture of membranes, *not* with oxytocin induction. **EV, RE/KN, 6, PhI, Pharmacological and parenteral therapies**

14. **(2)** A 30 min whirlpool bath is expected to increase this woman's cervical dilatation an additional 2–3 cm. Relief from discomfort and general body relaxation reduce the woman's anxiety, which decreases adrenaline production. An increase in oxytocin and endorphins occurs. Labor is facilitated, *not* slowed (**1**), unless she is in the latent phase of the first stage. The woman's labor is monitored continuously; if birth is imminent (**3**), she is removed from the bath. The whirlpool bath has a *positive* effect on the labor pattern and cervical dilatation (**4**). **IMP, COM, 3, HPM, Health promotion and maintenance**

15. **(1)** The woman will probably be taken to the birth room when the vertex is seen at the introitus with contractions; at this point, there is usually still time to move a woman who is a nullipara. Options **2**, **3**, and **4** are incorrect since birth may still be *hours* away. **IMP, RE/KN, 5, HPM, Health promotion and maintenance**

16. **(4)** She turns inward into herself. Only conversation directed at her should be initiated now; she perceives all she hears as pertaining to her. She does become more dependent (**1**), but she is an *adult* and should be treated as such. No woman is "demanding" in labor (**2**)—there is only the woman whose needs have not been met. She may become more irritable (**3**), but should *never be left alone*. To leave her alone would be abandonment (legally speaking). **PL, RE/KN, 5, PsI, Psychosocial integrity**

17. **(3)** During the early first stage of labor (2 cm dilatation), in most cases, the FHR is assessed every 30 min, if labor is progressing to the active phase and when membranes rupture. Blood pressure (**1**) is assessed every hour. Vaginal examination (**2**) is performed as *necessary* to identify progress of labor. Temperature (**4**) is usually assessed every 4 hr; it may be assessed every 2 hr if membranes are ruptured. **IMP, RE/KN, 5, HPM, Health promotion and maintenance**

18. **(4)** The woman needs to know that someone is in control and requires firm, direct coaching with demonstration of breathing techniques. Leaving the room (**1**) is abandonment, and can be seen by the woman as punishment for her "inappropriate" behavior. Suggesting pain medication (**2**) may be interpreted by the woman that the coach has no confidence in her; it also does not acknowledge the woman's perception of discomfort. Saying that "it will soon be over" (**3**) may be false reassurance; it is always difficult to predict the time of birth ("soon" can be interpreted as 5 min!). This response also fails to acknowledge the woman's perception of discomfort. **IMP, ANL, 7, PsI, Psychosocial integrity**

19. **(1)** The litmus (pH) paper turns dark blue when exposed to an alkaline fluid such as amniotic fluid. The paper does *not* turn yellow (**2**), olive (**3**), or white (**4**) in the presence of amniotic fluid. **EV, RE/KN, 5, HPM, Health promotion and maintenance**

20. **(3)** The side-lying position relieves supine hypotension by reducing compression of the vena cava and aorta. The woman may faint if she rises quickly (**1 and 4**). Oxygen (**2**) is not needed, and would be of little value as long as the major vessels remain compressed. **IMP, COM, 3, PhI, Reduction of risk potential**

21. **(3)** A side effect of epidural anesthesia is maternal hypotension, and therefore the nurse should check the BP *immediately* after administration of the drug. FHR deceleration (**1**) would be *caused* by a drop in maternal BP, putting the fetus at risk for hypoxia; therefore, the maternal BP is the *priority*. The maternal heart rate (**2**) is *not* affected. Although contraction strength and frequency (**4**) *may* decrease, the effect of maternal BP on *fetal oxygenation* is the *main concern*. **AS, ANL, 6, PhI, Pharmacological and parenteral therapies**

22. **(2)** The reason for the previous cesarean in this case was breech presentation, which is not present now. The women described in the other options would not be good candidates for VBAC. In option **1**, the vertical incision through the uterus, and subsequent scar, is considered to weaken the uterus and compromise its ability to withstand stretching and contracting. In option **3**, original cause for the previous cesarean (fetopelvic disproportion) may remain. In option **4**, the infant may acquire herpes during passage through an infected birth canal. **PL, RE/KN, 5, HPM, Health promotion and maintenance**

23. **(4)** The situation describes an *early deceleration*, one that "mirrors" the contraction by falling as the contraction increases and returning to the baseline as the contraction decreases. Early decelerations are caused by the baby's vagal response to fetal head compression. These decelerations are thought to be *benign* with good fetal outcome and show little or

no response to interventions geared to increase fetal oxygen. The nurse should simply document these baseline changes and continue to observe the fetal heart pattern. The measures in options **1**, **2**, and **3** are taken in times of *fetal distress* and are therefore *inappropriate* and *ineffective* in this case. **AN, SYN, 5, HPM, Health promotion and maintenance**

24. **(4)** The FHR is best heard through the fetus' back; with vertex presentation and with the fetal occiput to the mother's right, the fetal back is also on the mother's right side and in the lower quadrant. The fetus would have to be left sacrum anterior (LSA) for the FHR to be in the mother's LUQ **(1)**. The fetus would have to be right sacrum anterior (RSA) for the FHR to be in the mother's RUQ **(2)**. The fetus would have to be left occiput anterior (LOA) for the FHR to be in the mother's LLQ **(3)**. **AS, COM, 5, HPM, Health promotion and maintenance**

25. **(2)** Minimizing the amount of edema at this time (*immediately* after birth) will reduce discomfort later. Freezing **(1)** *destroys* tissues. The purpose of applying cold is *not to distract* **(3)**; distraction does little to decrease discomfort. Ice packs (covered) *decrease, not* increase **(4)**, circulation to the area. **PL, APP, 1, SECE, PhI, Reduction of risk potential**

26. **(4)** During the first hour, every 15 min x 4, the nurse assesses: BP, heart rate, respiration, lochia, fundal tone and position, *bladder filling*, perineum, recovery from medications, and reaction to birth experience; temperature is assessed at 1 hr. If complications occur, the frequency and number of assessments are adjusted, prn. The fundus **(1)** and BP **(2)** are checked every *15 min* x 4; then every 30 min x 2; then per hospital protocol if the assessments reveal no complications. The temperature **(3)** is checked *once* at the end of the first hour and then per hospital protocol if the values remain within normal limits. **AS, ANL, 5, HPM, Health promotion and maintenance**

27. **(2)** This assessment is the only one that could diagnose prolapse of the umbilical cord that may not be visible in the vagina or at the vaginal orifice or palpable with vaginal examination. If the cord is prolapsed out of the vagina, keep it warm and moist with continuous applications of warm, sterile saline compresses. Option **1** is incorrect because the fluid needs to be assessed, but that is done *following* assessment of the FHR. Option **3** is incorrect because the FHR is the *only* way to diagnose whether the fetus is being well oxygenated; a prolapsed cord may not be visible. Option **4** is incorrect because this may be indicated, but is not the *priority* action. **AN, ANL, 5, PhI, Reduction of risk potential**

28. **(2)** With false labor, the intensity of contractions lessens with walking. The other options all describe the contractions of *true* labor: intervals are regular **(1)** and shorten gradually **(3)**, and duration increases **(4)**. **AN, APP, 5, HPM, Health promotion and maintenance**

29. **(4)** The nurse needs to intervene immediately when a coach is heard to say, "Push with your mouth closed and no noise!" because this pushing method encourages the Valsalva maneuver with cardiovascular risks and other sequelae. Encouraging relaxation between contractions **(1)** and semi-Fowler's (or side-lying) position **(2)** *is appropriate* at this time. Short bursts of pushing when the woman feels the urge to push **(3)** are effective for the *second* stage of labor. **EV, SYN, 5, HPM, Health promotion and maintenance**

30. **(2)** The fetal monitor readings are consistent with early (head compression) deceleration; continue to monitor per standard. Options **1**, **3**, and **4** are incorrect because this is *not an ominous pattern.* **EV, SYN, 5, PhI, Reduction of risk potential**

31. **(4)** With the breech in the fundus, the fetus must be vertex; nodulations (elbows, hands, knees, feet) on the mother's left mean that the fetal back must be in the mother's right flank. LSP **(1)** means that the fetus is breech (the head is in the fundus) and the nodulations would be felt over the entire maternal abdomen since the fetal back would be to the mother's back. RSA **(2)** means that the fetus is breech and the nodulations would not be easily felt; the fetal back would be in the anterior of the mother's abdomen. LOP **(3)** means that the vertex is presenting but the nodulations would be easily felt all over the maternal abdomen; the fetal back would be to the maternal back. **EV, APP, 5, HPM, Health promotion and maintenance**

# Complications During the Intrapartal Period

## Chapter Outline

## 🔑 Key Points

- Dystocia results from differences in the normal relationships among the *six* essential factors of labor.
- Uterine contractility is *increased* by oxytocin and prostaglandin, and *decreased* by tocolytic agents.
- *Medical emergencies* can occur *secondary to dystocia*: disseminated intravascular coagulopathy (DIC), adult respiratory distress syndrome (ARDS), thrombophlebitis, cardiac decompensation.
- *Management* of preterm labor includes: prenatal education of signs and symptoms, home monitoring and therapy, tocolysis, and, in the event that tocolysis is not possible, stimulation of fetal lung maturity.

## Key Words

Adult respiratory distress syndrome (ARDS)

Amniotic fluid (pulmonary) embolus

Dystocia

Macrosomia

Prolapsed umbilical cord

Tocolysis

Uterine rupture

## General Aspects

I. **Pathophysiology**: interference with normal processes and patterns of labor/birth result in maternal and/or fetal jeopardy (e.g., *preterm labor*, *dysfunctional* labor patterns; *prolonged* [> 24 hr] labor; *hemorrhage: uterine rupture/inversion, amniotic fluid embolus*).

II. **Etiology/risk factors:**

A. *Preterm labor*—unknown.

B. *Dysfunctional labor* (**dystocia**: see **p. 131–132**)

1. Physiologic response to anxiety/fear/pain →results in release of catecholamines, increasing physical/psychological stress → myometrial dysfunction; painful and ineffectual labor.

2. *Iatrogenic factors*: premature or excessive analgesia, particularly during latent phase.

3. *Maternal factors*:
    a. Pelvic contractures.
    b. Uterine tumors (e.g., myomas, carcinoma).
    c. Congenital uterine anomalies (e.g., bicornate uterus).
    d. Pathologic contraction ring (*Bandl's* ring).
    e. Rigid cervix, cervical stenosis/stricture.
    f. Hypertonic/hypotonic contractions.
    g. Prolonged rupture of membranes. **NOTE**: *Intrauterine infection* may have caused rupture of membranes, or may follow rupture.
    h. Prolonged first or second stage.
    i. Medical conditions: diabetes, hypertension.

4. *Fetal factors*:
    a. Macrosomia (large for gestational age).
    b. Malposition/malpresentation.
    c. Congenital anomaly (e.g., hydrocephalus, anencephaly).

 d. Multi-fetal gestation (e.g., interlocking twins).
 e. Prolapsed cord.
 f. Postterm.
 5. *Placental factors*:
 a. Placenta previa.
 b. Inadequate placental function with contractions.
 c. Abruptio placentae.
 d. Placenta accreta.
 6. Physical restrictions: when confined to bed, *flat position*, etc.

**III. Assessment**
 A. Prenatal history, physical examination, laboratory and other *diagnostic test* results (e.g., ultrasound, nonstress test [NST]).
 B. Emotional status.
 ☞ C. Vital signs, fetal heart rate (FHR).
 D. Labor assessment:
 1. *Preadmission events*: contractions, membranes, etc.
 2. *Physical examination*: lung status, edema, rashes, respiratory conditions, etc.
 ☞ 3. *Contraction pattern*: frequency, duration, intensity.
 ☞ 4. *Leopold's* maneuvers (abdominal palpation): presentation, position (identification of presenting part, the fetal lie, and attitude), degree of descent into the pelvis, and location of point of maximal impulse (PMI) of FHR in relation to maternal abdomen.
 ☞ 5. *Vaginal examination*: presentation, position, station; cervical effacement, dilatation; status of membranes; fullness of rectum.
 E. Collection of specimens: urine, blood; assessment of amniotic fluid from vaginal vault (color, character, amount).
 F. Assessment for **risk factors** in labor—warning signs:
 1. *Contractions*: intrauterine pressure 75 mm Hg, or greater (by intrauterine pressure catheter [IUPC]), lasting 90 sec or longer, occurring at intervals of less than 2 min.
 2. *FHR*: bradycardia, tachycardia, or persistent decreased variability; irregular; absence of.
 3. *Vaginal discharge*: meconium stained or bloody; foul smelling; persistent bright or dark red.
 4. *Prolapsed umbilical cord*.
 5. Arrest in progress of *cervical dilatation/ effacement* and/or descent of the fetus (see **Length of Labor, Chapter 4, p. 120**).
 6. *Maternal temperature*: 100.4° F (38° C) or greater.

**IV. Analysis/nursing diagnosis**
 A. *Anxiety/fear* for self and infant related to implications of prolonged or complicated labor/ birth.

 B. *Pain* related to hypertonic contractions/ dysfunctional labor.
 C. *Individual coping impairment* related to physical/ psychological stress of complicated labor/birth, lowered pain threshold secondary to fatigue.
 D. *Injury risk* related to prolonged rupture of membranes, infection.
 E. *Fluid volume deficit* related to excessive blood loss secondary to placenta previa, abruptio placentae, Couvelaire uterus, disseminated intravascular coagulopathy (DIC).

**V. Nursing care plan/implementation**
 A. Goal: *minimize physical/psychological stress during labor/birth*. Assist woman to cope effectively.
 1. Reinforce relaxation techniques.
 2. Support couple's effective coping techniques/mechanisms.
 3. Meet woman's comfort needs.
 B. Goal: *emotional support*.
 1. Encourage verbalization of anxiety/fear/ concerns.
 2. Explain all procedures—to minimize anxiety/fear, encourage cooperation/ participation in care.
 3. Provide quiet environment conducive to rest.
 ☞ C. Goal: *continuous monitoring of maternal-fetal status and progress through labor*—to identify early signs of dysfunctional labor, fetal distress; facilitate prompt, effective treatment of emerging complications.
 D. Goal: *minimize effects of complicated labor on mother, fetus*.
 1. *Position* change: *lateral Sims'*—to reduce compression of inferior vena cava and descending aorta.
 ☞ 2. Oxygen per mask, as indicated.
 3. Institute interventions appropriate to emerging problems (see specific disorder).

**VI. Evaluation/outcome criteria**
 A. Woman has successful birth of viable infant.
 B. Maternal/infant status stable, satisfactory.

# Disorders Affecting Protective Functions: *Preterm Labor*

**Definition**: preterm labor occurs after 20 wk gestation and before beginning of week 38.

 I. **Pathophysiology**: physiologic events of labor (i.e., contractions, spontaneous rupture of membranes, cervical effacement/dilatation) occur before completion of normal, term gestation.

 II. **Etiology**: unknown. *Theory*: may be due to fetal factors released when placental function begins to diminish and intrauterine environment is hostile to continuing fetal well-being.

## III. Coexisting disorders:

A. Infections that may cause premature rupture of membranes (PROM).

B. PROM of unknown etiology.

C. Hypertension (pre-eclampsia/eclampsia).

D. Uterine overdistention:
1. Polyhydramnios.
2. Large baby.
3. Multi-fetal gestation.

E. Maternal diabetes, renal or cardiovascular disorder.

F. Severe maternal illness (e.g., pneumonia, acute pyelonephritis, urinary tract infection [UTI]).

G. Abnormal placentation:
1. Placenta previa.
2. Abruptio placentae.

H. Fetal death.

I. Incompetent cervical os (small percentage).

J. Uterine anomalies (rare):
1. Intrauterine septum.
2. Bicornate uterus.

K. Uterine fibroids.

## IV. Prevention:

A. *Primary*—close obstetric supervision; education in warning signs/symptoms of preterm labor:
1. Dull lower backache that radiates like a wave to the front of the abdomen (characteristic of a true labor contraction).
2. Contractions every 10 min for 2 hr even after position changes and drinking some glasses of water; low back pain and light bloody discharge ("*bloody show*").
3. Constant menstrual-like cramping low in the abdomen.
4. Pelvic pressure extending to the back and thighs.

B. *Secondary*—prompt, effective treatment of associated disorders (see **III** above).

C. *Tertiary*—suppression of preterm labor.
1. Bedrest.
2. *Position*: side lying—to promote placental perfusion.
3. Hydration.
4. Pharmacologic (may require "informed consent"; follow hospital protocol). *Beta-adrenergic* agents to reduce sensitivity of uterine myometrium to oxytocic and prostaglandin stimulation; increase blood flow to uterus.
5. May be maintained at home with adequate follow-up and health teaching.

## V. Contraindications for suppression—labor is *not* suppressed in presence of:

A. Placenta previa or abruptio placentae.

B. Chorioamnionitis.

C. Erythroblastosis fetalis.

D. Severe pre-eclampsia.

E. Severe diabetes (e.g., "brittle").

F. Increasing placental insufficiency.

G. Ruptured membranes (depends on cause and if sepsis).

## VI. Assessment

A. Maternal vital signs. Response to medication:
1. Hypotension.
2. Tachycardia, arrhythmia.
3. Dyspnea, chest pain.
4. Nausea and vomiting.

B. Signs of infection:
1. Increased temperature.
2. Tachycardia.
3. Diaphoresis.
4. Malaise.
5. Increased baseline fetal heart rate.

C. Contractions: frequency, duration, strength.

D. Emotional status—signs of denial, guilt, anxiety, exhaustion.

E. Signs of continuing and progressing labor. NOTE: vaginal examination *only* if indicated by other signs of continuing labor progress.
1. Effacement.
2. Dilatation.
3. Station.

F. Status of membranes.

G. Fetal heart rate, activity (continuous monitoring).

H. Fetal fibronectin—swab of vagina/cervix to determine if woman is at higher risk for preterm labor.

## VII. Analysis/nursing diagnosis

A. *Anxiety/fear* related to possible outcome.

B. *Self-esteem disturbance* related to feelings of guilt, failure.

C. *Physical mobility impairment* related to imposed bedrest.

D. *Knowledge deficit* related to medication side effects.

E. *Individual coping impairment* related to possible outcome.

F. *Gas exchange impairment* related to side effects of medication (circulatory overload; pulmonary edema).

G. *Diversional activity deficit* related to imposed bedrest, decreased environmental stimuli.

H. *Urinary elimination alteration* related to bedrest.

I. *Constipation* related to bedrest.

## VIII. Nursing care plan/implementation

A. Goal: *tocolysis* (inhibition) of uterine activity.
1. Administer tocolytic medications as ordered—*ritodrine (Yutopar)*, *terbutaline*, or *magnesium sulfat*e. (Recent evidence suggests magnesium sulfate may be ineffective in suppressing preterm labor).

B. Goal: *safeguard status*.
1. Continuous maternal-fetal monitoring.

2. Maternal *position*: *side lying* to increase placental perfusion, and prevent supine hypotension.

3. I&O—to identify early signs of possible circulatory overload.

4. Report **warning signs/symptoms** of tocolysis promptly to physician:
   a. Maternal pulse of 110 or more.
   b. Diastolic pressure of 60 mm Hg or less.
   c. Respirations of 25 or more; crackles (rales).
   d. Complaint of shortness of breath and chest tightness.*
   e. Contractions: increasing frequency, strength, or duration or cessation of contractions.
   f. Intermittent back and thigh pain.
   g. Rupture of membranes.
   h. Vaginal bleeding.
   i. Fetal distress, e.g., tachycardia, 180 beats/min or more.
   j. Laboratory results: hyperglycemia, hyperkalemia.

5. Give **antidote**, per order: *propranolol*, 1 mg, for beta-mimetic drugs toxicity, (e.g., *ritodrine, terbutaline*); or *calcium gluconate* or *calcium chloride*, 1 g for IV injection given over 3 min period for magnesium sulfate toxicity.

6. Goal: **health teaching**. Home care: preterm labor.
   a. Teaching about medications: dosage ordered, etc.
   b. Teaching about signs/symptoms of toxicity to report **STAT**: severe dizziness, drowsiness, headache, nervousness, restlessness; severe muscle cramps and weakness; continuous nausea and vomiting; dyspnea; pulmonary edema, respirations of 25/min or more; continuous palpitations, chest pain.
   c. Teaching about *side-lying position* for resting.
   d. Teach/practice stress reduction/relaxation techniques.
   e. Make appropriate referrals, if assistance is needed in the home (e.g., child care).

C. Goal: *comfort measures*.
   1. Basic hygienic care—bath, mouth care, cold washcloth to face, perineal care.
   2. Backrub, linen change—to promote relaxation.

D. Goal: *emotional support*.
   1. Encourage verbalization of guilt feelings, anxiety, fear, concerns; provide factual information.
   2. Support positive self-concept.
   3. Keep informed of progress.

E. Goal: *provide quiet diversion* (e.g. television, reading materials, handcrafts).

F. Goal: **health teaching.**
   1. Explain, discuss proposed management to suppress preterm labor.
   2. Describe, discuss side effects of medication.
   3. Explain rationale for bedrest, position.

## If Labor Continues to Progress

I. Goal: *facilitate infant survival.*
   A. Administer *betamethasone*, as ordered, 48 hr before birth—to increase/stimulate production of pulmonary surfactant.
   B. Notify perinatal team—to increase chances for fetal survival, ensure prompt, expert management of neonate and provide information and support to parents.
   C. Monitor progress of labor to identify signs of impending birth. NOTE: May give birth before complete (10 cm) dilatation.
   D. Consider transfer to high-risk facility.
   E. Prepare for birth.

II. Goal: *emotional support.*
   A. Do *not* leave woman (or couple) alone.
   B. Encourage verbalization of anxiety, fear, concern.
   C. Explain all procedures.

III. Goal: *comfort measures.* NOTE: Analgesics may be **contraindicated**—to prevent depression of fetus/neonate.

IV. Goal: *support effective coping techniques.*
   A. Encourage/support childbirth techniques—coach, as necessary; discourage hyperventilation.

V. Goal: **health teaching** for *preterm birth.*
   A. Discuss need for episiotomy, possibility of outlet forceps-assisted birth—to reduce stress on fetal head, *or*
   B. Prepare for cesarean birth—to reduce possibility of fetal intraventricular hemorrhage (very premature infant).
   C. Rationale for avoiding use of medications to reduce contraction pain.

## Immediate Care of Neonate

I. Goal: *safeguard status.*
   A. Stabilize environmental temperature—to prevent chilling (isolette or other controlled-temperature bed).
   B. Suction, oxygen, as needed; may need intubation.
   C. Parenteral fluids, as ordered—to support normal acid-base balance, pH; administer *antibiotics*, as necessary.
   D. Arrange transport to high-risk facility, as necessary.

*Alert: If a steroid, such as *betamethasone* (*Celestone, Solup*), is used (to stimulate fetal lung maturity) in conjunction with beta-mimetic drugs (e.g., *ritodrine, terbutaline*), **risk for cardiac decompensation is greatly increased.** (Maternal HR: ≥ 140 beats/min; continuous palpitations, chest pain.)

II. Goal: *continuous monitoring of status*
☞ A. Electronic monitors—to observe respiratory and cardiac functions.
〰 B. Blood samples—to monitor blood gases, pH, hypoglycemia.

## Postpartum Care

I. Goal: *emotional support.*
A. Facilitate attachment.
B. If couple, foster sense of mutual experience and closeness.
C. Help her/them maintain a positive self-image.
D. Encourage touching of infant before transport to nursery or high-risk facility; father/partner may accompany infant and report back to mother.
E. Encourage early contact—to facilitate mother's need to ventilate her feelings.
F. Assist parent(s) with grieving process if necessary.
G. Refer to support group if necessary.

⋈ II. **Evaluation/outcome criteria:** The woman:
A. Verbalizes understanding of medical/nursing recommendations and treatments.
B. Complies with medical/nursing regimen.
C. Experiences no discomfort from side effects of therapy.
D. Experiences successful outcome—labor inhibited.
E. Carries pregnancy to successful termination.
F. If preterm birth occurs, copes effectively with outcome (physiologically compromised neonate, neonatal demise).

# Grief and Childbearing Experience

The loss of a pregnancy or a newborn, or the birth of a physiologically compromised child (premature, congenital disorder), is a crisis situation. The unexpected outcome can cause the parent(s) to suffer a sense of loss of self-esteem, self-concept, positive body image, feelings of worth (see **Table 3.6, p. 73**).

⋈ I. **Assessment**
A. Response to loss of the "fantasy child"/real child:
1. *Behavioral*—anger, hostility, depression, disinterest in activities of daily living, withdrawal.
2. *Biophysical*—somatic complaints (stomach pain, malaise, anorexia, nausea).
3. *Cognitive*—feelings of guilt.
B. Knowledge/understanding/perception of situation.
C. Coping abilities, mechanisms.
D. Support system.

⋈ II. **Analysis/nursing diagnosis**
A. *Family coping impairment* related to psychological stress associated with fear for infant, guilt feelings, impact on self-image.

B. *Individual coping impairment* related to anxiety, stress.
C. *Family coping impairment* related to disturbance in intrafamily relations secondary to individual coping deficits, recriminations.
D. *Parenting alteration* related to lack of effective bonding secondary to emotional separation from infant, feelings of guilt.
E. *Dysfunctional grieving* related to guilt feelings, impact of loss on self-concept.
F. *Body image disturbance, self-esteem, role performance alteration* related to perceived failure to complete gestational task and produce perfect, healthy infant; associated with sleep deprivation.
G. *Social isolation* related to severe coping deficit, dysfunctional grieving, disturbance in self-esteem.

⋈ III. **Nursing care plan/implementation**
A. Goal: *emotional support.*
1. Provide privacy; encourage open expression/verbalization of feelings, fears, concerns, perceptions.
2. Crisis intervention techniques.
B. Goal: *facilitate bonding, effective coping, and/or anticipatory grieving processes.*
1. Encourage contact and participation in care of infant who is premature or compromised.
2. Keep informed of infant's status.
3. Provide realistic data.
🏠 C. Goal: **health teaching.**
1. Clarify misperceptions, as appropriate.
☞ 2. Discuss, demonstrate infant care techniques (e.g., feeding infant who has cleft lip and/or palate).
3. Refer to appropriate community resources.

⋈ IV. **Evaluation/outcome criteria:** The parent:
A. Verbalizes recognition and acceptance of diagnosis.
B. Verbalizes understanding of relevant information regarding treatment, prognosis.
C. Makes informed decision regarding infant care.
D. Demonstrates comfort and increasing participation in care of neonate.
E. Shows evidence of bonding (eye contact, cuddles, calls infant by name).

# Disorders Affecting Comfort, Rest, Mobility: *Dystocia*

I. **Definition:** difficult labor, birth.
💡 II. **Etiology: the six "P's"**
A. **Position** (*maternal*).
B. **Psychological** response (*maternal*).
C. **Placenta**—*previa, abruptio* (see **Chapter 3, p. 78-79, 81, 84**).

D. **Power**: forces of labor (uterine contractions, use of abdominal muscles):
  1. Premature analgesia/anesthesia.
  2. Uterine overdistention (multifetal pregnancy, fetal macrosomia).
  3. Uterine myomas.
E. **Passageway**: resistance of cervix, pelvic structures:
  1. Rigid cervix.
  2. Distended bladder.
  3. Distended rectum.
  4. Dimensions of the bony pelvis: pelvic contractures.
F. **Passenger**: accommodation of the presenting part to pelvic diameters:
  1. Fetal malposition/malpresentation:
     a. Transverse lie.
     b. Face, brow presentation.
     c. Breech presentation.
     d. Cephalopelvic disproportion (CPD) or fetopelvic disproportion (FPD).
  2. Fetal anomalies.
     a. Hydrocephalus.
     b. Conjoined ("Siamese") twins.
     c. Myelomeningocele.
  3. Fetal size.

**III. Hazards**
A. *Maternal:*
  1. Fatigue, exhaustion, dehydration—due to prolonged labor.
  2. Lowered pain threshold, loss of control—due to prolonged labor, continued uterine contractions, anxiety, fatigue, lack of sleep.
  3. Intrauterine infection—due to prolonged rupture of membranes and frequent vaginal examinations.
  4. Uterine rupture—due to obstructed labor or hyperstimulation.
  5. Cervical, vaginal, perineal lacerations—due to obstetric interventions.
  6. Postpartum hemorrhage—due to uterine atony and/or trauma.
B. *Fetal:*
  1. Hypoxia, anoxia, demise—due to decreased oxygen concentration in cord blood.
  2. Intracranial hemorrhage—due to changing intracranial pressure.

## Hypertonic Dysfunction

I. **Pathophysiology**: increased resting tone of uterine myometrium; diminished refractory period; prolonged latent phase (see **Figure 5.1**).
  A. *Nullipara*—more than 20 hr.
  B. *Multipara*—more than 14 hr.
II. **Etiology**: unknown. *Theory*—ectopic initiation of incoordinate uterine contractions.

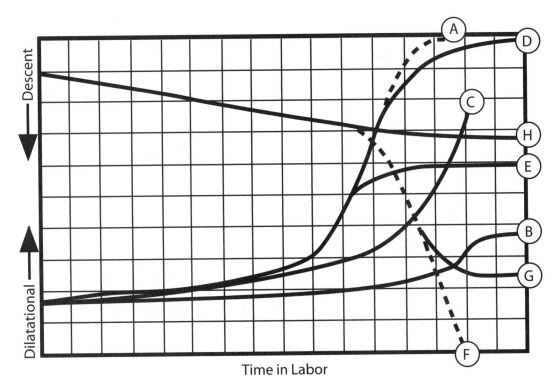

**FIGURE 5.1** Graph showing **types of abnormal labor**. (**A**) Normal labor curve. (**B**) Prolonged latent phase. (**C**) Protracted active-phase dilation. (**D**) Prolonged deceleration phase. (**E**) Secondary arrest of dilatation. (**F**) Normal descent. (**G**) Protracted descent. (**H**) Arrest of descent.

III. **Assessment**

A. Onset—early labor (latent phase).

B. Contractions:

1. Continuous fundal tension, incomplete relaxation.

2. Painful.

3. Ineffectual—no effacement or dilatation.

C. Signs of fetal distress:

1. Meconium-stained amniotic fluid.

2. Fetal heart rate irregularities.

D. Maternal vital signs.

E. Emotional status.

F. *Medical* evaluation *procedures*: vaginal examination, ultrasonography—to rule out CPD.

IV. **Analysis/nursing diagnosis**

A. *Pain* related to hypertonic contractions, incomplete uterine relaxation.

B. *Anxiety/fear* for self and infant related to strong, painful contractions without evidence of progress.

C. *Individual coping impairment* related to fatigue, exhaustion, anxiety, tension, fear.

D. *Gas exchange* (fetal) *impairment* related to incomplete relaxation of uterus.

E. *Sleep pattern disturbance* related to prolonged ineffectual labor.

V. **Nursing care plan/implementation**

A. *Medical management.*

1. Short-acting barbiturates (see **Table 4.3, p. 104**)—to encourage rest, relaxation.

2. Intravenous fluids—to restore/maintain hydration and fluid-electrolyte balance.

3. If CPD, cesarean birth.

B. *Nursing management.*

1. Goal: *emotional support*—assist coping with fear, pain, discouragement.

a. Encourage verbalization of anxiety, fear, concerns.

b. Explain all procedures.

c. Reassure. Keep couple informed of progress.

2. Goal: *comfort measures.*

a. *Position*: *Side lying*—to promote relaxation and placental perfusion.

b. Bath, backrub, linen change, clean environment.

c. Environment: quiet, darkened room—to minimize stimuli and encourage relaxation, warmth.

d. Encourage voiding—to relieve bladder distention; to test urine for ketones.

3. Goal: *prevent infection.* Strict aseptic technique.

4. Goal: *prepare for cesarean birth if necessary.*

VI. **Evaluation/outcome criteria:** The woman:

A. Relaxes, sleeps, establishes normal labor pattern.

B. Demonstrates no signs of fetal distress.

C. Successfully completes uneventful labor.

## *Hypotonic Dysfunction During Labor*

I. **Pathophysiology**: after normal labor at onset, contractions diminish in frequency, duration, and strength; lowered uterine resting tone; cervical effacement and dilatation slows/ceases.

II. **Etiology/risk factors:**

A. Premature or excessive analgesia/anesthesia (*caudal* or *epidural* block).

B. CPD.

C. Overdistention (polyhydramnios, fetal macrosomia, multifetal pregnancy).

D. Fetal malposition/malpresentation.

E. Maternal fear/anxiety.

III. **Assessment**

A. Onset—may occur in latent phase; most common during active phase.

B. Contractions—normal previously, now demonstrate:

1. Decreased frequency.

2. Shorter duration.

3. Diminished intensity (mild to moderate).

4. Less uncomfortable.

C. Cervical changes—slow or cease.

D. Signs of fetal distress—rare.

1. Usually occur late in labor due to infection secondary to prolonged rupture of membranes.

2. Tachycardia.

E. Maternal vital signs may indicate infection (↑ temperature).

F. *Medical* diagnosis—*procedures*: vaginal examination, ultrasonography—to rule out CPD (most common cause).

IV. **Analysis/nursing diagnosis**

A. *Knowledge deficit* related to limited exposure to information.

B. *Anxiety/fear* related to failure to progress as anticipated; fear for fetus.

C. *Injury risk* (infection) related to prolonged labor and/or ruptured membranes.

V. **Nursing care plan/implementation**

A. *Medical management.*

1. Amniotomy—artificial rupture of membranes.

2. Oxytocin augmentation of labor—intravenous infusion of *oxytocin* to increase frequency, duration, strength, and efficiency of uterine contractions (see **Induction of labor, p. 115–117**).

3. If CPD, cesarean birth.

B. *Nursing management.*

1. Goals: *emotional support, comfort measures, prevent infection*—as for **Hypertonic dysfunction** (see V. B. p. 133).

2. Other—see **Induction of labor, p. 117.**

VI. **Evaluation/outcome criteria:** The woman:

A. Reestablishes normal labor pattern.

B. Experiences successful birth of viable infant.

# Disorders Affecting Fluid-Gas Transport: *Maternal*

## Uterine Rupture

I. **Pathophysiology**: stress on uterine muscle exceeds its ability to stretch.

II. **Etiology/risk factors:**
   A. Overdistention—due to large baby, multifetal gestation, polyhramnios.
   B. Old scars—due to previous cesarean births or uterine surgery.
   C. Contractions against CPD, fetal malpresentation, pathologic retraction ring (*Bandl's*).
   D. Injudicious obstetrics—malapplication of forceps (or application without full effacement/dilatation).
   E. Tetanic contraction—due to hypersensitivity to oxytocin (or excessive dosage) during induction/augmentation of labor.

III. **Assessment**
   A. Identify predisposing factors early.
   B. *Complete uterine rupture:*
      1. Pain: sudden, sharp, abdominal; followed by cessation of contractions; tender abdomen.
      2. Signs of shock; vaginal bleeding.
      3. Fetal heart tones–absent.
      4. Presenting part—not palpable on vaginal examination.
   C. *Incomplete rupture:*
      1. Contractions: continue, accompanied by abdominal pain and failure to dilate.
      2. Signs of shock.
      3. May demonstrate vaginal bleeding.
      4. Fetal heart tones—absent.

IV. **Prognosis**
   A. Maternal—guarded.
   B. Fetal—grave.

V. **Analysis/nursing diagnosis**
   A. *Pain* related to rupture of uterine muscle.
   B. *Fluid volume deficit* related to massive blood loss secondary to uterine rupture.
   C. *Anxiety/fear* related to concern for self, fetus.
   D. *Tissue perfusion alteration* related to blood loss secondary to uterine rupture.
   E. *Urinary elimination alteration* related to necessary conservation of intravascular fluid secondary to blood loss.
   F. *Anticipatory grieving* related to expected loss of fetus; inability to have more children.

VI. **Nursing care plan/implementation**
   A. *Medical management.*
      1. Surgical—laparotomy, hysterectomy.
      2. Replace blood loss—transfusion, packed cells.
      3. Reduce possibility of infection with antibiotics.
   B. *Nursing management.*
      1. Goal: *safeguard status.*
         a. Report *immediately*; mobilize staff.
         b. Prepare for immediate laparotomy.
         c. Oxygen per mask—to increase circulating oxygen level.
         d. Order **STAT** type and cross-match for blood—to replace blood loss.
         e. Establish intravenous line—to infuse fluids, blood, medications.
         f. Insert indwelling catheter—to deflate bladder.
         g. Abdominal prep—to remove hair, bacteria.
         h. Surgical permit (informed consent) for hysterectomy.
      2. Goal: *emotional support.* Allay anxiety (woman and family).
         a. Encourage verbalization of fears, anxiety, concerns.
         b. Explain all procedures.
         c. Keep family informed of progress.

VII. **Evaluation/outcome criteria**
   A. Woman experiences successful termination of emergency; minimal blood loss.
   B. Woman's postoperative status is stable.

## Amniotic Fluid (Pulmonary) Embolus

I. **Pathophysiology**: *acute cor pulmonale*—due to embolus blocking vessels in pulmonary circulation; *massive hemorrhage*—due to DIC resulting from entrance of thromboplastinlike material into bloodstream.

II. **Etiology**: amniotic fluid (with any meconium, lanugo, or vernix) enters maternal circulation through open venous sinuses at placental site; travels to pulmonary arterioles.
   A. Rare.
   B. Associated with: tumultuous labor, abruptio placentae, rupture of membranes.

III. **Prognosis—carries a high rate of maternal mortality.**

IV. **Assessment**
   A. May occur during labor, at time of rupture of membranes, or immediately postpartum.
   B. Sudden dyspnea, tachypnea, and cyanosis; apprehension.
   C. Chest pain; pleuritic pain.
   D. Hypotension, tachycardia.
   E. Frothy sputum.
   F. Signs of DIC:
      1. Purpura—local hemorrhage.
      2. Increased vaginal bleeding—massive.
      3. Rapid onset of shock.

✳ G. Signs of **adult respiratory distress syndrome (ARDS):**
1. Pale color; diaphoresis; dyspnea; cyanosis, nonresponsive to nasal oxygen or intermittent positive pressure breathing.
2. Apprehension; disorientation
3. Distended neck veins.
4. Pulse rate increased.
5. History of dystocia: labor with failure to progress, difficult forceps-assisted birth, amniotic fluid (pulmonary) embolus.

⋈ V. **Analysis/nursing diagnosis**
A. *Gas exchange impairment* related to pulmonary edema.
B. *Fluid volume deficit* related to DIC.
C. *Anxiety/fear for self and fetus* related to severity of symptoms, perception of jeopardy.

⋈ VI. **Nursing care plan/implementation**
A. *Medical management.*
◯ 1. IV *heparin*, whole *blood.*
2. Birth: immediate, by forceps, if possible.
◯ 3. *Digitalize*, as necessary.
B. **Nursing management.**
☞ 1. Goal: *assist ventilation.*
a. *Position*: *semi-Fowler's* for breathing comfort.
b. Oxygen under positive pressure and emergency equipment should be readily available.
c. Suction, prn.
2. Goal: *facilitate/expedite administration of fluids, medications, blood.*
☞ a. Establish intravenous line with large-bore needle.
◯ b. Administer *heparin*, fluids, as ordered.
☞ 3. Goal: *restore cardiopulmonary function, if needed.* Cardiopulmonary resuscitation techniques.
4. Goal: *emotional support* of woman, family.
a. Reassurance and coaching in relaxation techniques to lessen anxiety.
b. Explain all procedures.
c. Keep informed of status.

⋈ VII. **Evaluation/outcome criteria**
A. Dyspnea relieved.
B. Bleeding controlled.
C. Successful birth of viable infant.
D. Uneventful postpartum course.

# Disorders Affecting Fluid-Gas Transport: *Fetal*

## Fetus in Jeopardy—General Aspects

I. **Pathophysiology**: maternal hypoxemia, anemia, ketoacidosis, Rh isoimmunization, or decreased uteroplacental perfusion.

II. **Etiology/risk factors:** *maternal*:
A. Pre-eclampsia/eclampsia.
B. Heart disease.
C. Diabetes.
D. Rh or ABO incompatibility.
E. Insufficient uteroplacental/cord circulation due to:
1. Maternal hypotension/hypertension.
2. Cord compression:
a. Prolapsed.
b. Knotted.
c. Nuchal.
3. Hemorrhage; anemia.
4. Placental problem:
a. Malformation of the placenta/cord.
b. Premature "aging" of placenta.
c. Placental infarcts.
d. Abruptio placentae.
e. Placenta previa.
F. Postterm gestation.
G. Maternal infection.
H. Polyhydramnios.
I. Hypertonic uterine contractions.
1. PROM with chorioamnionitis.
2. Dystocia (e.g., from CPD).

⋈ III. **Assessment**—*intrapartal*
〰⊕ A. Amniotic fluid examination—at/or after rupture of membranes. *Signs of fetal distress*: meconium-stained, vertex presentation due to relaxation of fetal anal sphincter secondary to hypoxia/anoxia. NOTE: Fetus "gasps" in utero—may aspirate meconium and amniotic fluid.
⚡ B. Fetal activity:
1. Hyperactivity—due to hypoxemia, *elevated* carbon dioxide.
2. Cessation—possible fetal death.
〰 C. *Methods of monitoring* FHR:
1. Stethoscope or fetoscope.
2. Phonocardiography with microphone application.
3. Internal fetal electrode—attached directly to fetus through dilated cervix after membranes ruptured.
4. Doppler probe using ultrasound flow.
5. Cardiotocograph—transducer on maternal abdomen transmits sound.

☞ D. *Abnormal* FHR patterns (see **Figure 4.5, p. 103**):
1. Persistent irregularity.
2. Persistent tachycardia of 160 or more beats/min.
3. Persistent bradycardia of 100 or fewer beats/min.
4. *Early deceleration*—due to vagal response to head compression.
5. *Late deceleration*—due to uteroplacental insufficiency.
6. *Variable deceleration*—due to cord compression.
7. Decreased or loss of variability in FHR pattern.

◄► IV. **Analysis/nursing diagnosis**
A. *Gas exchange impairment (fetal)*, related to decreased placental perfusion/insufficient cord circulation.
B. *Tissue perfusion alteration* related to hemolytic anemia.
C. *Fetal injury risk* related to hypoxia.

## Prolapsed Umbilical Cord

(See **Figure 5.2**)

I. **Pathophysiology**: cord descent in advance of presenting part; compression interrupts blood flow, exchange of fetal-maternal gases → fetal hypoxia, anoxia, death (if unrelieved).

II. **Etiology/risk factors:**
A. Spontaneous or artificial rupture of membranes before presenting part is engaged.
B. Excessive force of escaping fluid, as in *polyhydramnios.*
C. *Malposition*—breech, compound presentation, transverse lie.
D. *Preterm* or small-for-gestational-age (SGA) fetus—allows space for cord descent.

◄► III. **Assessment**
A. Visualization of cord outside (or inside) vagina.
B. Palpation of pulsating mass on vaginal examination.
C. Fetal distress—variable deceleration and persistent bradycardia.

◄► IV. **Analysis/nursing diagnosis**
A. *Gas exchange impairment (fetal)*, related to interruption of blood flow from placenta/fetus.
B. *Anxiety/fear (maternal)*, related to knowledge of fetal jeopardy.

◄► V. **Nursing care plan/implementation**
A. Goal: *reduce pressure on cord.*
1. *Position: knee to chest; lateral* modified *Sims'* with hips *elevated;* modified *Trendelenburg.*
2. With gloved hand, support fetal presenting part off cord.
B. Goal: *increase maternal-fetal oxygenation;* give
☞ oxygen per mask (8–10 L/min).
C. Goal: *protect exposed cord;* cover cord with warm
☞ sterile wet saline dressing.

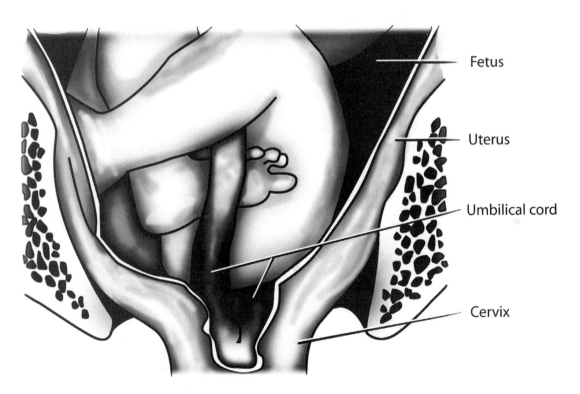

**FIGURE 5.2 PROLAPSED UMBILICAL CORD**

Fetus

Uterus

Umbilical cord

Cervix

D. Goal: *identify fetal response* to above measures, reduce threat to fetal survival: monitor FHR continuously.

E. Goal: *expedite termination of threat to fetus*; prepare for immediate vaginal/cesarean birth.

F. Goal: *support mother and significant other* by staying with them and explaining.

**VI. Evaluation/outcome criteria**

A. FHR returns to normal rate and pattern.

B. Uncomplicated birth of viable infant.

# Summary of Warning Signs During Labor

I. *Contractions*—strong, every 2 min or less, lasting 90 sec or more; poor relaxation between contractions.

II. Sudden sharp abdominal *pain* followed by *boardlike abdomen* and *shock*—abruptio placentae or uterine rupture.

III. Marked *vaginal bleeding*.

IV. *FHR periodic pattern decelerations*—late, variable, absent (see **Figure 4.5, p. 103**).

V. Baseline:
A. Bradycardia (< 100 beats/min).
B. Tachycardia (> 160 beats/min).

VI. *Amniotic fluid:*
A. Amount: excessive; diminished.
B. Odor.
C. Color: meconium stained; port-wine; yellow.
D. 24 hr or more since rupture of membranes.

VII. *Maternal hypotension.*

# Summary

Complications during the intrapartal period have both physical and emotional sequelae. The mother (family) faces life-threatening hazards. A long and difficult labor is both physically and emotionally draining. These difficulties and fatigue may negatively affect a new parent's initial response to the newborn. The family may face short-term or long-term grief reactions if the outcome is tragic. The nurse's care-taking skills are important: the ability to assist the mother (family) to develop/maintain effective individual coping and a sense of self-worth.

# Study and Memory Aids

**Definition: Tocolysis—From Greek:**

*toco-, toko-* = a combining form meaning childbirth, labor
*lysis* = to break down or dissolve

**Definition: Dystocia—From Greek:**

*dys-* = a prefix meaning abnormal, diseased; difficult, painful, faulty
*toco-, toko-* = a combining form meaning childbirth, labor

**Dystocia—Etiology: "Six P's"**

**P**osition
**P**sychological response
**P**lacenta
**P**ower
**P**assageway
**P**assenger

# Questions

1. Brethine (*Terbutaline*) SQ is chosen as the beta-adrenergic agent to treat a woman's preterm labor. Which common *maternal* side effect can the nurse expect?
   1. Hypoglycemia.
   2. Decreased reflexes.
   3. Tachycardia.
   4. Hyperkalemia.

2. A woman is hospitalized for preterm labor at 28 wk. She is given betamethasone (*Celestone, Solupan*). She asks the nurse what the drug is for. The nurse's explanation should be based on the knowledge that the drug is used to:
   1. Treat fetal respiratory distress syndrome (RDS).
   2. Prevent chorioamnionitis.
   3. Promote fetal pulmonary maturity.
   4. Increase uteroplacental exchange.

3. A woman is in labor with a large fetus. She experiences sudden, sharp abdominal pain, which is followed by a cessation of contractions and a tender abdomen. The nurse notifies the physician **STAT** because these signs and symptoms indicate:
   1. Abruptio placentae.
   2. Placenta previa.
   3. Uterine rupture.
   4. Uterine inversion.

4. The nurse is legally obligated to recognize the types of fetal heart rate (FHR) tracings on electronic fetal monitor strips. The nurse recognizes a late FHR deceleration as:
   1. A transitory decrease of FHR below baseline, concurrent with uterine contractions.
   2. An abrupt transitory decrease in FHR that varies in duration, intensity, and timing related to onset of contractions.
   3. A transitory decrease in FHR below baseline rate, starting at peak of contraction and lasting beyond end of contraction.
   4. An FHR below 120 beats/min lasting longer than 10 min.

5. The nurse is legally obligated to recognize the types of fetal heart rate (FHR) tracings on electronic fetal monitor strips. The nurse recognizes a variable FHR deceleration as:
   1. A transitory decrease of FHR below baseline, concurrent with contractions.
   2. A transitory decrease in FHR below baseline rate, starting at peak of contraction and lasting beyond end of contraction.
   3. An FHR below 120 beats/min lasting longer than 10 min.
   4. An abrupt transitory decrease in FHR that varies in duration, intensity, and timing related to onset of contractions.

6. Heart failure (HF) is one cause of maternal mortality during labor. Under what condition must the maternity nurse be on the alert for development of HF in a healthy woman in labor?
   1. During a long second stage of labor with prolonged bearing down.
   2. If the woman becomes exhausted during a difficult (dystotic) labor.
   3. Secondary to other therapy, such as tocolysis and use of betamethasone.
   4. Secondary to other therapy, such as use of prostaglandins to augment/induce labor.

7. A woman in preterm labor is undergoing tocolysis and has shown signs/symptoms of toxicity. The nurse prepares and administers the antidote for terbutaline toxicity, which is:
   1. *Yutopar*, 1mg.
   2. Calcium gluconate, 10 mg.
   3. Inderal, 0.5 mg.
   4. Naloxone hydrochloride (*Narcan*).

8. The nurse will discontinue ritodrine tocolysis for a woman in premature labor, and notify the physician in the presence of which clinical occurrence?
   1. Maternal pulse of 104 and regular.
   2. Maternal blood pressure of 140/68.
   3. The woman complains of shortness of breath and chest tightness.
   4. The woman complains of palpitations.

9. The nurse's plan of care must include an alert for possible complications that can arise from therapeutic interventions. The nurse bases care on the knowledge that a woman who is a healthy primigravida in preterm labor is at increased risk for cardiac decompensation if she:
   1. Receives betamethasone during tocolysis.
   2. Has a prolonged second stage of labor.
   3. Becomes fatigued during a 24 hr labor.
   4. Receives IV fluids and sucks on ice chips.

10. Preterm labor/birth give rise to physical, emotional, and financial stress for the family and possible physical/intellectual/sensory impairment for the child; therefore, nurses assure that all women who are pregnant know and have a list of signs and symptoms that indicate preterm labor. Which symptoms reported to the nurse by a woman who is pregnant are likely due to preterm labor?
    1. Irregular contractions during the day, groin pain, heavy discharge.
    2. Abdominal pain, occasional contractions, mucousy discharge.
    3. Pelvic pressure, contractions during position changes, watery discharge.
    4. Contractions every 10 min for 2 hr, low back pain, light bloody discharge.

11. The labor and birth room nurse notes that moments after a woman's membranes rupture, she becomes dyspneic, tachypneic, and apprehensive, and she is experiencing pleuritic pain. The nurse suspects:
    1. Placenta abruptio.
    2. Placenta previa.
    3. Imminent birth.
    4. Amniotic fluid embolus.

12. A 17-year-old, para 0-0-0-0, is admitted at 38 wk gestation and diagnosed with mild pre-eclampsia. Her condition stabilizes and induction of labor is begun with *Pitocin*. Cervical dilation is 2 cm and effacement is 70%. Amniotomy is done and scalp electrode and intrauterine contraction monitors are inserted. Which nursing action would be inappropriate?
    1. Promote rest by checking on her less frequently.
    2. Position her in lateral decubitus position.
    3. Monitor intake and output hourly.
    4. Observe for blood pressure changes related to *Pitocin*.

13. The nurse knows that oxytocin stimulation of labor must be discontinued immediately if which danger sign occurs?
    1. Contractions last 60 sec and occur every 3 min.
    2. FHR is 182 beats/min for longer than 10 min.
    3. FHR falls from 138 to 128 beats/min with contractions.
    4. The woman complains of discomfort with contractions.

14. For 3 hr, a woman in labor has stayed at 6 cm dilated, station (vertex) with molding extending to +2 station. The physician orders *Pitocin* augmentation of labor. The nurse's responsibility is to:
    1. Assist in initiating induction.
    2. "Piggy-back" IV fluid containing *Pitocin*.
    3. Start an accurate record.
    4. Challenge the order.

15. A woman is admitted to the hospital in early labor; her membranes ruptured before admission. The nurse anticipates that the physician will order "bedrest" if assessment shows:
    1. Cervical dilatation: 3 cm.
    2. Effacement: 90%.
    3. Station: –2.
    4. Contractions every 3 min, lasting 30 sec.

16. Complications can occur at any time when a woman is in labor. All nurses must be ready to intervene for emergencies such as prolapsed umbilical cord. The nurse knows that the primary goal of emergency care given when prolapsed cord occurs during labor is to:
    1. Prevent cold air from prematurely stimulating fetal respiration.
    2. Apply water to the cord to prevent it from drying while it is still pulsating.
    3. Stimulate and restore circulation in the cord by vasodilation.
    4. Prevent or relieve pressure on the umbilical cord.

17. During a woman's labor, the nurse must be alert for life-threatening umbilical cord prolapse, especially:
    1. During the second stage of labor.
    2. When the woman is ambulatory.
    3. When the presenting part is not engaged in the pelvic brim.
    4. If the amniotic sac is intact.

18. In addition to changing the mother's position, what other independent nursing intervention is indicated when the umbilical cord is prolapsed out of the vagina?
    1. Wash the cord immediately with warm antiseptic solution and replace it into the vagina.
    2. Cover the cord with a wet sterile sponge.
    3. Keep the cord warm and moist with continuous applications of warm sterile saline compresses.
    4. Apply a clamp to the exposed cord and cover with a sterile towel.

19. When a woman is admitted to the labor area with a questionable diagnosis of placenta previa or abruptio placentae, which admission procedure would the nurse omit?
    1. Giving an enema.
    2. Collecting a urine specimen.
    3. Starting an IV infusion.
    4. Leopold's maneuvers.

# Answers/Rationale

1. **(3)** Tachycardia is a side effect of terbutaline. The findings in options **1**, **2**, and **4** are *not* among the common side effects of this drug. **EV, RE/KN, 6, PhI, Pharmacological and parenteral therapies.**

2. **(3)** Corticosteroids have been found to hasten production of surfactant in fetal lungs. This drug is used to *prevent* RDS, not treat it (**1**). This drug does *not* prevent infection of the fetal membranes, or chorioamnionitis (**2**), and it does not affect uteroplacental exchange (**4**). **PL, RE/KN, 5, PhI, Pharmacological and parenteral therapies.**

3. **(3)** These signs and symptoms describe uterine rupture, which occurs when the stress on the uterine muscle exceeds its ability to stretch, e.g., overdistention with a large fetus or fetuses, previous cesarean births, tetanic contractions (secondary to *Pitocin* induction/augmentation of labor). The uterus remains contracted (tone is increased) with abruptio (**1**), but rupture does *not* occur. Signs and symptoms of placenta previa (**2**) include painless bright-red bleeding; uterine tone is within *normal* limits. Inversion (**4**), turning inside out, does *not* occur during *labor*; it may occur after the baby's birth if the cord is pulled to try to remove the placenta before it is detached from the uterine wall. **IMP, APP, 3, PhI, Physiological adaptation.**

4. **(3)** A late FHR deceleration is defined as a transitory decrease in FHR below baseline rate, starting at peak of contraction and lasting beyond end of contraction. The other options describe *early* FHR deceleration (**1**), *variable* FHR deceleration (**2**), and FHR *bradycardia* (**4**). **AN, RE/KN, 5, PhI, Reduction of risk potential.**

5. **(4)** Variable FHR decelerations are abrupt transitory decelerations that vary in duration, intensity, and timing related to onset of contractions. The other options describe *early* FHR deceleration (**1**), *late* FHR deceleration (**2**), and FHR *bradycardia* (**3**). **AN, RE/KN, 5, PhI, Reduction of risk potential.**

---

**Key to Codes**

**Nursing process: AS**, assessment; **AN**, analysis; **PL**, planning; **IMP**, implementation; **EV**, evaluation. (See **Appendix J** for explanation of nursing process steps.)

**Cognitive level: RE/KN**, recall/knowledge; **COM**, comprehension; **APP**, application; **ANL**, analysis; **EVL**, evaluation; **SYN**, synthesis. (See **Appendix J** for explanation.)

**Category of human function: 1**, protective; **2**, sensory-perceptual; **3**, comfort, rest, activity, and mobility; **4**, nutrition; **5**, growth and development; **6**, fluid-gas transport; **7**, psychosocial-cultural; **8**, elimination. (See **Appendix L** for explanation.)

**Client need: SECE**, safe, effective care environment; **HPM**, health promotion and maintenance; **PsI**, psychosocial integrity; **PhI**, physiological integrity. (See **Appendix M** for explanation.)

**Client subneed:** See **Appendix M** for explanation.

6. (3) Therapy such as use of a beta-mimetic (ritodrine, terbutaline) for tocolysis and the use of betamethasone (*Celestone, Solup*) to stimulate fetal lung development (production of surfactant) increases a healthy woman's risk of heart failure. A woman who is healthy will become exhausted with a long labor (1), but heart failure will not develop because of it. Neither a difficult labor in itself (2) nor use of prostaglandins (4) predisposes the woman who is healthy to heart failure. **EV, RE/KN, 6, PhI, Pharmacological and parenteral therapies.**

7. (3) Inderal, 0.5 mg, is the antidote for terbutaline toxicity. *Yutopar* (1) is similar in action to terbutaline. Calcium gluconate (2) is the antidote for magnesium sulfate toxicity. *Narcan* (4) is the antidote for narcosis and depressed respirations. **IMP, RE/KN, 1, PhI, Pharmacological and parenteral therapies.**

8. (3) Shortness of breath and chest tightness are symptoms of cardiac decompensation. In addition, be especially alert for heart failure if a steroid such as betamethasone (*Celestone, Solup*) is used to stimulate fetal lung maturity. The antidote for ritodrine hydrochloride (*Yutopar*) is propranolol, 1 mg. A maternal pulse of 130 exceeds the therapeutic range. The findings in 1, 2, and 4 represent side effects of ritodrine therapy, but remain within *acceptable* normal limits. **IMP, COM, 6, PhI, Pharmacological and parenteral therapies.**

9. (1) A corticosteroid such as betamethasone (*Celestone, Solup*, used to stimulate fetal lung maturity) plus a beta-mimetic drug such as ritodrine or terbutaline (used for tocolysis, stopping preterm labor) increases risk of cardiac decompensation. Signs/symptoms: shortness of breath, chest tightness; P ≥ 140; R ≥ 25. *None* of the situations in options 2, 3, and 4 leads to cardiac decompensation in the woman who is both healthy and pregnant. **IMP, RE/KN, 6, PhI, Physiological adaptation.**

10. (4) Contractions occurring every 10 min for 2 hr (even after position changes and drinking glasses of water), low back pain, and light bloody discharge (bloody show) are common signs of true labor. Other symptoms of preterm labor include: constant menstrual-like cramping low in the abdomen, dull lower backache that radiates like a wave to the front of the abdomen, and pelvic pressure extending to the back and thighs. Option 1 is incorrect because irregular contractions throughout the day, pain in the groin, and heavy vaginal discharge (leukorrhea) are common in *normal* pregnancy. Option 2 is incorrect because abdominal pain is *not* a sign of preterm labor and needs to be further evaluated; occasional contractions and mucousy discharge are commonly seen in *normal* pregnancy. Option 3 is incorrect because pelvic pressure could result from a baby that is low-lying, and contractions can be stimulated by position changes; watery discharge could be due to ruptured membranes (amniotic fluid), and does need to be assessed more

thoroughly. **EV, APP, 5, HPM, Health promotion and maintenance.**

11. (4) These signs suggest amniotic fluid embolism. This can also follow placental separation after the birth of the baby. Immediate recognition of the condition is important for timely, prompt intervention. DIC and adult respiratory distress syndrome (ARDS) are possible sequelae. *None* of the conditions in options 1, 2, and 3 would cause this type of client response. **EV, ANL, 6, PhI, Physiological adaptation.**

12. (1) This woman who is critically ill now has an additional medication with powerful side effects that must be monitored regularly; it would be inappropriate to monitor her *less* frequently. The actions in options 2, 3, and 4 *are all proper* nursing measures for a woman who is hypertensive and undergoing induction of labor. **IMP, ANL, 3, SECE, Management of care.**

13. (2) Persistent tachycardia (acceleration) is one sign of fetal distress. The findings in options 1, 3, and 4 are all within *normal* range. **EV, ANL, 1, PhI, Physiological adaptation.**

14. (4) The data suggest that the labor may be complicated by cephalopelvic disproportion (CPD). Augmenting labor with exogenous oxytocin may serve to wedge the presenting part deeper into the maternal pelvis and severely compromise the fetus. Labor should not be augmented as ordered (1 and 2) under these conditions, since CPD may be present. While maintaining an accurate record (3) is important, the nurse needs to *challenge* this order, not just document it. **IMP, ANL, 1, SECE, Management of care.**

15. (3) Station at −2 means that the presenting part of the fetus is high enough to allow the umbilical cord to slip down in front of the presenting part. Cervical dilatation (1), effacement (2), and contractions (4) are *irrelevant* to umbilical cord prolapse. NOTE: When membranes rupture, the nurse's primary responsibility is to assess for FHRs, since the umbilical cord can be "washed down" at the time the membranes rupture. **EV, ANL, 1, HPM, Health promotion and maintenance.**

16. (4) Compression of the umbilical cord compromises fetal oxygenation and, therefore, fetal well-being. Cold air (1) does not enter the uterus via the vagina following rupture of membranes. The cord should be kept moist with sterile warm *saline* compresses, *not water* (2), to prevent it from drying. (Maintenance of *pulsation* is a goal since it indicates that fetal circulation continues.) Vasodilation (3) does *not* occur during cord compression; if the cord is external to the vagina, *vasoconstriction* will occur if it is not kept warm and moist, secondary to the effect on Wharton's jelly, which surrounds the vessels in the cord (on exposure to cold, the jelly expands and constricts the vessels in the cord, since the covering of the cord is not elastic and cannot expand). **PL, ANL, 6, PhI, Reduction of risk potential.**

**17. (3)** The umbilical cord can slip past the presenting part *before* it engages snugly in the pelvic brim. There is no room for the cord to slip past the full-term fetus during the *second* stage **(1)**. Women *can* be ambulatory **(2)** when membranes are intact or after the presenting part has engaged, when prolapse is *not* likely. Sufficient amniotic fluid in an intact sac **(4)** cushions the umbilical cord. **AS, RE/KN, 6, PhI, Reduction of risk potential.**

**18. (3)** This action maintains cord integrity; warmth prevents Wharton's jelly from expanding and closing off umbilical blood vessels. The actions in options **1** and **2** do not protect the cord. Clamping the cord **(4)** cuts off any uteroplacental-fetal circulation, and the fetus will die. **IMP, ANL, 1, PhI, Reduction of risk potential.**

**19. (1)** Giving an enema may result in dislodging a low-lying placenta, and severe hemorrhage may follow. Touching the cervix through the rectal and vaginal mucosas causes reflex uterine contractions, which result in cervical changes. These changes (dilatation and effacement) pull up and away from the low-lying placenta, thus dislodging it from its implantation site. A urine analysis **(2)** *is* appropriate for admission to a labor floor to rule out infection. Starting an intravenous infusion **(3)** on admission *is* appropriate for someone who is bleeding and when anesthesia and surgical intervention may be required. Leopold's maneuvers **(4)** *could* assist in diagnosing an abnormally high fetus (commonly seen when the placenta occupies the lower uterine segment) and the general tone of the uterus (muscle tone is unaffected by placenta previa; it is increased in the presence of abruptio placentae). In addition, a blood specimen is obtained to assess for low platelets, a sign of DIC, which can occur with abruptio placentae. **IMP, ANL, 6, SECE, Management of care.**

# The Postpartal Period

## Chapter Outline

- Key Points
- Key Words
- Biologic Foundations
  - Uterine Involution
  - Birth Canal
  - Abdominal Wall
  - Cardiovascular System
  - Urinary Tract
  - Integument (Skin)
  - Legs
  - Weight
  - Menstruation and Ovarian Function

- Nursing Management
  - Pharmacology: Medications to Stimulate Uterine Tone
- Psychological/Behavioral Changes
- Breastfeeding and Lactation
- Formula Feeding
- Critical Path/Case Management
- Home Care Following Early Discharge
- Summary
- Study and Memory Aids
- Questions
- Answers/Rationale

## 🔑 Key Points

- Following expulsion of the placenta, *levels of estrogen and progesterone fall rapidly*, resulting in many of the *anatomic and physiologic changes* in the postpartum period.

- "Motherliness" can be exhibited by either parent.

- The interactional structure of a family must be restructured with the addition of the new member.

- The biggest differences between Western and non-Western beliefs and practices in childbearing occur in the *postpartal* period and require sensitive and knowledgeable consideration in the nursing plan of care.

- Careful assessment is essential in order to detect any deviations from the norm, to provide comfort measures for the relief of discomfort or pain, and to guard against injury and/or infection in the care of the newborn and mother.

## Key Words

"After pains"

Autolysis

"Baby blues"

Colostrum

Critical path/case management

Engorgement (breast)

Homan's sign

Home care

Involution

Let-down reflex

Lochia

    Rubra

    Serosa

    Alba

Oxytocic medications

Puerperium ("fourth trimester")

Telephone follow-up

"Warm lines"/help lines

## Biologic Foundations

**General overview**: This review of the normal physiologic and psychological changes occurring during the postpartal period—the "fourth trimester" (birth to 6 wk after)—provides the database necessary for assessing the woman's progress through involution, planning and implementing care, anticipatory guidance, health teaching, and evaluating the results. Emerging problems are identified by comparing the woman's status against established standards.

### Uterine Involution

**Definiton**: integrated processes by which the uterus returns to nonpregnant size, shape, and consistency.

▶ I.  **Assessment**

    A. *Contractions* ("after pains")—shorten muscles, close venous sinuses, restore normal tone.

       1.  Frequency, intensity, and discomfort decrease after first 24 hr.

2. More common in women who are multiparas, and after birth of a large baby; primiparous uterus remains contracted.

3. Increased by breastfeeding.

B. *Autolysis*—breakdown and excretion of muscle protein (decreasing size of myometrial cells).

   1. *Lochia*—sloughing of decidua (the upper 2 layers of the endometrium, leaving the basal layer to regenerate the endometrium) and blood. See **F** below.

C. Formation of *new endometrium*—4–6 wk until placental site healed; heals without scarring.

D. *Cervix*.

   1. *Immediately* following birth—bruised, small tears; admits one hand.

   2. *Eighteen hr* after birth—becomes shorter, firmer; regains normal shape.

   3. *One wk* postpartum—admits two fingers.

   4. Never returns fully to prepregnant state

      a. Parous os is wider and not perfectly round.

      b. Lacerations heal as scars radiating out from the os.

E. *Fundal height and consistency*.

   1. *After birth*—at umbilicus; size and consistency of firm grapefruit.

   2. *Day 1* (first 12 hr—one finger breadth (about 1 cm) above umbilicus.

   3. Descends by one fingerbreadth (about 1 cm) *daily* until day 10.

   4. *Day 10*—behind symphysis pubis, nonpalpable.

F. *Lochia*.

   1. *Character*:

      a. *Rubra* (red): from birth to about *day 3 or 4*; consists of: blood endometrial decidua, bacteria, fetal lanugo, vernix, small shreds of placental tissue and membranes.

      b. *Serosa* (pink to brown): apparent about *day 3 until about day 7*. The amount of blood decreases; the placental site exudes serous material and lymph.

      c. *Alba* (creamy yellowish-white to gray-white): appears during *second* or *third* wk. As endometrial epithelialization progresses, the amount of lochia decreases markedly and takes on a seromucinous consistency. Cessation of flow occurs at about 6 wk. It contains numerous leukocytes and bacteria.

   2. *Amount*: scant, light, moderate, or heavy.

      a. Moderate: 4–8 pads/d (*average* 6 pads/d).

      b. Following cesarean birth: less lochia—due to manipulation during surgery.

   3. *Odor*: normal lochia has characteristic "fleshy" odor; foul odor is characteristic of infection.

4. *Clots*: normal: a few small clots, most commonly on arising—due to pooling in vagina. NOTE: Clots and *heavy* bleeding

! are associated with uterine atony, retained placental fragments.

# Birth Canal

I. **Characteristic changes:**

   A. *Vagina*—never returns fully to prepregnant state

      1. First few weeks postpartum: thin-walled, due to lack of estrogen; few rugae.

      2. Week 3: Rugae may reappear.

      3. Hymen—if torn, may heal.

   B. *Pelvic floor*.

      1. Immediately after birth: infiltrated with blood, stretched, torn.

      2. Month 6: Considerable tone regained.

   C. *Perineum* (see **REEDA, p. 118**).

      1. Immediately following birth: edematous; may have episiotomy (or repaired lacerations); hemorrhoids.

      2. Healing, incisional line clean; no separation.

      3. Hematoma: blood in connective tissue beneath skin; complains of pain, unrelieved by mild analgesia or heat; perineal distention; painful, tense, fluctuant mass.

# Abdominal Wall

I. **Characteristic changes:**

   A. Overdistention during pregnancy may cause: rupture of elastic fibers, persistent striae, and diastasis of the rectus muscles.

   B. Usually takes 6–8 wk to retrogress, dependent on previous muscle tone, obesity, and amount of distention during pregnancy.

   C. Strenuous exercises discouraged until 8 wk postpartum.

# Cardiovascular System

I. **Characteristic changes:**

   A. Immediately after birth—*increased* cardiac load, due to:

      1. Return of uterine blood flow to general circulation.

      2. Diuresis of excess interstitial fluid.

   B. Volume—returns to prepregnant state (4 L) in about 3 wk. Major reduction—during first week, due to diuresis and diaphoresis.

   C. Blood values (see **Table 2.2, p. 28**).

      1. High WBC during labor (25,000/mL); drops to normal level in first few days.

      2. Week 1—Hgb, RBC, Hct, elevated fibrinogen return to normal.

D. Blood coagulation.

1. During *labor*: rapid consumption of clotting factors.
2. During *postpartum*: increased consumption of clotting factors. Hypercoagulability maintained during first few days postpartum; predisposes to thrombophlebitis, ! pulmonary embolism.

II. **Assessment:**

A. **Potential (maternal) cardiac complications**—vital signs:

1. *Temperature—elevated* in:
   a. Excessive blood loss, dehydration, exhaustion, infection.
   b. Puerperal infection: 100.4° F (38° C) after first day postpartum.
2. *Pulse*—physiologic *bradycardia* (50–70) common through second day postpartum; may persist 7–10 days; etiology: unknown. *Tachycardia*—associated with: excessive blood loss, dehydration, exhaustion, infection.
3. *Blood pressure*—generally unchanged; *elevation*—associated with: pre-eclampsia, essential hypertension, pain.

## Urinary Tract

I. **Characteristic changes:**

A. *Output*—increased due to diuresis (12 hr–5 days postpartum); daily output to 3000 mL.

B. *Urine constituents*:

1. Sugar—primarily lactose.
2. Acetonuria—after prolonged labor; dehydration.
3. Proteinuria—first 3 days in response to the catalytic process of involution.

C. Dilatation of ureters—subsides in first few weeks.

II. **Assessment:**

! A. **Potential complications**—measure first few voidings, palpate bladder to determine emptying

1. Edema, trauma, and/or anesthesia may lead to retention with overflow.
2. *Overdistended bladder*—common cause of excessive uterine bleeding in immediate postpartum.

## Integument (skin)

I. **Characteristic changes:**

A. *Striae*—persist as silvery or brownish lines.
B. *Diastasis recti abdominis*—some midline separation may persist.
C. *Diaphoresis*—excessive perspiration for first few (approximately 5) days.
D. Breast changes—see **Nursing Management I. C. Breasts, p. 145.**

## Legs

I. **Characteristic changes:**

A. Should have no redness, tenderness, local areas of increased skin temperature, or edema.
B. May have some soreness from birth position.
C. *Homans' sign* should be negative (no calf pain when knee is extended and gentle pressure applied to dorsiflex the foot).

## Weight

I. **Characteristic changes:**

A. Initial weight loss—fetus, placenta, amniotic fluid, excess tissue fluid.
B. Weighs more than in prepregnant state (weight maintained in breasts).
C. Week 6—weight loss is individualized.

## Menstruation and Ovarian Function

I. **Characteristic changes:**

A. First menstrual cycle may be anovulatory.
B. *Nonnursing*—ovulation at 4–6 wk; menstruation at 6–8 wk.
C. *Nursing*—anovulatory period varies (39 days to 6 mo or more); same for duration of lactation; contraceptive value: *very unreliable.*

# Nursing Management

I. **Assessment**—minimum of twice daily

A. Vital signs.
B. Emotional status, response to baby.
C. *Breasts*

1. Observe: size, symmetry, placement and condition of nipples, leakage of colostrum.
   a. Although one breast is usually larger than the other, breasts are essentially symmetrical in shape.
   b. Nipples: in breast midline, erectile, intact (no signs of fissure).
   c. Bilateral leakage of colostrum is common.
2. Note: reddened areas, elevations, supernumerary nipples, inverted nipples, cracks.
3. Observe for signs of (normal) *engorgement* (i.e., tenderness, distention, prominent veins). Transient; normally occurs shortly before lactation is established—due to venous and lymphatic stasis.
4. Palpate for: local heat, edema, tenderness, ! swelling (*signs of localized infection*).

D. Fundus, lochia, perineum.
E. Voiding and bowel function.

*(continued on p. 147)*

## PHARMACOLOGY BOX 6.1 ⬭ MEDICATIONS TO STIMULATE UTERINE TONE

| Drug/Dosage | Indication/Action | ▶◀ Assessment: Side Effects | ▶◀ Nursing Management |
|---|---|---|---|
| **Carboprost** | | | |
| Hemabate (*Prostin*/M15); *oxytocic, prostaglandin* IM injection: 1 ampule (250 mcg); onset within minutes; *intramyometrial* injection (by physician *only*), ½–2 ampules (125–500 mcg) diluted with 10 mL saline (injected *transabdominally* into anterior wall of uterus); onset within minute | Treat uterine atony and uterine inversion: stimulate rapid, sustained uterine contractions | **!** *Severe hypertension* (systolic > 170 mm Hg or diastolic > 100 mm Hg) Diarrhea commonly seen with dosage above 1 ampule **!** Possible bronchoconstriction and wheezing | Review client history: *avoid* use in clients with severe symptomatic asthma Observe for adverse reactions Monitor BP Store in refrigerator |
| **Cytotec** | | | |
| (*synthetic prostaglandin*) E1 analog PO or rectally: 400–600 mcg | Treat uterine atony | More common: abdominal or stomach pain (mild); diarrhea Less common or rare: constipation; cramps, gas; headache; heartburn, indigestion, nausea and/or vomiting | Observe for adverse reaction Increased diarrhea when magnesium is being administered |
| **Ergonovine** | | | |
| USP, NF (*Ergotrate maleate*); oxytocic, ergot alkaloid Oral: 0.2–0.4 mg q 6–12 h for 48 hr; onset in 6–15 min IM injection: 0.2 mg (1 mL) if nausea precludes oral preparation; onset "in a few minutes" *Initial* response: firm, tetanic contraction *Subsequent* response: alternating minor relaxations and contractions for 1 ½ hr; then vigorous rhythmic contractions for 3–4 hr after injection | Treat uterine atony: stimulate prolonged *nonphasic* uterine contractions | *Hypertension:* **!** Severe hypertensive episodes may occur if woman is hypertensive, or receiving vasoconstrictors. *Hypersensitivity:* Nausea, vomiting Sudden change in BP, pulse | *Assess for hypertension before administering!* Monitor for changes in BP, pulse Store in cool place |
| **Methylergonovine** | | | |
| NF (*Methergine*); *oxytocic, ergot alkaloid* and congener of lysergic acid (LSD) Oral: 0.2 mg tab, q 6–8 h for maximum of 1 wk; onset in 5–10 min IM injection: 0.2 mg (1 mL) q 2–4 h; onset in 2–5 min IV infusion (*emergency only*): 0.2 mg (1 mL) *slowly over 60 sec*; onset immediate | Treat uterine atony: stimulate rapid, sustained tetanic uterine contractions Treat subinvolution of uterus | Nausea, vomiting *Transient hypertension* (has only minimum vasoconstrictive effect) CNS effects: dizziness, headache, tinnitus Diaphoresis Palpitations Temporary chest pains | *Avoid* administering about the time woman receives analgesic such ⬭ as *oxycodone* and *aspirin* (Percodan)—may result in **!** hallucinations Monitor BP Store in cool place away from light |

*(continued)*

## PHARMACOLOGY BOX 6.1 ⊂⊃ MEDICATIONS TO STIMULATE UTERINE TONE (continued)

| Drug/Dosage | Indication/Action | ◀ Assessment: Side Effects | ◀ Nursing Management |
|---|---|---|---|
| **Oxytocin Injection** | | | |
| USP (*Pitocin, Syntocinon, Uteracon*); oxytocic, synthetic posterior pituitary hormone<br>IV injection: 10 U/mL; onset in 1 min<br>IV infusion: 10–40 U/1000 mL 5% dextrose or physiologic electrolyte solution<br>IM injection: 3–10 U; onset in 3–7 min; duration 30–60 min | Treat uterine atony: stimulate *phasic* uterine muscle contraction<br>Assist breastfeeding: promote milk-ejection (let-down) reflex, facilitate flow of milk during engorgement | *Hypertension,* if client is concurrently receiving ⊂⊃ *ephedrine, methoxamine,* or other vasopressors<br>*Hypersensitivity* | Monitor for return of atony when effect wears off<br>Store in cool place |

F. Legs (see **p. 145**).

G. Signs of complications (see **Maternal warning signs, p. 148**).

◀ **II. Analysis/nursing diagnosis:** (See **Analysis/nursing diagnosis during the fourth stage of labor, p. 111**).

◀ **III. Nursing care plan/implementation**

  A. Goal: *safety* (prevent hemorrhage).

    1. Review prenatal and labor/birth history to identify *predisposing factors*:

      a. Previous history of bleeding after birth.

      b. Large baby (or twins, triplets, etc.), polyhydramnios.

      c. Saddle-block anesthesia.

      d. Long difficult labor (dystocia).

      e. Intrauterine infection.

      f. Grand multipara.

    2. Take *precautionary* measures:

      a. Remind woman to keep bladder empty so that "living ligature" can contract.

      b. Keep uterus empty of clots.

      c. Provide gentle massage, prn, to allow uterus maximum capacity to contract well.

  ⊂⊃ 3. Administer oxytocic medications, prn. (See **Pharmacology Box 6.1**.)

  B. Goal: *comfort measures.*

  ☞ 1. Perineal care—to promote healing, prevent infection.

  ☞ 2. Sitz baths—to promote healing.

  ⊂⊃ 3. Apply topical *anesthetics,* witch hazel, epifoam to episiotomy area, hemorrhoids.

  ⊂⊃ 4. Administer mild *analgesia,* as ordered.

    5. Instruct in tensing buttocks on position change—to reduce stress on suture line, discomfort.

  ☞ 6. Breast care: *bottle-feeding* mother.

      a. Wash daily with clear water and mild soap.

      b. Support with well-fitting brassiere.

      c. For engorgement:

    ☞ (1) Prevent with tight binder.

  ☞ ⊂⊃ (2) Treat with ice pack and mild *analgesic.*

    (3) *Avoid* nipple stimulation.

    d. See also **Breastfeeding and lactation, p. 149–150**.

  C. Goal: *encourage normal bowel function* (normal to take 1–3 days for function to resume).

  ⊂⊃ 1. Administer stool softeners, as ordered.

    2. Encourage ambulation.

  🍎 3. Increase *dietary fiber* (salads, fresh fruit, vegetables, bran cereals).

    4. Provide adequate *fluid* intake.

  ▥ D. Goal: **health teaching.** *Discharge planning.*

  ☞ 1. Reinforce appropriate perineal self-care.

  ✋ 2. Reinforce handwashing (see **Nursing actions during the fourth stage of labor, p. 111–112**).

  ☞ 3. *Infant care.*

    a. Bathing, cord care, circumcision care, diapering.

    b. Feeding, burping.

    c. Assessment—temperature, skin color, newborn rash, jaundice.

    d. Normal stool cycle and voiding pattern.

    e. Common sleep/activity patterns.

  🚦 f. Newborn warning signs to report **immediately:**

    (1) Diarrhea, constipation.

    (2) Colic, vomiting.

    (3) Fever.

    (4) Signs of inflammation and/or infection at cord stump.

    (5) Bleeding at circumcision site.

    (6) Rash, jaundice.

    (7) Deviation from normal patterns.

    4. *Self-care.*

    a. Adequate rest, nutrition, hydration.

    b. Breast self-examination; wear bra to support breasts, and promote comfort.

    c. Normal process of involution; lochial patterns.

5. Resumption of *sexual intercourse.*
   a. Sexual intercourse can be resumed by end of third or fourth postbirth week if bleeding has stopped and the episiotomy is healed.
   b. Physiologic reactions to sexual stimulation for the first three postbirth months are reduced in both rapidity and intensity of response.
   c. For first 6 weeks to 6 months, vagina does not lubricate well because steroid hormone depletion following birth inhibits the vasocongestive response to sexual tension.
   d. Use of a water-soluble gel (K-Y), or a contraceptive cream or jelly is recommended for lubrication.
   e. Vaginal tenderness may be present.
      (1) To relax vagina and identify possible areas of discomfort, partner can be instructed to insert one or more clean, lubricated fingers into vagina and rotate them.
      (2) Coital position of comfort is chosen in which woman can control depth of penile penetration, e.g., side-by-side or female-superior.
   f. Presence of baby influences postbirth sexual relationship.
      (1) A common concern is that baby will hear them.
      (2) Sexual response cycle may be interrupted by hearing the baby cry or move, leaving both partners frustrated and unsatisfied.
      (3) Fatigue from child care affects desire.
6. Postbirth *contraception.*
   a. Explain that time interval varies as to first postpartal ovulation.
   b. Family planning options may resume if desired (see **Table 1.2, p. 10–12**)
      (1) If not breastfeeding, oral contraceptives after first menstrual period (low dose given to breastfeeding mothers).
      (2) Use of IUD or diaphragm decided at postpartal check-up.
      (3) Emphasize need to recheck size and fit of diaphragm.
      (4) Other options: condom plus spermicides.
7. *Exercises*—to restore muscle tone, relieve tension
   a. Mild exercise during first few weeks
      (1) Deep abdominal breathing.
      (2) Supine head-raising.
      (3) Stretching from head to toe.
      (4) Pelvic tilt.
      (5) *Kegel's*—to regain perineal muscle tone (see **p. 40**).
   b. Strenuous exercises (sit-ups, leg lifts—deferred until later in postpartum.
8. **Maternal warning signs to report STAT**
   a. *Vaginal discharge*: prolonged lochia rubra; excessive lochia or vaginal discharge; foul-smelling lochia or vaginal discharge; recurrence of bright-red vaginal bleeding after lochia has changed to rust color.
   b. Pelvic or perineal *pain.*
   c. *Fever*, with or without chills.
   d. Burning sensation during urination (*dysuria*); inability to urinate.
   e. Swollen area on *leg* that is painful, red, or hot to the touch.
   f. Localized swelling or a painful, hot area on the *breast.*
   g. See also *Home care following early discharge*, **p. 152-153**.

E. Goal: *anticipatory guidance*—discharge planning: Mothers may be discharged earlier in their postpartum recovery—(24 hr after birth if asymptomatic). See discussion at end of this chapter, *Critical path/case management* (**p. 151–152**), and *Home care following early discharge* (**p. 152-153**).
   1. Discuss, assist in organizing time schedule. Nap, when possible, when infant asleep—to minimize fatigue.
   2. Common maternal emotional/behavior changes, feelings:
      a. Jealous of infant; guilt feelings.
      b. *"Baby blues"*—due to hormonal fluctuations, fatigue, change of lifestyle.
      c. Feelings of inadequacy.
   3. Discuss support groups, aid in identifying supportive people.

**IV. Evaluation/outcome criteria**
A. Woman experiences normal, uncomplicated postpartal period. All assessment findings within normal limits.
B. Woman returns demonstrations of appropriate self-care measures/techniques:
   1. Perineal care, pad change, handwashing.
   2. Breast care, breast self-examination.
C. Woman verbalizes understanding of:
   1. Need for adequate rest and diversion.
   2. Appropriate time for resumption of intercourse and exercise.
   3. Appropriate nutritional intake to meet needs (own and, if breastfeeding, infant).
   4. Signs to be reported immediately.
   5. Returns demonstration of appropriate infant care measures.
   6. Evidences beginning comfort and increasing confidence in parenting role.

**V. Postpartal assessment**—6 wk or less after birth:
    A. Weight, vital signs, urine for protein, complete blood count.
    B. Breast examination—lactating or not.
    C. Pelvic examination—involution and position of uterus; perineal healing; tone of pelvic floor.
    D. Desire for selection of method of contraception.

# Psychological/Behavioral Changes

**Focus**: *achievement of developmental tasks*—progress in assumption of maternal role

**I. Assessment**
    A. *Taking-in* phase*—1–3 days following birth.
        1. Talkative; verbally relives labor/birth experience.
        2. Passive, dependent, concerned with own needs (eating, sleeping, elimination).
    B. *Taking-hold* phase*—day 3 → 2 wk.
        1. Impatient to control own bodily functions, care for self.
        2. Expresses interest/concern in learning how to care for baby (desire to assume "mothering" role).
        3. Responds to positive reinforcement.
    C. *Letting-go* phase*—mother "lets go" of former self-concept, role, lifestyle; begins to integrate new role and self-concept as "mother."
        1. Feelings of insecurity, inadequacy.
        2. Hesitancy in approaching infant-care tasks.
    D. *"Baby blues"*—may appear on day 4 or 5. (NOTE: Often, father/partner experiences same feelings.)
        1. Thought to result from fatigue (sleep deprivation), realization of need for role change, recognition of new responsibilities.
        2. Mild depression; cries without provocation.
        3. Frightened—intimidated by own perceptions of responsibilities.
    E. Lag in experiencing "maternal feelings"—usually resolved within 6 wk.
        1. May contribute to "baby blues."
        2. Guilt regarding lack of "maternal feelings."
        3. Diminished by prompt bonding experience.
    F. *Attachment*: a feeling of affection or loyalty that binds one person to another. Occurs at critical periods, e.g., birth or adoption; it is unique, specific, and enduring.
    G. *Bonding*: describes the initial mutual attraction between people, such as between parent and child, at first meeting.

**II. Analysis/nursing diagnosis**
    A. *Family coping impairment* related to achieving developmental tasks.
    B. *Situational low self-esteem* related to perceived inadequacy in acceptance of maternal role.
    C. *Individual coping impairment* related to "baby blues," lag in experiencing maternal feelings.

**III. Nursing care plan/implementation**
    A. *Taking-in.* Goal: *emotional support.*
        1. Encourage verbalization of labor/birth experiences; compliment parents on "how well" they did.
        2. Explore feelings of disappointment, if any.
        3. Meet dependency needs; comment on appearance, hair, personal gowns.
        4. Encourage rooming in.
    B. Goal: **health teaching.** *Taking-hold.*
        1. Discuss self-care, postpartal physiologic/psychological changes.
        2. Demonstrate infant care; mother returns demonstration.

**IV. Evaluation/outcome criteria**
    A. Woman demonstrates beginning comfort in maternal role.
    B. Woman develops confidence and competence in infant care.
    C. Woman expresses satisfaction with self, infant; eager to return home.
    D. Woman is successful in breastfeeding. (Tension inhibits let-down reflex; baby nurses poorly.)

# Breastfeeding and Lactation

**I. Biologic foundations**
    A. *Antepartal* alterations:
        1. High estrogen/progesterone levels—stimulate proliferation and development of breast ducts.
        2. High progesterone levels—also → development of mammary lobules and alveoli.
    B. *Postpartum* alterations:
        1. Rapid drop in estrogen/progesterone levels.
        2. Increased secretion of **prolactin**—stimulates alveolar cells → milk.
        3. Suckling—stimulates release of **oxytocin** → contraction of ducts → milk ejection (*let-down reflex*).
        4. *Engorgement*—due to venous and lymphatic stasis:
            a. Immediately precedes lactation.
            b. Lasts about 24 hr.
            c. Frequent feeding reduces engorgement.

**II. Assessment**
    A. *Colostrum* (yellowish fluid)—continues for first 2–3 days; may have some antibiotic, immunologic, and nutritive value.
    B. Milk (bluish-white, thin, consistency)—secreted on about third day.

---

* This section is based on a study written by Reva Rubin.

**III. Analysis/nursing diagnosis**

A. *Knowledge deficit* related to breastfeeding techniques.

B. *Pain* related to engorgement.

C. *Personal identity disturbance* related to problems in breastfeeding.

D. *Sleep pattern disturbance* related to discomfort and/or infant care needs.

**IV. Nursing care plan/implementation**

A. Goal: *promote successful breastfeeding*

1. Encourage first feeding right after giving birth.

2. Encourage emptying both breasts at each feeding and before engorgement to stimulate milk production, prevent mastitis.

3. Encourage rest, relaxation, fluids.

4. *Nutritional* counseling (see **Chapter 2, p. 36–39, 55**).

    a. Additional 500 calories/d (per baby; i.e., for twins, mother increases intake by 1000 calories). May be supplied by: one extra pint of milk, one extra egg, and one extra serving of meat, citrus fruit, and vegetable.

    b. Drink to satisfy thirst.

B. Goal: *prevent or relieve engorgement.*

1. Pain: relieved by warm packs, emptying breasts.

2. Suggest she wear good, supportive bra.

3. Administer *analgesics*, as ordered/necessary.

C. Goal: **health teaching.**

1. Instruct, demonstrate rooting reflex and putting infant to breast. Infant must grasp nipple and areola over location of milk sinuses.

2. Demonstrate *burping* techniques, what to do if infant chokes; removing infant from breast.

3. Instruct in *basic nipple care.*

    a. Use good handwashing.

    b. Nurse on each breast making sure areola is in mouth, alternating position of infant.

    c. Alternate "beginning" breast.

    d. Break suction before removing infant from breast.

    e. Air-dry nipples after each feeding and apply lanolin if abraded. NOTE: Creams, lotions, and ointments block secretion of a natural bacteriostatic oil by Montgomery's glands—and infant may refuse breast until it is washed. Instead, expressed milk may be massaged gently around nipple.

    f. Provide daily hygiene of breasts.

4. Instruct in care of *cracked or fissured nipples.*

    a. Encourage and support mothers.

    b. Air-dry nipples after each feeding.

    c. Use nipple shield if nipples extremely sore.

    d. Discontinue nursing for 48 hr; maintain milk supply by expressing milk with pump.

5. Discuss *avoiding* use of any drugs except under medical supervision—may affect infant or suppress lactation.

6. Discuss possibility of sexual stimulation during breastfeeding.

    a. Validate normalcy and acceptability.

    b. NOTE: During orgasm, milk may squirt from nipples.

7. Explain that contraceptive value of nursing is unpredictable; the time that ovulation is inhibited varies widely.

8. Explain *contraindications to breastfeeding*:

    a. Active tuberculosis.

    b. Severe chronic maternal disease.

    c. Mastitis (temporary interruption may be necessary).

    d. Breast cancer.

    e. Severe cleft lip or palate in newborn (may pump and give in special bottles).

    f. HIV-positive status; AIDS.

**V. Evaluation/outcome criteria**

A. Woman verbalizes understanding of breastfeeding techniques, nutritional requirements for successful lactation.

B. Woman successfully demonstrates breastfeeding; infant nurses well.

C. Woman demonstrates appropriate burping techniques; clears excessive mucus from infant's mouth without incident.

D. Woman verbalizes understanding of basic breast-care techniques:

1. Self-examination.

2. Clear water bath.

3. Drying nipples after bathing, feeding.

4. Care of cracked or irritated nipples.

# Formula Feeding

I. A successful alternative to breast feeding in certain instances.

A. Parental choice.

B. Maternal active infection, e.g., tuberculosis, syphilitic breast lesions, AIDS or HIV positive.

C. Adoption.

II. **Feeding skills.**

A. Baby needs to be wide awake.

B. During feedings, parent should assume an *en face* position, hold infant closely and securely; parent can talk, sing or just enjoy a time of peaceful relaxation with baby.

C. Hold bottle like a pencil so that fluid fills the nipple to *avoid* air bubbles.

D. A tight bottle cap and small nipple hole makes infant work very hard so that he or she may fall asleep before satiation. The bubbles in the bottle are tiny. *Solution*: loosen the bottle cap and enlarge nipple hole.

E. If, as the baby sucks, the bubbles in the bottle are large, too much air is entering the baby and stomach cramping and regurgitation may occur. *Solution*: tighten the bottle cap.

F. *Signs that baby has had enough*: baby falls asleep, turns head aside, ceases to suck; baby voids six or more times per day.

G. *Test temperature* of formula on back of feeder's hand; if comfortably warm, it is correct temperature.

H. To *test size of nipple hole*, hold bottle of formula upside down. Formula should drip. If hole is too big, formula runs in a stream; if too little, bottle needs to be shaken to get a drop.

I. Most newborns need to be *"burped"* or *"bubbled"*. Burp before feeding, then after every ounce of formula.

J. To *feed* baby, place the nipple in the infant's mouth over the tongue to rest against the roof of the mouth; this stimulates the sucking reflex.

K. Baby's stools are soft but formed, yellow with a characteristic odor; usually stool is passed during feeding or immediately after. Change diaper immediately because stool is irritating to baby's skin.

III. **Safety tips.**

A. **Never** prop the bottle—nipple may fall against the throat and block the air, or baby could drown in the formula or aspirate any that is regurgitated. If continued in later months, bottle propping has been implicated in causing *nursing bottle caries* or decay of teeth from continuous bathing of teeth with carbohydrate-containing fluid.

B. **Never** leave baby alone while feeding until he or she is old enough to remove bottle from the mouth.

C. At end of feeding and burping, place baby in crib on *right side* so air can come up easily.

# Critical Path/Case Management

**Definition**: *Critical path* refers to the exact timing of all key incidents that must occur to achieve the standard outcomes within the DRG-specific length of stay. *"Key incidents"* refers to physical, emotional, and teaching and discharge planning needs.

I. **Critical Path/Case Management**

A. Developed to implement care needed by clients who have a time limit for hospital stay: 24–48 hr for most new mothers.

B. Examples: nursing responsibilities for a 24 hr stay.

1. *Between 3 and 8 hr after birth:*
   a. Assist with ambulation.
   b. Teach (and observe return demonstration of, prn): self-perineal care, handwashing, assessment and massage of uterine fundus, assessment of lochia character and amount.
   c. Teach about newborn (and observe return demonstration, prn): holding, techniques for positioning for feeding and burping.

2. *During second 8 hr period:*
   a. *Maternal self-care*: teach (and observe return demonstration, prn) about: diet, activity/rest, elimination, sitz bath, medication.
   b. *Newborn care*: teach (and observe return demonstration, prn) about: diaper changes, cord care, circumcision care, feedings and burping.
   c. *Parental concerns*: teach about bonding and attachment; normal newborn characteristics including crying; use of water feedings, pacifiers, and suckling patterns.

3. *During third 8 hr period*: teach/review *warning signs* for mother and newborn to report stat; observe *return demonstration* of infant bath, cord care, circumcision care; refer, prn, e.g., lactation consultant; teach *safety*, e.g., baby positioning, car seat, need for baby to be attended to at all times and no propping of baby bottles; discuss *sibling* rivalry. Provide *anticipatory guidance* regarding baby's crying, sneezing, jaundice, etc.

C. *Implications*: During any one shift, a nurse's assignment may include: a mother who has newly delivered and needs frequent checks; women in different 8 hr periods after giving birth; new admissions, discharges; and the occasional emergency (e.g., hemorrhage, convulsion); in addition, the nurse may be caring for clients who are prenatal with various medical conditions.

D. Standard plans of care and check lists to individualize care to meet woman's unique needs.

1. Standard care plan check lists: lochia, fundus, etc.
2. A check list for each woman to fill out indicating her particular teaching priorities; e.g., woman may prefer to learn about infant illness first, etc. (Woman must be able to read and comprehend; provide lists in woman's language, prn.)

## II. Criteria for early discharge:

### Mother:

- *Uncomplicated* pregnancy, labor, birth and postpartum course.
- The mother's knowledge, ability, and confidence to provide adequate care for her infant including: breastfeeding or bottle feeding, elimination patterns, *infant care* basics, infant *safety*, and ability to recognize signs of illness and common infant problems, particularly *jaundice*.
- Maternal *syphilis*, *hepatitis B* surface antigen, and GBS (group B strep) status have been checked.
- *Social* and *environmental* factors should be examined including: home environment, social support, history of child abuse or neglect and drug use.

### Infant:

- *The infant's vital signs* within normal ranges and stable for the last 12 hours, including a respiratory rate < 60 per minute, a heart rate 100 to 160 beats per minute and axillary temperature of 36.5° to 37.4° C (97.7° to 99.3° F), in an open crib with appropriate clothing.
- No abnormalities requiring continued hospitalization.
- The infant has *urinated and passed* at least *one stool* spontaneously.
- The infant has completed at least 2 *successful feedings* and the infant is able to coordinate *sucking, swallowing, and breathing* while feeding.
- No evidence of excessive bleeding at the *circumcision site* for at least 2 hours.
- *Infant screening tests* in accordance with state regulations, including cord or infant blood type and *direct Coombs'* test results, including *hearing* screening and newborn screen for *inborn metabolic disorders*.

Early discharge (< 48 hours after birth) for infants who are at term and healthy can be accomplished, but it does not mean that it is appropriate for every mother and infant. Each mother-infant dyad should be evaluated individually to determine the optimal time of discharge. The timing of discharge should be the decision of the physician caring for the infant.

*Source*: Adapted from Committee on Fetus and Newborn, *Hospital Stay for Healthy Term Newborns*, Pediatrics 113 (5) 1436.

## III. Maternal warning signs: Mother (family) is given a postpartum discharge list of signs that require reporting STAT:

| Breasts | Redness, heat, pain, cracked and fissured nipples, inverted nipples |
| --- | --- |
| Elimination | *Urine*: inability to void, urgency, frequency, dysuria; *bowel*: constipation, diarrhea |
| Energy level | Lethargy, extreme fatigue |
| Legs | Painful, reddened area; warmth on posterior aspect of calf; pain when ambulating |
| Lochia | Odor: heavy, foul, > 1 pad soaked in one hour |
| Perineum | Pronounced edema, not intact; signs of infection; marked discomfort |
| Pulse | Tachycardia |
| Rest | Inability to rest or sleep |
| Temperature | More than 100.4° F (38° C) *after* the first 24 hr. |
| Uterus | Deviated from the midline, boggy, tender |

# 🏠 Home Care Following Early Discharge

**Definition**: service developed in response to consumers' need for continued assistance following early discharge from hospital to meet limits of DRG-specific length of stay (legislation was enacted to provide up to 48 hours after delivery; mother may choose earlier discharge with follow-up as needed).

## I. Reason for care:

A. The most critical period for a new mother is the *first* 24 hr, specifically because of her need to be monitored for *postpartum hemorrhage*.

B. The need for services occurs when the new mother is asked to return home, often to her full responsibilities, following 9 mo of gestation; has experienced hours of physical/emotional stress of labor; has not had adequate sleep/rest while in the hospital; needs to learn about self-care, recover physically, learn about baby care, and begin attachment/bonding and integrating the new addition with her (their) family structure.

## II. Assessment, (initial)

A. Review of woman's progress through her critical path and what remains to be done; what are her preferences for teaching?

B. Components of discharge planning covered before discharge; what remains to be done (or redone)?

## III. Services offered:

A. Home visits—planned collaboratively with family.

B. Telephone follow-up:

1. Assessment.
2. Health teaching.
3. Identify complications to facilitate timely interventions, including referrals.

C. "Warm" line/help line: not a "crisis" hot line; provides consultation for crisis prevention on such issues as: postpartum depression, the infant's crying, care of hemorrhoids, breastfeeding or suppression of lactation, etc.

D. Support groups (e.g., LaLeche League).

IV. **Care providers:** many home care services are developed and implemented with nurse practitioners who are experts in nursing; telephone follow-up and "warm" lines/help lines may by staffed by knowledgeable volunteers as well.

## Breastfeeding Foundations

Prolactin → milk production
Oxytocin → milk ejection

## Postpartum Home Care—Services with Early Discharge

Home visits
Telephone follow-up
"Warm" line/help line
Support groups

# Summary

The nurse's knowledge of the postpartum client's physical, emotional, and social needs lays the foundation for the nursing process with the woman (and family) during this period, the *"fourth trimester"* of the childbearing cycle. The nurse's skill and dedication are put to the test in trying to achieve high standards of care within the time limits of the DRG-specific requirements. To that end, nurses have developed *critical paths, early discharge classes* and discharge plans, *check lists,* and *home care services* (e.g., telephone follow-up, "warm" lines/help lines) and support groups. Used individually or in combination, these services are effective in preventing crises and facilitating physiologic and psychological adjustments in the postpartum period.

## Study and Memory Aids

### Definition

Decidua—from Latin, "cast off" or "shed"

### Normal Lochia—Assessment

Rubra:        Birth—day 3 or 4
Serosa:       Days 3 → 7
Alba:         Week 2 → 6

### Hemorrhage Prevention—Goal

Hemorrhage remains the No. 1 cause of maternal mortality.

### Psychological/Behavioral Changes—Maternal Role-Taking (Reva Rubin)

Taking-in
↓
Taking-hold
↓
Letting-go

# Questions

1. Postbirth, a new mother begins to bleed excessively. The *first* nursing action is to:
   1. Start an IV with *Pitocin.*
   2. Administer the oxytocic order per os.
   3. Massage the fundus until firm.
   4. Assess for lacerations.

2. A young mother is concerned because someone told her that her uterus weighs 2 pounds now, but will get smaller by "involution." She wonders if involution is a form of weight loss that she can use to lose weight in general. The nurse's response is based on knowledge that uterine involution is accomplished by:
   1. Autolysis.
   2. Inversion.
   3. Regeneration of the three layers of the endometrium.
   4. Scarring at the placental site.

3. In assessing involution of the woman's uterus, the nurse determines that it is normal involution when the uterus is:
   1. Firm, 3 cm above the umbilicus.
   2. Firm, below the umbilicus, in the midline.
   3. Slightly boggy, 2 cm above the umbilicus.
   4. Slightly boggy, below the umbilicus, in the midline.

4. The nurse applies a covered ice pack to a new mother's episiotomy area several hours after childbirth to reduce discomfort by:
   1. Numbing the area to increase comfort.
   2. Minimizing the amount of edema.
   3. Helping her focus on the cold rather than on the pain.
   4. Increasing circulation to the area for more rapid healing.

5. A new mother complains of "afterpains." The nurse's *first* action is to:
   1. Administer ordered analgesics.
   2. Advise her to stop breastfeeding until "afterpains" cease.
   3. Encourage relaxation and breathing exercises.
   4. Assess her for bladder filling.

6. The nurse gathers the following data: a woman gave birth to a daughter instead of a much-desired son. Now, the morning after giving birth, she seems withdrawn, is staying in bed and staring at the wall. Analysis indicates that which action is necessary?
   1. No action, since this is a natural "let-down" after giving birth.
   2. Referral for psychiatric consult.
   3. Reassurance that her baby is beautiful and healthy.
   4. Helping the mother to verbalize her disappointment.

7. In the "taking-hold" phase of postpartum recovery, the nurse can expect the new mother to:
   1. Express concern about her behavior during labor.
   2. State she will assume full care of the baby "tomorrow."
   3. Order extra helpings of food at each mealtime.
   4. Ask to take care of her baby herself.

8. During a postpartum home visit to a new mother on the day after discharge, the nurse's most therapeutic teaching intervention regarding sexual activity is to explain that:
   1. She should use vaseline for lubrication.
   2. She may begin sexual intercourse any time after the first week.
   3. She should use the woman-superior position when resuming sexual intercourse.
   4. She can expect to have the same speed and intensity of response to sexual stimulation as she had before pregnancy.

9. The nurse is teaching a lactation class. A woman confides that she is surprised to learn from the nurse that one of the following is *not* related to successful breastfeeding. That one factor is:
   1. Maternal nutrition.
   2. Rest and relaxation.
   3. Breast size.
   4. Father's/partner's attitude.

10. A new mother tells the nurse, "I want to breastfeed as long as I can because I don't want to use contraceptives." The nurse's best response would be:
    1. "That's right. While breastfeeding, you will not ovulate."
    2. "You do not need to worry as long as you do not menstruate."
    3. "Wait to resume intercourse until your periods start, then use the symptothermal method of contraception."
    4. "It is best to use some type of contraceptive, like foam and condoms."

11. Nursing care for a new mother with engorged breasts who is not breastfeeding includes:
    1. Frequent manual expression of milk, ice bags, analgesics.
    2. Pumping breasts, restriction of fluids, ice bags.

3. Firm support, ice bags, analgesics.
4. Application of a tight binder, administering drugs to suppress lactation.

12. Which is the appropriate *initial* nursing action for a woman with an elevated temperature 4 hr after vaginal birth?
    1. Push fluids by mouth (PO).
    2. Do nothing, since it is a normal finding this soon after giving birth.
    3. Check physician's orders for medication for infection.
    4. Medicate her for pain, since temperature elevation is one sign of pain.

13. Around the third postpartum day, the nurse would describe normal lochia as:
    1. Rubra.
    2. Alba.
    3. Serosa.
    4. Menstra.

14. A woman gave birth 1 ½ hr ago. She is alert and physically active in bed. She states that she needs to urinate. The nurse's *most therapeutic* response is:
    1. "I'll walk you to the bathroom and stay with you."
    2. "You can get up any time you want to, now."
    3. "Make sure you wash your hands before and after, and wipe yourself once with each tissue, from front to back."
    4. "Lean forward a little as you void. This will keep the urine off your stitches and be more comfortable."

15. Which laboratory finding would the nurse note as normal for a new mother following birth?
    1. A drop in hematocrit.
    2. A drop in white blood cell count.
    3. Trace to 1+ proteinuria.
    4. A decrease in coagulation factors.

16. Which new mother would the nurse expect to be an acceptable candidate for safe early discharge?
    1. 17 hr after vaginal birth, third-degree perineal laceration, hemoglobin 12 g.
    2. 32 hr after cesarean birth, voiding and ambulating.
    3. 12 hr after vaginal birth, temperature 100° F, scant lochia rubra.
    4. 28 hr after vaginal birth, membranes ruptured 30 hr before birth, spinal headache.

17. Early discharge following birth carries with it the caution that assessment parameters should be within normal limits for the number of postpartum hours. Which nursing assessment finding would require a delay of a planned discharge at 24 hr postpartum?
    1. Lochia rubra, moderate.
    2. Fundus at umbilicus, firm.
    3. Pulse 62.
    4. Three voidings in 14 hr, total 490 mL.

18. During the fourth stage of labor, which client-centered goal is accurately stated and *takes priority*?
    1. Perineal edema is prevented by application of a covered ice pack.
    2. The woman will verbalize increased comfort.
    3. The woman will saturate no more than one peripad per hour.
    4. The woman is encouraged to void.

19. The postpartum nurse plans nursing care based on the knowledge that in the immediate postpartum period, the most serious consequence likely to occur from bladder distention is:
    1. A urinary tract infection.
    2. Excessive uterine bleeding.
    3. Afterpains.
    4. Bladder wall atony.

20. Which condition would alert the nurse to a possible postbirth hemorrhage?
    1. Precipitate birth.
    2. A full stomach.
    3. Preterm birth.
    4. Pudendal block anesthesia.

21. The nurse is especially alert for postpartum hemorrhage in the woman who:
    1. Had numerous vaginal examinations during labor.
    2. Was recently catheterized for bladder distention.
    3. Gave birth following a 26 hr labor augmented with exogenous oxytocin.
    4. Has diabetes mellitus, well controlled.

22. A woman who gave birth 8 hr ago appears anxious and says she feels "light-headed." A perineal pad has been in place for 15 min and contains clots and a heavy flow of lochia rubra. Which action would the nurse take *first*?
    1. Call the physician.
    2. Assess her vital signs.
    3. Get supplies to start an IV.
    4. Lift both of her legs high.

23. To safely administer ergonovine (*Ergotrate*) or methylergonovine (*Methergine*) to a woman who is postpartum, the nurse should know the woman's:
    1. Blood pressure.
    2. Pulse.
    3. Blood type and Rh.
    4. Method of feeding.

24. During an in-service presentation, nurses are discussing their beliefs about rubella vaccination. The nurse in charge knows that intervention is needed when some of the nurses state that:
    1. Women allergic to duck eggs may develop a hypersensitivity reaction.
    2. Mothers who are lactating should not receive the live attenuated virus.

    3. A transient arthralgia or rash may develop, but is benign.
    4. Women should practice contraception for 2–3 mo after vaccination.

25. A mother is feeding formula to her newborn. She says that he seems to get full fast and that he has regurgitated some of the formula already. She adds, "Maybe I just don't know how to feed him." As the baby sucks on the nipple, large bubbles are seen in the bottle. The nurse suggests:
    1. "Tighten the bottle cap a little."
    2. "Hold the baby in a more upright position."
    3. "Bubble (burp) him after every half ounce."
    4. "Let me show you how. Then you can try again."

26. A nurse breastfeeding her 6-wk-old infant has returned to work in the newborn nursery. She notices that her nipples leak milk whenever she hears any newborn cry. A more experienced nurse suggests that the new mother (like all women who are lactating) needs to wear a breast pad because the let-down reflex in the woman who is lactating is stimulated by:
    1. Oxytocin.
    2. Estradiol.
    3. Pregnanediol.
    4. Luteinizing hormone (LH).

27. Which statement by a mother who is breastfeeding shows correct understanding of the nurse's initial instructions?
    1. "I'll call softly to him to get him to turn toward the breast."
    2. "A 15 min application of ice, followed by the electric pump and nursing, repeated until my breasts soften, will help my engorgement."
    3. "Tapping the baby on the cheek will make him let go of the nipple."
    4. "He will need to be fed less often than a formula-fed baby."

---

**Key to Codes**

**Nursing process: AS,** assessment; **AN,** analysis; **PL,** planning; **IMP,** implementation; **EV,** evaluation. (See **Appendix J** for explanation of nursing process steps.)

**Cognitive level: RE/KN,** recall/knowledge; **COM,** comprehension; **APP,** application; **ANL,** analysis; **EVL,** evaluation; **SYN,** synthesis. (See **Appendix J** for explanation.)

**Category of human function: 1,** protective; **2,** sensory-perceptual; **3,** comfort, rest, activity, and mobility; **4,** nutrition; **5,** growth and development; **6,** fluid-gas transport; **7,** psychosocial-cultural; **8,** elimination. (See **Appendix L** for explanation.)

**Client need: SECE,** safe, effective care environment; **HPM,** health promotion and maintenance; **PsI,** psychosocial integrity; **PhI,** physiological integrity; . (See **Appendix M** for explanation.)

**Client subneed:** See **Appendix M** for explanation.

# Answers/Rationale

1. **(3)** The nurse should massage the fundus until firm and expel any clots. If bladder is filling, ask her to void. Then reassess for continued uterine tone. If bleeding is excessive or uterine tone cannot be maintained, *then* an IV with the ordered amount of *Pitocin* (usually 40 mcg in 1000 mL Ringer's solution) is started (1); this may need to be done by another nurse while the first nurse continues to compress the relaxed uterus. Option **2** is incorrect because any oral preparation requires time to contract the uterus, and is *given* only if uterine tone is not maintained by other means. Assessment for internal vaginal/perineal lacerations (4) may be warranted if continued bleeding is noted *after* the fundus is firmed with gentle massage. **IMP, ANL, 6, HPM, Health promotion and maintenance.**

2. **(1)** Involution is accomplished by autolysis of some tissue, contraction of stretched muscle fibers, and sloughing of the decidua. Inversion (2) is the turning inside-out of the uterus. Only the upper two-thirds of the endometrium are regenerated, *not* the bottom layer (3). *No* scarring of the placental site (4) takes place because regeneration occurs upward from the bottom third of the endometrium. **IMP, RE/KN, 5, HPM, Health promotion and maintenance.**

3. **(2)** Firm, below the umbilicus, in the midline describes the uterus in normal involution. In option 1, the fundus is *high*, possibly indicating a filling bladder, which could soon cause the uterus to relax and hemorrhage to occur. A boggy fundus (3 and 4) indicates uterine *atony*, the No. 1 cause of postpartum hemorrhage. **EV, APP, 5, HPM, Health promotion and maintenance.**

4. **(1)** Numbing the area will increase comfort *several hours* after birth. After the first 2 hr, ice packs have *little* effect on edema formation (2). Distraction (3) does *not* decrease discomfort. Ice packs *decrease* circulation to the area, rather than increasing it (4). **PL, COM, 3, PhI, Basic care and comfort**

5. **(4)** A filling bladder presses up on the lower uterine segment, causing the uterus to relax; the uterus tries to maintain tone by contracting. Analgesics (1) are appropriate only after other comfort measures fail. Mild analgesics given 40 min before the mother breastfeeds, and reassurance that this discomfort is transitory (about 2 days), usually is sufficient for most women. Cessation of breastfeeding (2) is *not* warranted. Encouraging relaxation and breathing exercises (3) is appropriate only *after* ensuring an empty bladder. **IMP, ANL, 3, PhI, Basic care and comfort**

6. **(4)** The nurse should help the mother to verbalize her disappointment. The new mother must accept the reality of the child who was born and let go of the fantasy (or dream) child that she held during the pregnancy. Sometimes, the woman is disappointed and must resolve this response before she can bond with the newborn. This woman's response is *not* suggestive of the natural "letdown" after giving birth or of "baby blues" (1). A psychiatric referral (2) is *not* necessary at *this* time. The response in option 3 does *not* address the new mother's *feelings* at this time; it may be viewed as a "put-down" by the new mother. **PL, APP, 7, PsI, Psychosocial integrity**

7. **(4)** Asking to take care of her baby herself indicates that she has moved out of the "taking-in" phase and into the "taking-hold" phase (per Reva Rubin). The behaviors in options 1, 2, and 3 are all *expected* of a new mother in the "*taking-in*" phase. NOTE: Progression through these phases is not seen today primarily because many women are discharged within hours (6–24) after giving birth. **EV, APP, 7, PsI, Psychosocial integrity**

8. **(3)** The woman-superior position is more comfortable for the woman since she can control the depth and angle of penile penetration. Option 1 is incorrect because petroleum jelly (vaseline) may clog pores or damage condoms or diaphragms. In the postpartum period hormone-poor vaginal mucosa does not provide good lubrication, so dyspareunia is common; the woman should use contraceptive cream (which provides both contraception and lubrication) or a water-soluble product (such as K-Y Jelly). Option 2 is incorrect because most couples are ready to resume sexual intercourse after healing occurs and when lochia stops, usually by about 3 wk postpartum. Option 4 is incorrect because the woman's physiologic response is *slower* and less intense during the early postpartum period. **IMP, APP, 3, HPM, Health promotion and maintenance**

9. **(3)** Breast size is not related to successful lactation. Breast size is genetically determined and is related to amount of fat in the breast. The factors in options 1, 2, and 4 all *are* directly related to the new mother's success with lactation. **AN, RE/KN, 4, HPM, Health promotion and maintenance**

10. **(4)** Breastfeeding is unreliable as a contraceptive method. Foam can be recommended, since the postpartum hormone-poor mucosa does not provide good lubrication and dyspareunia is common; foam with nonoxynol-9 has an antimicrobial action as well as contraceptive value. Condoms decrease the likelihood of transmission of sexually transmitted disease as well as provide contraception. Option 1 is incorrect because some women who breastfeed *have* been known to ovulate as early as the 39th day after giving birth. Option 2 is incorrect because women ovulate before menstruation, and therefore conception *may* occur even before the first menstruation. Option 3 is incorrect because people are usually ready to resume intercourse *sooner* than the time menstruation resumes. Also, although the symptothermal method does provide one method to determine when ovulation resumes, it has a higher failure rate than use of spermicide and condoms. **IMP, COM, 5, HPM, Health promotion and maintenance**

11. (3) Firm support, ice bags, and analgesics may be all that are required for comfort during the transient period (24–36 hr) of engorgement. Emptying the breasts (1 and 2) is the stimulus that is needed for the *continued production* of milk. A tight binder (4) is uncomfortable, and there are no universally accepted antilactogenic drugs (*Parlodel* was taken off the market early in 1995). **IMP, COM, 3, PhI, Basic care and comfort**

12. (2) An elevated temperature is secondary to the work and dehydrating effects of labor and birth. It would only be cause for concern in the presence of *other* signs of infection. She should take only sips of water to meet thirst; if she takes gulps or takes large amounts of water rapidly (1), she may vomit! Elevated temperature, by itself, does not indicate the need for medication (3 and 4). **IMP, ANL, 5, HPM, Health promotion and maintenance**

13. (3) Lochia serosa is usually seen by the third postpartum day. The amount of blood decreases, and the placental site exudes serous material and lymph. Lochia rubra (1) is red and made up of blood, endometrial decidua, and fetal lanugo, vernix, and sometimes meconium and small shreds of placental tissue and membranes; it is usually seen for the *first* 2 days. Lochia alba (2) usually appears about the *third week*. As endometrial epithelialization progresses, the amount of lochia decreases markedly and takes on a seromucinous consistency and a gray-white color. Cessation of lochial flow occurs at about 6 wk. There is *no such word* as menstra (4). **AS, RE/KN, 5, HPM, Health promotion and maintenance**

14. (1) The nurse should accompany the new mother, due to the dangers of hypotension and fainting caused by splanchnic engorgement (excessive filling or pooling of blood within the visceral vasculature that occurs following the removal of pressure from the abdomen, and happens after the birth of a baby). Option 2 is incorrect because this suggests that she get up on her own; instead, the nurse should *accompany* the woman for her first ambulation to decrease the possibility of her fainting and falling. Option 3 is incorrect because although this hygiene measure is correct to prevent infection, it is more important to maintain client safety during her first ambulation. Option 4 is incorrect because this action would indeed be advisable for increasing comfort during voiding if stitches are painful, but it is *more important* to protect her from falling during her first ambulation. **IMP, APP, 1, PhI, Basic care and comfort**

15. (3) Proteinuria, trace to 1+, is a common finding for 1–2 days after a woman gives birth, as a result of the catalytic processes of involution (autolysis, or self-digestion, and breakdown of excess protein in the uterine muscle cells). Hematocrit may *rise* for a short time in normal postpartum cases, rather than drop (1), because there is a greater loss in plasma volume than in blood cells during the first 72 hr. An *increase* in white blood cells (leukocytosis

of pregnancy), averaging about 12,000 mcg/L (20,000–25,000), is normal during pregnancy, rather than a decrease (2). An extensive *activation* of blood-clotting factors occurs after childbirth, rather than a decrease (4). **AS, RE/KN, 8, PhI, Reduction of risk potential**

16. (3) This mother meets the criteria for early discharge at 12 hr after vaginal birth: slight temperature elevation (100° F, 37.8° C) is expected as a normal consequence of labor (an elevation of 100.4° F, 38° C or less is acceptable); lochia is within normal range. The woman should have an intact perineum, *without* third- or fourth-degree perineal laceration (1), to qualify for early discharge. A cesarean birth (2) constitutes a "*complicated* birth"; the usual postoperative stay is 2–3 days. Another *deterrent* to early discharge is premature rupture of membranes (4). **AN, COM, 1, SECE, Management of care**

17. (4) 490 mL total output is *insufficient*. The new mother should be experiencing diuresis at this time, voiding about 3000 mL/24 hr on the first postpartum day, as her water metabolism reverts to the nonpregnant state. The findings in options 1, 2, and 3 all *are* within normal limits at this time. **EV, ANL, 8, HPM, Health promotion and maintenance**

18. (3) The woman who saturates one or more peripads in 1 hr is in danger; postpartum hemorrhage is commonly defined as 500 mL/first 24 hr. Uterine atony is the most common cause of hemorrhage during the fourth stage; hemorrhage remains one of the most life-threatening complications worldwide for new mothers. While the goals in options 1, 2, and 4 are desirable, they do *not directly* relate to a threat to life and well-being, such as hemorrhage, and do not take priority.

NOTE: An accurately stated goal contains three elements: who, what, within what time limits. *Who* = the woman; *what* = will saturate no more than one peripad; *what time period* = 1 hr. **PL, ANL, 6, HPM, Health promotion and maintenance**

19. (2) A full bladder presses on the lower uterine segment and raises the uterus in the abdomen; therefore, the living ligature of the uterine fundus cannot contract and excessive uterine bleeding can occur. A distended bladder alone does *not* cause urinary tract infection (1) *immediately*; uterine atony is the *immediate* consequence. Afterpains (3) are caused by uterine contractions (which *prevent* excessive uterine bleeding). Repeated and prolonged bladder distention does cause bladder wall atony (4); however, the *immediate* danger is that even with the first distention, *uterine atony* can occur. **PL, ANL, 6, PhI, Physiological adaptation**

20. **(1)** Precipitate birth causes the uterus to become very tired, so that it does not contract well, resulting in increased risk of hemorrhage. Precipitate birth is birth following very rapid labor. The labor—from the beginning of cervical dilatation and effacement to full dilatation and birth—is 3 hr in length or less. (Rapid labor/birth can also result in lacerations of the cervix, lower uterine segment, vagina, and perineum.) A full stomach **(2)** does *not* cause postbirth hemorrhage. Preterm birth **(3)** is *not* a cause of postbirth hemorrhage. Pudendal block anesthesia **(4)** does *not* affect uterine muscle tone; the living ligature is not affected by this anesthesia. **AN, COM, 6, PhI, Physiological adaptation**

21. **(3)** Constant, prolonged stimulation of any muscle leads to fatigue in that muscle; uterine atony and hemorrhage can result from a 26 hr, augmented labor. Numerous vaginal examinations during labor **(1)** can predispose the woman to postpartum ("childbed") fever, but are *not* considered a precipitating factor in postpartum hemorrhage. Catheterization to keep the bladder empty **(2)** is a preventive measure *against* postpartum uterine atony and hemorrhage. A woman with well-controlled diabetes **(4)** usually has a baby whose weight is average for gestational age (AGA) and does *not* experience hydramnios (that is, her uterus has not been overdistended; her muscle tone, and therefore her risk of hemorrhage, should be *similar to that of other* women who are postpartum). **AN, ANL, 6, HPM, Health promotion and maintenance**

22. **(4)** Blood flow to the head and heart can be improved by lifting her legs. Then the nurse massages the fundus while calling for help verbally or by pressing the emergency button. Calling the physician first **(1)** would *delay* therapeutic intervention. Assessing her vital signs first **(2)** would *delay* therapeutic intervention; the nurse already knows that the woman's blood pressure has fallen since she complained of light-headedness and is anxious. Getting supplies first **(3)** to start an IV would *delay* therapeutic intervention; a second nurse would start the IV, etc. **IMP, ANL, 6, PhI, Physiological adaptation**

23. **(1)** Ergot products, used to contract the uterus, cause vasoconstriction and can raise blood pressure. Therefore, they are not given to women who have high blood pressure from any cause. Pulse **(2)**, blood type and Rh, **(3)** and method of feeding **(4)** are *not relevant* when safely administering an ergot product to increase uterine tone. **AS, COM, 6, PhI, Pharmacological and parenteral therapies**

24. **(2)** Mothers who are lactating *can* receive the live attenuated virus. The statements in options **1, 3,** and **4** are all *true* regarding rubella vaccination during the early postpartum period and therefore intervention is *not* needed.

NOTE: If the woman receiving rubella vaccination is also Rh negative and is a candidate for RhoGAM, she should be tested within 3 mo to determine if the vaccination "took." The RhoGAM may prevent the vaccination from "taking" and she will not be immune to rubella. Rubella vaccination would then need to be repeated. **EV, RE/KN, 1, SECE, Safety and infection control**

25. **(1)** A loose cap allows too much air into the bottle. The air bubbles result in a feeling of fullness and discomfort; regurgitation is common. The large bubbles are responsible in this situation, *not* positioning **(2)**. Although frequent burping **(3)** is appropriate, it does *not* resolve the problem of air bubbles. The comment in option **4** is a *put-down* for the mother, implying that the nurse "knows better." **IMP, COM, 4, HPM, Health promotion and maintenance**

26. **(1)** Oxytocin, produced by the posterior pituitary, stimulates the let-down reflex. Stimuli (infant's sucking, mother's emotions) stimulate the hypothalamus, which then stimulates the pituitary gland. Estradiol **(2)**, produced by the ovary, is the most potent naturally occurring human hormone in women; estrogen *prepares* the breasts for lactation. Pregnanediol **(3)** is a biologically *inactive* compound found in the urine of women during pregnancy or the secretory phase of the menstrual cycle; it is produced by the reduction of progesterone. LH **(4)**, produced by the anterior pituitary, stimulates secretion of sex hormones by the ovary; it is involved in the *maturation of ova.* **IMP, RE/KN, 5, HPM, Health promotion and maintenance**

27. **(2)** Covered ice packs for no more than 15 min, followed by the electric pump and nursing (repeat as necessary) until the breasts are softened, is one treatment for engorgement in mothers who are breastfeeding. Application of warm, moist heat may help lessen the engorgement; however, most mothers' breasts are so swollen that heat only brings more blood to an already congested area. Newborn infants do *not* respond to voice **(1)**; the mother needs to bring the baby to the breast with a nipple touching the cheek or lips to elicit the rooting reflex. To break the suction **(3)**, the mother needs to gently insert her finger into the corner of the baby's mouth between the gums; pulling the baby away without breaking suction can be painful and lead to sore nipples. Babies who are breastfed often feed *more* frequently than babies who are formula-fed, *not* less frequently **(4)**. **EV, EVL, 4, HPM, Health promotion and maintenance**

# Complications During the Postpartal Period

---

## 🔑 Key Points

- Postpartum hemorrhage is the most common and most serious type of excessive maternal blood loss; *causes*: uterine atony; lacerations of the birth canal; subinvolution of placental site, retained placental tissue, or infection.

- Clotting disorders—hypofibrinogenemia and disseminated intravascular coagulation (DIC) are associated with a number of pregnancy-related conditions.

- Postpartum infection is a significant cause of maternal morbidity; its origin may be a *continuation* from the antepartum period or a *result* of intrapartal events.

- Sequelae of childbirth trauma include: alterations in pelvic support, uterine displacement, and genital fistulas.

**General overview:** Postpartum complications arise from many sources. Some problems that the new mother may experience in the postpartum period result from h*igh-risk medical conditions* that *predate* the pregnancy (e.g., heart disease, diabetes mellitus, and infections). Others have *antecedents during* pregnancy (e.g., pre-eclampsia/eclampsia and HELLP syndrome). Intrapartum events can give rise to postpartum infections (e.g., placenta previa, or a long, difficult labor with many vaginal examinations). These conditions have been covered in previous chapters.

## Key Words

Disseminated intravascular coagulation (DIC)

Hypofibrinogenemia

Postpartum hemorrhage

    Uterine atony

    Lacerations

    Subinvolution

Postpartum infection

    "Childbed fever"

    Endometritis

    Pelvic cellulitis or parametritis

    Perineal infection

    Mastitis

    Thrombophlebitis

Postpartum psychosis

Sheehan's syndrome

# Disorders Affecting Fluid–Gas Transport

## Postpartum Hemorrhage

**Definition**: loss of 500 mL of blood or more during first 24 hr postpartum in *vaginal* birth; 1000 mL in *cesarean* birth.

I. **Pathophysiology**: excessive loss of blood secondary to trauma, decreased uterine contractility → hypovolemia.

II. **Etiology/risk factors** (in order of frequency):

A. Uterine atony.

1. Uterine overdistention (multiple pregnancy, polyhydramnios, fetal macrosomia).
2. Multiparity.
3. Prolonged or precipitous labor.
4. Anesthesia—general or regional (particularly saddle block).
5. Myomata (fibroids).
6. Oxytocin induction of labor.
7. Overmassage of uterus in postpartum.
8. Distended bladder.

B. Lacerations—cervical, vagina, perineal.

C. Retained placental fragments—usually delayed postpartum hemorrhage.

D. Hematoma—deep pelvic, vaginal, or episiotomy site.

III. **Assessment** (review *warning signs*, **Chapter 6, p. 152**)

A. *Uterus*: boggy, flaccid; excessive vaginal bleeding (dark; seepage, large clots)—due to uterine atony, retained placental fragments.

B. **Signs of shock**: air hunger; anxiety/ apprehension, tachycardia, tachypnea, hypotension.

C. *Blood values* (admission and postpartal): Hgb, Hct, clotting time.

D. Estimated *blood loss*: during labor/birth; in early postpartum.

E. *Pain*: vulvar, vaginal, perineal.

F. *Perineum*: distended—due to edema; discoloration—due to hematoma.

G. *Vaginal hematoma*: "feeling of fullness"; assessed when woman is *side lying* with knees drawn up, bearing down; a dark purple-blue mass seen at the vaginal introitus is characteristic. Woman may also complain of rectal pressure.

H. *Lacerations*: bright-red vaginal bleeding with firm fundus.

IV. **Analysis/nursing diagnosis**

A. *Fluid volume deficit* related to excessive blood loss secondary to uterine atony, retained placental fragments.

B. *Anxiety/fear* related to unexpected complication.

C. *Tissue perfusion alteration* related to decreased oxygenation secondary to blood loss.

D. *Activity intolerance* related to fatigue.

V. **Nursing care plan/implementation**

A. *Medical management.*

1. Intravenous oxytocin infusion; intravenous or oral ergot preparations (*ergonovine* [*Ergotrate Maleate*], *methylergonovine* [*Methergine*]); *carboprost* (*Prostin/M15*), *Hemabate*, an *oxytocic*; *prostaglandin*. (See **Pharmacology Box 6.1**).

2. *Lab tests*: clotting time, platelet count, fibrinogen level, hemoglobin, hematocrit, CBC.

3. Type and cross-match for blood replacement.

4. Surgical:

a. Repair of lacerations.
b. Evacuation, ligation of hematoma.
c. Curettage—retained placental fragments.

B. *Nursing management.*

1. Goal: *minimize blood loss.*

a. Notify physician promptly of abnormal assessment findings.
b. Order laboratory work **STAT**, as directed—to determine blood loss and etiology.
c. Fundal massage.
d. Administer medications to stimulate uterine tone.

2. Goal: *stabilize status.*

a. Establish IV line—to enable administration of medications and rapid absorption/action. Administer *whole blood* (with larger catheter).
b. Administer medications, as ordered—to control bleeding, combat shock.
c. Prepare for surgery, as ordered.

3. Goal: *prevent infection.* Strict aseptic technique; use *standard precautions*.

4. Goal: *continual monitoring.* Vital signs, bleeding (do pad count or weigh pads), fundal status.

5. Goal: *prevent sequelae (Sheehan's syndrome)*—hypopituitarism following an infarct of the pituitary following postpartum hemorrage.

6. Goal: **health teaching**. After episode: reinforce appropriate perineal care and handwashing techniques.

VI. **Evaluation/outcome criteria**: The woman's:

A. Vital signs are stable.

B. Bleeding has diminished or is absent.

C. Assessment findings are within normal limits.

## Subinvolution

**Definition**: delayed return of uterus to normal size, shape, position.

I. **Pathophysiology**: inability of inflamed uterus (endometritis) to contract effectively → incomplete uterine involution; failure of contractions to effect closure of vessels in site of placental attachment → bleeding.

II. **Etiology/risk factors**:

A. Premature or prolonged rupture of membranes (PROM) with secondary amnionitis, endometritis.

B. Retained placental fragments.

C. Oxytocin stimulation or augmentation of labor of overdistended uterine muscle may interfere with involution.

III. **Assessment**

A. *Uterus*: large, flabby; lack of uterine tone; failure to progressively shrink.

B. *Discharge*: persistent lochia; painless fresh bleeding, hemorrhagic episodes.

IV. **Analysis/nursing diagnosis**

A. *Pain* related to tender, inflamed uterus secondary to endometritis.

B. *Anxiety/fear* related to change in physical status.

C. *Knowledge deficit* related to diagnosis, treatment, prognosis.

D. *Injury risk* related to infection.

E. *Fluid volume deficit* related to excessive bleeding.

V. **Nursing care plan/implementation**

A. *Medical management*

1. Surgical (curettage)—to remove placental fragments.

2. *Antibiotic* therapy—to treat intrauterine infection.

3. *Oxytocics*—to stimulate/enhance uterine contractions.

B. *Nursing management*

1. Have woman void or catheterize; massage uterus gently.

2. Goal: **health teaching.**
   a. Explain condition and treatment.
   b. Describe, demonstrate perineal care, pad change, handwashing.

3. Goal: *emotional support.* Encourage verbalization of anxiety regarding recovery, separation from newborn.

4. Goal: *promote healing.*
   a. Encourage rest, compliance with medical/nursing regimen.
   b. Administer *oxytocics, antibiotics,* as ordered.

VI. **Evaluation/outcome criteria:** The woman:

A. Verbalizes understanding of condition and treatment.

B. Complies with medical/nursing regimen.

C. Demonstrates normal involutional progress.

D. Has assessment findings (vital signs, fundal height and consistency, lochial discharge) that are within normal limits.

E. Expresses satisfaction with care.

# Hypofibrinogenemia

I. **Pathophysiology:** decreased clotting factors, fibrinogen; may be accompanied by disseminated intravascular coagulation (DIC).

II. **Etiology/risk factors:**

A. Missed abortion (retained dead fetus syndrome).

B. Fetal death, delayed emptying of uterine contents.

C. Abruptio placentae; Couvelaire uterus.

D. Amniotic fluid (pulmonary) embolism.

E. Hypertension.

III. **Assessment**

A. Observe for bleeding from injection sites, epistaxis, purpura.

B. See DIC *assessment* (**p. 162**).

C. Maternal vital signs, color.

D. I&O.

E. *Diagnostic laboratory tests*:

1. Thrombin clot test—**important**: size and persistence of clot.
2. Prothrombin time (PT)—*prolonged.*
3. Bleeding time—*prolonged.*
4. Platelet count—*decreased.*
5. Activated partial thromboplastin time—*prolonged.*
6. Fibrinogen (factor I concentration)—*decreased.*
7. Fibrin degradation products—*present.*

IV. **Analysis/nursing diagnosis**

A. *Fluid volume deficit* related to uncontrolled bleeding secondary to coagulopathy.

B. *Anxiety/fear* related to unexpected critical emergency.

C. *Tissue perfusion alteration* related to decreased oxygenation secondary to blood loss.

V. **Nursing care plan/implementation**

A. *Medical management.*

1. Replace platelets.
2. Replace blood loss.
3. IV *heparin*—to inhibit conversion of fibrinogen to fibrin.

B. *Nursing management.*

1. Goal: *continuous monitoring.*
   a. Vital signs.
   b. I&O hourly.
   c. Skin: color, emergence of petechiae.
   d. Note, measure (as possible), record and report blood loss.

2. Goal: *control blood loss.*
   a. Establish IV line, administer fluids or blood products as ordered.
   b. *Position: side-lying*—to maintain blood supply to vital organs.

3. Goal: *emotional support.*
   a. Encourage verbalization of anxiety, fear, concerns.
   b. Explain all procedures.
   c. Remain with woman continuously.
   d. Keep woman and family informed.

**VI. Evaluation/outcome criteria:** The woman's:

A. Bleeding is controlled.

B. Laboratory studies are returning to normal values.

C. Status is stable.

## Disseminated Intravascular Coagulation (DIC):

**Definition**: diffuse or widespread coagulation initially within arterioles and capillaries leading to hemorrhage.

I. **Pathophysiology**: activation of coagulation system from tissue injury → fibrin, microthrombin form in brain, kidneys, lungs → microinfarcts, tissue necrosis → red blood cells, *platelets*, prothrombin, other clotting factors trapped, destroyed in process → excessive clotting → release of fibrin split products → inhibition of platelet clotting → bleeding.

II. **Etiology/risk factors:**

A. Obstetric complications (see **Hypofibrinogenemia, etiology, p. 161**).

B. Neoplastic disease.

C. Low perfusion states, e.g., severe pre-eclampsia.

III. **Assessment**—*objective data*:

A. Skin, mucous membranes: petechiae, ecchymosis.

B. Extremities (fingers, toes): cyanosis.

C. Bleeding: venipuncture sites, wound, oral, rectal, vaginal.

D. Urine output: oliguria → anuria.

E. Level of consciousness: convulsions, coma.

F. Laboratory data: *prolonged*—PT (> 15 sec); *decreased*—platelets, fibrinogen level.

IV. **Analysis/nursing diagnosis**

A. *Tissue perfusion alteration* related to peripheral microthrombi.

B. *Injury risk* (death) related to bleeding.

C. *Skin impairment risk* related to ischemia.

D. *Urinary elimination alteration* related to renal tubular necrosis.

VI. **Nursing care plan/implementation**

A. Goal: *prevent and detect further bleeding*.

1. Carry out nursing measures designed to alleviate underlying problem (e.g., shock, birth of fetus).

2. Medications: *heparin* SO$_4$ IV, 1000 U/hr, if ordered, to reverse abnormal clotting (controversial).

3. IVs: blood to lessen shock; platelets, cryoprecipitate, fresh plasma to restore clotting factors, fibrinogen.

4. Observe: vital signs, *central venous pressure* (CVP) (normal 5–15 mm Hg), *pulmonary artery pressure* (PAP) (normal 20–30 systolic and 8–12 diastolic), and *intake and output* for signs of shock or fluid overload from frequent infusions; specimens for *occult blood* (urine, stool).

5. Precautions: *avoid* IM injections if possible; apply pressure 5 min to venipuncture sites; *no* rectal temperatures.

VI. **Evaluation/outcome criteria**

A. Clotting mechanism restored (increased platelets, normal PT).

B. Renal function restored (urine output > 30 mL/hr).

C. Circulation to fingers, toes; no cyanosis.

D. No irreversible damage from renal, cerebral, cardiac, or adrenal hemorrhage.

# Disorders Affecting Protective Functions

## Postpartum Infection (See Table 7.1, p. 163).

### General aspects

**Definition**: reproductive system infection occurring during the postpartal period.

I. **Pathophysiology**: bacterial invasion of birth canal; most common: localized infection of the lining of the uterus (**endometritis**).

II. **Etiology:**

A. Anaerobic nonhemolytic streptococci.

B. *Escherichia coli*.

C. *Chlamydia trachomatis* (bacteroides).

D. Staphylococci.

III. **Risk factors/predisposing conditions:**

A. Anemia.

B. Premature or prolonged rupture of membranes (PROM).

C. Prolonged labor.

D. Repeated vaginal examinations during labor.

E. Intrauterine manipulation—e.g., manual extraction of placenta.

F. Retained placental fragments.

G. Postpartum hemorrhage.

IV. **Assessment**

A. Fever 38° C (100.4° F) or more on two or more occasions after first 24 hr postpartum. *Warning: puerperal infection.*

B. Other signs of infection: pain, malaise, dysuria, subinvolution, foul odor to lochia.

V. **Analysis/nursing diagnosis**

A. *Fluid volume deficit* related to excessive blood loss, anemia.

B. *Knowledge deficit* related to danger signs of postpartum period.

C. *Injury risk* related to infection.

*(continued on p. 164)*

## TABLE 7.1 POSTPARTUM INFECTIONS

| Condition/Etiology | ► Assessment:Signs/Symptoms | ► Nursing Interventions |
|---|---|---|
| **Postpartum infection** | | |
| Traumatic labor and birth and postpartum hemorrhage make women more vulnerable to infection by such bacteria as nonhemolytic streptococci, *Escherichia coli*, and *Staphylococcus species* | 1. Dependent on location and severity of infection<br>2. Usually include fever, pain, swelling, and tenderness<br>3. Temperature ≥ 100.4° F (38° C) *after first 24 hr postbirth on 2 or more occasions* indicates puerperal infection ("childbed fever") | 1. *Monitor*:<br>   Signs and symptoms<br>   Drainage (e.g., uterine)<br>2. Obtain culture and sensitivity<br>3. Administer *antimicrobial* agents and *analgesic* agents<br>4. Ensure comfort; encourage rest<br>5. Use *standard precautions*<br>6. *Force fluids* and provide *high calorie diet*<br>7. Keep family informed of mother's and newborn's progress<br>8. Promote maternal-infant contact as soon as possible<br>9. Plan and implement discharge and follow-up care |
| **Endometritis** | | |
| Microorganisms invade placental site, and may spread to entire endometrium | 1. Fever<br>2. Chills<br>3. Anorexia<br>4. Malaise<br>5. Boggy uterus<br>6. Foul-smelling lochia<br>7. Uterine cramps | 1. Administer *antimicrobial* agents and *analgesic* agents<br>2. Encourage *Fowler's position* to promote drainage<br>3. *Force fluids*<br>4. Use *standard precautions* |
| **Pelvic cellulitis or parametritis** | | |
| Microorganisms spread via lymphatics and invade tissues surrounding uterus | 1. Fever<br>2. Chills<br>3. Lower abdominal pain<br>4. Tenderness | 1. Administer *antimicrobial* agents and *analgesic* agents<br>2. Encourage bedrest<br>3. *Force fluids* |
| **Perineal infection** | | |
| Trauma to perineum makes women more vulnerable to infection | 1. Localized pain<br>2. Fever<br>3. Swelling<br>4. Redness<br>5. Seropurulent drainage | 1. Administer *antimicrobial* agents and *analgesic* agents<br>2. Provide sitz baths or other heat/cold applications<br>3. Use *standard precautions* |
| **Mastitis** | | |
| Lesions or fissures on nipples allow entry of microorganisms (e.g., *Staphylococcus aureus*) from nose/mouth of infant or mother's unwashed hands (breast milk is a good medium for growth of organism) | 1. Marked engorgement<br>2. Pain<br>3. Chills<br>4. Fever<br>5. Tachycardia<br>! 6. If untreated, single or multiple breast abscesses may form | 1. Order culture and sensitivity studies of mother's milk<br>2. Administer *antimicrobial* agents and *analgesic* agents<br>3. Apply heat or cold therapy<br>4. Assist with incising and draining abscesses<br>5. Use *standard precautions* and perform meticulous handwashing |
| **Thrombophlebitis** | | |
| Infected pelvic or femoral thrombi<br>Increased tendency to clot formation during pregnancy !<br>Trauma to tissues<br>Hemorrhage decreases new mother's resistance to infection | 1. Pain<br>2. Chills and fever<br>3. *Femoral*: stiffness of affected area or part and *positive Homan's sign*<br>4. *Pelvic*: severe chills and wide fluctuations in temperature | *Femoral:*<br>1. Rest and *elevate* leg<br>2. Administer *antimicrobial* agents, *analgesic* agents, and *anticoagulants*<br>*Pelvic:*<br>1. Encourage bedrest<br>2. *Force fluids*<br>3. Administer *antimicrobial* agents and *anticoagulants* |

*Source*: ©Lagelquist, S. Davis's *NCLEX-RN® Success*, Philadelphia.

▶◀ **VI. Nursing care plan/implementation:** *prevention*

   A. Goal: *prevent anemia.*

      1. Minimize blood loss—accurate postpartal assessment and management of bleeding.

      🍎 2. *Diet*: *high* protein, *high* vitamin.

      💊 3. Vitamins, iron—suggest continuing prenatal pattern until postpartum check-up.

   B. Goal: *prevent entrance/transport of microorganisms.*

      ⚠ 1. Strict aseptic technique during labor, birth and postpartum (*standard precautions*).

      2. Minimize vaginal examinations during labor.

      ☞ 3. Perineal care.

   📖 C. Goal: **health teaching.**

      ✋ 1. Handwashing—before and after each pad change, after voiding and/or defecating.

      ☞ 2. Perineal care—wipe from front to back; use clear, warm water or mild antiseptic solution as a cascade; do *not* separate labia.

      ☞ 3. Maintain sterility of pads; apply from front to back.

      4. *Avoid* use of tampons until normal menstrual cycle resumes.

▶◀ **VII. Evaluation/outcome criteria**

   A. The woman's assessment findings are within normal limits.

      1. Vital signs.

      2. Rate of involution (fundal height, consistency).

      3. Lochia: character, amount, odor.

   B. The woman avoids infection.

## Endometritis—Infection of Lining of Uterus

   I. **Pathophysiology**: see *General aspects*, (**p. 162**).

   II. **Etiology**: most common: invasion by normal body flora (e.g., anaerobic streptococci).

   III. **Characteristics:**

      A. *Mild*, localized—asymptomatic, or low-grade fever.

      B. *Severe*—may lead to ascending infection, parametritis, pelvic abscess, pelvic thrombophlebitis.

      C. If remains localized, self-limiting; usually resolves within 10 days.

▶◀ **IV. Assessment**

   A. *Signs of infection*: fever, chills, malaise, anorexia, headache, backache.

   B. *Uterus*: large, boggy, extremely tender

      1. Subinvolution.

      2. Lochia: dark brown; foul odor.

▶◀ **V. Analysis/nursing diagnosis**

   A. *Anxiety/fear* related to effects on self and newborn.

   B. *Self-esteem disturbance and role performance alteration* related to inability to meet own expectations regarding parenting, secondary to unexpected hospitalization.

   C. *Pain* related to inflammation/infection.

   D. *Individual coping impairment* related to physical discomfort and psychological stress associated with self-concept disturbance; worry, guilt, concern regarding newborn at home.

   E. *Family processes alteration* with interruption of adjustment to altered life pattern related to postpartal infection/hospitalization.

▶◀ **VI. Nursing care plan/implementation**

   A. Goal: *prevent cross-contamination.*

      1. Contact-item isolation.

      ⚠ 2. Use *standard precautions*.

   B. Goal: *facilitate drainage.*

      1. Position: semi-Fowler's.

   🍎 C. Goal: *nutrition/hydration.*

      1. *Diet*: *high* calorie, *high* protein, *high* vitamin.

      2. Push *fluids* to 4000 mL/d (oral and/or IV, as ordered).

      3. I&O.

   D. Goal: *increase uterine tone/facilitate involution.*

      💊 1. Administer medications, as ordered (e.g., oxytocics, antibiotics).

   E. Goal: *minimize energy expenditure, as possible.*

      1. Bedrest.

      2. Maximize rest, comfort.

   F. Goal: *emotional support.*

      1. Encourage verbalization of anxiety, concerns.

      2. Keep informed of progress.

▶◀ **VII. Evaluation/outcome criteria:** The woman responds to medical/nursing regimen.

   A. Vital signs stable, within normal limits.

   B. All assessment findings within normal limits.

   C. Unable to recover organism from discharge.

## Urinary Tract Infections (UTIs)

   I. **Pathophysiology**: normal physiologic changes associated with pregnancy (e.g., ureteral dilatation) and the postpartal period (e.g., diuresis, increased bladder capacity with diminished sensitivity of stretch receptors) → increased susceptibility to bacterial invasion and growth → ascending infections (cystitis, pyelonephritis).

   II. **Etiology**: usually bacterial.

   III. **Risk factors:**

      A. Birth trauma to bladder, urethra, or meatus.

      B. Bladder hypotonia with retention (due to intrapartal anesthesia or trauma).

      C. Repeated or prolonged catheterization, or poor technique.

▶◀ **IV. Assessment**

   A. Maternal vital signs (fever, tachycardia).

   B. Dysuria, frequency (flank pain—with pyelonephritis).

   C. Feeling of "not emptying" bladder.

   D. Cloudy urine; frank pus.

V. **Analysis/nursing diagnosis**
  A. *Urinary elimination alteration* related to diuresis, dysuria, inflammation/infection.
  B. *Pain* related to dysuria secondary to cystitis.
  C. *Knowledge deficit* related to self-care (perineal care).

VI. **Nursing care plan/implementation**
  A. Goal: *minimize perineal edema.*
    1. Perineal ice pack in *fourth stage*—to limit swelling secondary to trauma, facilitate voiding.
    2. Perineal ice pack after *first 2 hr*—to provide comfort.
  B. Goal: *prevent overdistention of bladder.*
    1. Monitor level of fundus, lochia, bladder distention. (NOTE: Distended bladder displaces uterus, limits its ability to contract → boggy fundus → increased vaginal bleeding.)
    2. Encourage *fluids* and voiding; I&O.
    3. *Aseptic* technique for catheterization.
    4. Slow emptying of bladder on catheterization—to maintain tone.
  C. Goal: *identification of causative organism* to facilitate ordering of appropriate medication (*antibiotics*). Obtain clean-catch (or catheterized) specimen for culture and sensitivity.
  D. Goal: **health teaching.** See previous discussion re: fluids, general hygiene, diet, and medications.

VII. **Evaluation/outcome criteria:** The woman responds to medical/nursing regimen.
  A. Voiding: quantity sufficient (although small, frequent output may mean overflow with retention).
  B. Urine character: clear, amber, or straw-colored.
  C. Vital signs: within normal limits.
  D. No complaints of frequency, urgency, burning on urination, flank pain.

## Mastitis—Inflammation of Breast Tissue

I. **Pathophysiology:** local inflammatory response to bacterial invasion; suppuration may occur; organism can be recovered from breast milk.

II. **Etiology:** most common: *Staphylococcus aureus;* source—most common: infant's nose, throat.

III. **Assessment**
  A. Signs of infection (may occur several weeks postpartum):
    1. Fever.
    2. Chills.
    3. Tachycardia.
    4. Malaise.
    5. Abdominal pain.
  B. Breast:
    1. Reddened area(s).
    2. Localized/generalized swelling.
    3. Heat, tenderness, palpable mass.

IV. **Analysis/nursing diagnosis**
  A. *Skin integrity impairment* related to nipple fissures, cracks.
  B. *Pain* related to tender, inflamed tissue secondary to infection.
  C. *Body image, self-esteem disturbance* related to association of breastfeeding with female identity and role.
  D. *Anxiety/fear* related to sexuality; impact on breastfeeding, if any.

V. **Nursing care plan/implementation**
  A. Goal: *prevent infection.* **Health teaching** in early postpartum.
    1. Handwashing.
    2. Breast care—wash with warm water only (*no soap*)—to prevent removing protective body oils.
    3. Let breast milk dry on nipples to prevent drying of tissue.
    4. Clean bra (with no plastic pads or liners) to support breasts, reduce friction, minimize exposure to microorganisms.
    5. Good breastfeeding techniques (see **p. 149–150**).
    6. Alternate position of infant for nursing to change pressure areas.
  B. Goal: *comfort measures.*
    1. Encourage bra or binder—to support breasts, reduce pain from motion.
    2. Local heat or ice packs as ordered—to reduce engorgement, pain.
    3. Administer *analgesics*, as necessary.
  C. Goal: *emotional support.*
    1. Encourage verbalization of feelings, concerns.
    2. If breastfeeding discontinued, reassure woman that she will be able to resume breastfeeding.
  D. Goal: *promote healing.*
    1. Maintain lactation (if desired) by manual expression or breast pump, every 4 hr.
    2. Administer *antibiotics* as ordered.

VI. **Evaluation/outcome criteria:** The woman:
  A. Promptly responds to medical/nursing regimen.
    1. Symptoms subside.
    2. Assessment findings within normal limits.
  B. Successfully returns to breastfeeding.

## Thrombophlebitis

I. **Pathophysiology:** inflammation of a vein secondary to lodging of a clot.

II. **Etiology/risk factors:**
  A. Extension of endometritis with involvement of pelvic and femoral veins.
  B. Clot formation in pelvic veins following cesarean birth.

C. Clot formation in femoral (or other) veins secondary to poor circulation, compression, and venous stasis.

### III. Assessment
A. *Pelvic*—pain: abdominal or pelvic tenderness.
B. *Calf*—pain: positive *Homans'* sign (pain elicited by flexion of foot with knee extended).
C. *Femoral*:
   1. Pain.
   2. Malaise, fever, chills.
   3. Swelling.

### IV. Analysis/nursing diagnosis
A. *Pain* in affected region related to local inflammatory response.
B. *Anxiety/fear* related to outcome.
C. *Individual coping impairment* related to unexpected postpartum complications, hospitalization, separation from newborn.
D. *Physical mobility impairment* related to imposed bedrest to prevent the formation and dislodging of a clot (embolus).

### V. Nursing care plan/implementation
A. Goal: *prevent clot formation.*
   1. Encourage early ambulation.
   2. *Position*: *avoid* prolonged compression of popliteal space.
   3. Apply TED hose, and/or sequential compression stockings as ordered, preoperatively and/or postoperatively for cesarean birth or client at high risk of thrombophebitis.
B. Goal: *reduce threat of emboli.*
   1. *Bedrest*, with cradle to support bedding.
   2. Discourage massaging "leg cramps."
C. Goal: *prevent further clot formation.*
   1. Administer *anticoagulants*, as ordered.
D. Goal: *prevent infection.*
   1. Administer *antibiotics*, as ordered.
   2. Push *fluids*.
E. Goal: *facilitate clot resolution.* Heat therapy, as ordered.

### VI. Evaluation/outcome criteria: The woman responds to medical/nursing regimen.
A. Symptoms subside; all assessment findings within normal limits.
B. No evidence of further clot formation.

# Disorders Affecting Psychosocial–Cultural Functions

## Postpartum Psychosis

### I. General aspects
A. Can occur in both new parents.

B. Usually occurs within 2–4 wks of birth.
C. Increased incidence among single parents; 1–2% of mothers per 1,000 live births.
D. Most common symptomatology: affective disorders.
E. Psychiatric interventions required in small percentage of cases; if underlying cause unresolved, increased risk in subsequent pregnancies.

### II. Etiology/risk factors:
A. Unresolved role conflicts.
B. Unachieved normal development tasks.

### III. Assessment
A. Onset of postpartum psychosis is abrupt and occurs within days of childbirth.
B. *Symptoms* (early).
   1. May resemble *depression* (withdrawal) and then suddenly escalate to: delirium, hallucinations, anger toward self and baby, bizarre behavior, manifestations of *mania*, thoughts of hurting self or baby; paranoia.
   2. Loss of contact with reality.
   3. High suicide risk.
C. Differentiated from *postpartum depression.*
   1. Incidence: 7–20% of new mothers; within 6 mo after childbirth.
   2. Symptoms last > 2 wks; include at least 4 of the following: anorexia, weight loss, insomnia, neglect of personal hygiene; feelings of: worthlessness, guilt, fatigue, hypochondria; fear of harming baby; self destructive; loss of interest in usual activities; ↓ sex drive; psychomotor agitation.
   3. Contact with reality: intact, but can be disoriented.
D. Differentiated from "*baby blues*" (postpartum blues) because the "blues," usually transient and affecting 70–80% of women within 3–5 days after giving birth, (26% in adolescent mothers); periodic crying spells and is characterized by: feelings of loneliness or rejection, anxiety, confusion, restlessness, exhaustion, forgetfulness, and inability to sleep. Contact with reality is maintained consistently.

### IV. Analysis/nursing diagnosis
A. *Injury risk,* to self or child (abuse/neglect) related to postpartum psychosis.
B. *Individual coping impairment* related to perceived inability to meet role expectations ("mother") and ambivalence related to dependence/independence.
C. *Self-esteem disturbance and role performance alteration* related to "femaleness" and reaction to responsibility for care of newborn.
D. *Violence risk,* self-directed or directed at newborn related to anger or depression.
E. *Family coping impairment* related to lack of support system in early postpartum.

F. *Family processes alteration* related to psychological stress, interruption of bonding.

G. *Parenting alteration* related to hormonal changes and stress.

V. **Nursing care plan/implementation**

A. Goal: *emotional support.*

1. Encourage verbalization of feelings, fears, anxiety, concerns.

2. Support positive self-image, feelings of adequacy, self-worth.

   a. Reinforce appropriate comments and behaviors.

   b. Encourage active participation in self-care, comment on accomplishments.

   c. Reduce threat to self-image, fear of failure. Maintain support, gradually increase tasks.

B. Goal: *safeguard status of mother/newborn.*

1. Unobtrusive, protective environment.

2. Stay with woman when she is with infant.

C. Goal: *nutrition/hydration.*

1. Encourage selection of favorite foods—to aid security in decision making; counteract anorexia, refusal to eat by tempting appetite.

2. Push *fluids* (juices, soft drinks, milkshakes)—to maintain hydration.

D. Goal: *minimize stress, facilitate effective coping.*

1. Administer therapeutic medications, as ordered.

   a. Schizophrenia—*phenothiazines.*

   b. Depression—*mood elevators.*

   c. Manic behaviors—*sedatives, tranquilizers.*

VI. **Evaluation/outcome criteria:** The woman responds to medical/nursing regimen.

A. Increases interaction with infant.

B. Expresses interest in learning how to care for infant.

C. Evidences no agitation, depression.

D. Actively participates in caring for self and infant.

E. Demonstrates increasing comfort in mothering role.

F. Demonstrates positive family interactions.

# Sequelae to Trauma Sustained During Childbirth

I. **Pelvic relaxation:** a delayed, but direct, result of childbearing is the weakening and lengthening (overstretching of the supporting tissues of the perineum) of fascial supports of the pelvic organs. Symptoms most often appear during the perimenopausal period. Symptoms are related to the structure involved: urethra, bladder, uterus, vagina, cul-de-sac, or rectum. *Common symptoms*: pulling, dragging sensations, pressure, protrusions, fatigue, and low backache, and sometimes, urinary stress incontinence.

II. **Rectocele**: herniation or protrusion of the rectum into the posterior vaginal wall. (See **Figure 7.1**) *Complaints*: disturbance in bowel functioning, sensation of "bearing-down." Usually repaired surgically.

III. **Cystocele**: bladder hernia into the vagina is a sequel to injury to the vesicovaginal fascia. Often complicated by recurrent cystitis and ascending UTI. Often occurs along with rectocele. Complete emptying is difficult. (See **Figure 7.2**)

IV. **Urinary stress incontinence**: secondary to injury to bladder neck structures—angle between the urethra and the base of the bladder is lost or increased, if the supporting pubococcygeus muscle is injured. Mild stress incontinence may be relieved by strengthening the pubococcygeus muscle with *Kegel's* exercises.

V. **Uterine displacement**: uterine prolapse—falling, sinking, or sliding of the uterus from its normal position.

VI. **Pelvic fistula problems**: urethrovaginal, perineovaginal, vesicovaginal, rectovaginal, vesicocervical. **Health teaching** requires great sensitivity because the woman's reactions are often intense. The nurse suggests tactfully the hygienic practice of *douching and irrigating external perineal* structures with a deodorizing solution such as 1 tsp chlorine household bleach to 1 qt water. Before leaving the house, the woman can give herself *high enemas*, which provide temporary relief from oozing of fecal material in the preoperative period. Genitals should be thoroughly washed with unscented, un-colored, mild soap and warm water to *avoid* adding chemical irritation and/or allergy to her symptoms.

**FIGURE 7.1  RECTOCELE**

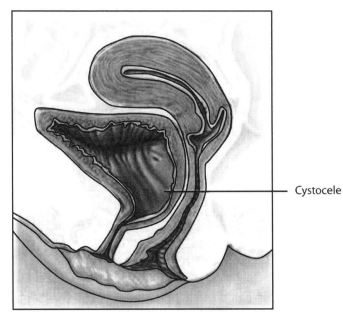

FIGURE 7.2 CYSTOCELE

# Summary

Nursing care of the new mother challenges the nurse with a variety of medical-surgical, psychiatric, and pediatric conditions. Disorders discussed in this chapter relate to *postpartum hemorrhage, infections, mental illness*, and *sequelae* to trauma sustained during childbirth. In addition, the nurse must confront the *sequelae* of conditions that arose during the *antepartum* (**Chapter** 3) and *intrapartum* periods (**Chapter** 5).

## 💡 Study and Memory Aids

### Postpartum Hemorrhage—Causes

Uterine atony
Lacerations
Retained placental fragments
Hematoma

### ❗ Postpartum Hemorrhage—Nursing Management: Alert

Ergot products and carboprost: monitor BP.

### ❗ Hypofibrinogenemia—Assessment

Check for predisposing conditions for DIC.

### UTI—Prevent Bladder Overdistention

❗ A full bladder → uterine atony → hemorrhage.

### Infections—Prevention

👐 HANDWASHING—for nurse *and* mother—cannot be overemphasized!

### Mild Stress Incontinence—Prevention

Remember Kegel's exercises!

# Questions

1. The nurse notes that a woman who is pregnant and has a rubella titer that is 1:6. This means that she:
   1. Has had rubella at some time in her life.
   2. Has just been exposed to rubella.
   3. Should receive rubella vaccination after giving birth.
   4. Must wait until she weans the baby before receiving vaccination for rubella.

2. After a woman has given birth, the nurse gives her Rho (Du) immune globulin before discharge, if needed, to prevent her from:
   1. Isoimmunization.
   2. Autoimmunization.
   3. Developing AB antibodies.
   4. Becoming Coombs negative.

3. Before administering RhoGAM (Rho [Du] immune globulin) to a new mother, the nurse explains that it is a drug that:
   1. Removes Rh+ antibodies from maternal blood.
   2. Destroys fetal Rho erythrocytes in maternal blood.
   3. Deactivates maternal Rh+ antibodies in fetal blood.
   4. Destroys fetal Rh+ erythrocytes in maternal blood.

4. A new mother, who is drug dependent, requests information about breastfeeding. The nurse's response is based on knowledge that breastfeeding:
   1. Should be encouraged, to increase bonding.
   2. Is encouraged, to wean the baby from the substance.
   3. May need to be discouraged.
   4. May be safe, because most substances do not pass into breast milk.

5. A mother who is lactating is worried and tells the nurse that she has been exposed to "some PCB" (polychlorinated biphenyl). Her breast milk is tested and found to have a trace of PCB. The nurse advises her to:
   1. Discontinue breastfeeding immediately.
   2. Avoid crash diets that mobilize her fat stores.
   3. Drink up to 2 liters of water every day to facilitate its elimination.
   4. Feel free to do whatever she wishes regarding breastfeeding, fluid intake, and diet.

6. At 8 hr postpartum, a new mother has an oral temperature of 100° F. The nurse's evaluation of her status is:
   1. Anemia.
   2. Breast engorgement.
   3. Dehydration.
   4. Infection.

7. After a long and difficult labor, a woman had a spontaneous vaginal birth, assisted with low forceps. Since she is at risk for postpartum infection, for which sign should the nurse watch?
   1. Laboratory value: increased RBC sedimentation rate.
   2. Decreased pulse rate.
   3. Decreased lochia flow.
   4. Temperature: 38° C (100.4° F) 30 hr postpartum.

8. The postpartum recovery room nurse recognizes that a new mother is particularly vulnerable to postpartum hemorrhage if she:
   1. Is an older primipara.
   2. Experienced polyhydramnios during pregnancy and labor.
   3. Experienced a third stage that lasted 30 min.
   4. Gained excessive weight during pregnancy.

9. Before developing a plan of care for a woman who has just given birth, the nurse reviews her pregnancy and intrapartal record to identify possible risk factors. The nursing plan of care is based on knowledge that the most common cause of postpartum hemorrhage is:
   1. Lacerations of the birth canal.
   2. Subinvolution of the placental site.
   3. Retained placental fragments.
   4. Uterine atony.

10. All of the following are appropriate nursing interventions for uterine atony. The *initial* intervention should be:
    1. Expulsion of clots.
    2. Gentle massage until the fundus is firm.
    3. Administration of an oxytocic medication.
    4. Ambulation to empty the urinary bladder.

11. A nursing plan of care includes therapeutic interventions for common conditions expected when a woman has just given birth. After evaluating results of unsuccessful nonpharmacologic measures to restore uterine tone, the nurse can expect to prepare and administer:
    1. Cervidil.
    2. Methergine (methylergonovine maleate).
    3. Vitamin K (AquaMEPHYTON).
    4. RhoGAM (Rho [Du] immune globulin).

12. During a woman's first hour postbirth, the nurse notices a continuous trickle of bright-red vaginal bleeding; the fundus remains firm. Based on analysis of these data, the nurse:
    1. Does nothing; this is normal.
    2. Prepares the woman for exploration of her vaginal vault for possible lacerations.
    3. Administers an oxytocic medication to stimulate the living ligature in the lower uterine segment.
    4. Examines the woman for possible vaginal hematoma.

13. The nurse would *not* administer Rho(Du) immune globulin to a new mother if:
    1. The mother is Rho(Du) negative.
    2. The infant is Rho(Du) positive.
    3. Coombs' test on the cord blood is negative.
    4. Coombs' test on the mother's blood is positive.

14. A woman has just arrived at the emergency department after suffering a spontaneous miscarriage at home. Which assessment data alerts the nurse that this woman may be a candidate for receiving Rho(Du) immune globulin?
    1. Woman is Rh negative; pregnancy of 11 wk gestation.
    2. Woman's religion forbids the use of blood products.
    3. Woman is Rh negative and states that the father is also Rh negative.
    4. Woman's Coombs' test is positive.

15. The nurse would help expel intrauterine blood and clots from a woman who is postpartum by using:
    1. Gentle pressure on a firm fundus, supporting the base of the uterus just above the symphysis.
    2. Vigorous massage of the boggy uterus, supporting the base of the uterus just above the symphysis.
    3. Firm pressure downward on the uterine fundus, in the direction of the vagina.
    4. Gentle pressure on the boggy fundus in the direction of the vagina.

16. A new mother was discharged 24 h after giving birth. Eight hours later, she calls the maternity unit concerned about a "flabby womb" (uterus) that doesn't contract well and episodes of painless bleeding." The nurse's response is based on knowledge that the mother:
    1. Is describing *uterine atony*, which is managed with keeping the bladder empty, gentle massage, and expulsion of clots.
    2. Is describing *subinvolution*, which is managed with curettage, antibiotics, and oxytocin.
    3. Is describing *hypofibrinogenemia*, which is managed with IV infusion of heparin, platelets, and blood.
    4. Is describing *normal involution*, which is managed with rest and reassurance.

# Answers/Rationale

1. **(3)** Rubella immunity is present if the titer is 1:8 or higher; because her titer is 1:6, this woman should receive rubella vaccination after giving birth. A titer of 1:6 indicates a *lack* of immunity, *not exposure* to rubella or a *history* of the disease (**1** and **2**). Breastfeeding (**4**) *can* continue after vaccination. NOTE: Before vaccination, the woman may be asked to sign an informed consent and verbalize that she understands that she must refrain from conceiving before 3 mo after vaccination, since rubella is teratogenic. Immune response may be inhibited if the woman has also received RhoGAM; her rubella titer must be rechecked at 3 mo to confirm that she has indeed developed antibodies against rubella, and she may need to be revaccinated. **EV, COM, 1, HPM, Health promotion and maintenance**

2. **(1)** Isoimmunization refers to the development of sensitivity in the human to antigens commonly found in other humans. Autoimmunization (**2**) refers to the development of antibodies against constituents of one's own tissues (e.g., a man may develop antibodies against his own sperm). AB antibodies (**3**) refer to blood type, *not* to the Rh factor. The immune globulin is given to prevent her from becoming Coombs' *positive* (**4**), that is, to keep her from developing Rh antibodies. **PL, COM, 1, PhI, Pharmacological and parenteral therapies**

3. **(4)** RhoGAM destroys fetal Rh+ erythrocytes in maternal blood. Once the woman is sensitized to the Rh factor, *nothing* will remove the antibodies (**1**); she will continue to be Coombs' positive. It destroys fetal Rh+, *not* Rho RBCs (**2**). *Nothing* deactivates maternal antibodies to the Rh factor (**3**); antibodies in fetal blood can *only* be removed with an exchange blood transfusion. **PL, COM, 6, PhI, Pharmacological and parenteral therapies**

4. **(3)** Drugs used in substance abuse are not pure. The drugs are often mixed with a variety of other substances. The single or mixed combination of drugs is likely to pass into breast milk. Methods other than breastfeeding are to be used to encourage bonding (**1**). Babies are *not* weaned from the substance (**2**) by taking breastfeedings from their mothers who are drug-dependent. Most substances *do* pass into breast milk (**4**). **IMP, RE/KN, 4, HPM, Health promotion and maintenance**

5. **(2)** Crash diets mobilize fats (where PCB is stored). If the level in milk is *high*, then breastfeeding should be discontinued, but discontinuation is unnecessary at trace levels (**1**). Increased fluid intake (**3**) does *not* facilitate elimination of PCB. There is a recommended restriction (**4**): She should *avoid* crash diets. **IMP, APP, 4, SECE, Safety and infection control**

6. **(3)** The body attempts to rid itself of excess fluids, and fluids may be restricted during labor and birth; due to these dehydrating effects, the woman may develop a slight temperature elevation after giving birth. Anemia (**1**) and breast engorgement (**2**) (which would not occur until the *3rd* day) would *not* cause a rise in temperature. It is *too early* for a postpartum infection (**4**) to cause a rise in temperature. **AN, ANL, 6, PhI, Physiological adaptation**

7. **(4)** A temperature of 38°C within the first 10 postpartum days, *excluding the first 24 hr*, is an indication of postpartum infection, and should be investigated. An increased sedimentation rate (**1**) is seen in *normal* pregnancy/postpartum period (a *decreased* rate is a sign of infection in the woman who is not pregnant). The pulse (**2**) becomes *rapid*, weak, and easily compressible with infection. Lochia flow (**3**) *increases*. **EV, COM, 1, PhI, Reduction of risk potential**

8. **(2)** Polyhydramnios refers to amniotic fluid in excess of 1.5 liters; this excess fluid stretches the uterine muscle, decreasing its ability to retain its tone after birth. *None* of the histories in options **1**, **3**, and **4** reflects a probable cause of postpartum hemorrhage. **AN, APP, 6, HPM, Health promotion and maintenance**

9. **(4)** The *most* common cause of postpartum hemorrhage is uterine atony. Lacerations (**1**) constitute the *second* most common cause of postpartum hemorrhage, and retained placental fragments (**3**) are the *third* most common cause. Subinvolution of the placental site (**2**) is an *infrequent* cause of postpartum hemorrhage; it is characterized by persistent lochia and episodes of brisk, painless bleeding. **PL, RE/KN, 6, PhI, Physiological adaptation**

10. **(2)** Gentle massage will stimulate the living ligature to contract. Expulsion of clots (**1**) is only attempted *after* the fundus is firm; the lower part of the uterus is supported (with the nurse's other hand), to prevent turning the uterus inside out. Ambulation (**4**) to empty the bladder is the *third* step, after massage and expulsion of clots. An oxytocic (**3**) is given *only* when all other measures fail. **IMP, ANL, 6, PhI, Physiological adaptation**

---

**Key to Codes**

**Nursing process: AS**, assessment; **AN**, analysis; **PL**, planning; **IMP**, implementation; **EV**, evaluation. (See **Appendix J** for explanation of nursing process steps.)

**Cognitive level: RE/KN**, recall/knowledge; **COM**, comprehension; **APP**, application; **ANL**, analysis; **EVL**, evaluation; **SYN**, synthesis. (See **Appendix J** for explanation.)

**Category of human function: 1**, protective; **2**, sensory-perceptual; **3**, comfort, rest, activity, and mobility; **4**, nutrition; **5**, growth and development; **6**, fluid-gas transport; **7**, psychosocial-cultural; **8**, elimination. (See **Appendix L** for explanation.)

**Client need: SECE**, safe, effective care environment; **HPM**, health promotion and maintenance; **PsI**, psychosocial integrity; **PhI**, physiological integrity. (See **Appendix M** for explanation.)

**Client subneed:** See **Appendix M** for explanation.

11. **(2)** Methergine (*Ergotrate*, ergonovine maleate) has an oxytocic effect. Cervidil (**1**) is a cervical riping agent, *not* used for uterine tone *after* birth. Vitamin K (**3**) is given to *prevent hemolytic* disease in the newborn during the first 8 days of life (after that, the newborn's gut has sufficient bacteria to produce his or her own vitamin K). RhoGAM (**4**) is an immune globulin given to *mothers who are Rh-negative* who give birth to infants who are Rh-positive, and who are *Coombs' negative*, to prevent Rh immunization. **IMP, APP, 6, PhI, Pharmacological and parenteral therapies**

12. **(2)** This type of bleeding suggests vaginal lacerations. Option **1** is incorrect because this type of bleeding *requires* further investigation. Option **3** is incorrect because, if the fundus is already firm, she does *not* need an oxytocic medication. Option **4** is incorrect because hematomas result from bleeding into an enclosed space; *no external* bleeding would be evident. **IMP, APP, 1, PhI, Physiological adaptation**

13. **(4)** A positive Coombs' test means that the mother has been sensitized to the Rh factor; that is, she has already developed antibodies. A mother who is Rh-negative (**1**) may be a candidate for receiving Rho (Du) immune globulin. The mother who is Rh-negative who gives birth to a baby who is Rh-positive (**2**) *may* be a candidate to receive Rho (Du) immune globulin. A mother who is Rh-negative *may* be a candidate for receiving Rho (Du) immune globulin if a Coombs' test on her baby who is Rh-positive is negative (**3**). **AN, ANL, 1, PhI, Pharmacological and parenteral therapies**

14. **(1)** If the pregnancy is at 8 wk or more, the woman who is Rh-negative is a candidate for Rho (Du) immune globulin if she is Coombs' negative (no titer of antibodies), even if this was her first pregnancy. Rho (Du) immune globulin *is* a blood product (**2**); the woman must be informed of this fact so that she can decide for herself. (NOTE: The process of preparing the immune globulin destroys any infectious microorganism the donor may have.) If both parents are Rh negative (**3**) and she has never had a blood transfusion, she will probably *not* need the medication. If her Coombs' test is positive (**4**), she has already been sensitized to the Rh factor; since the medication *cannot* reverse the sensitization, no medication is given. **AN, ANL, 6, PhI, Pharmacological and parenteral therapies**

15. **(1)** Using gentle pressure on a firm fundus while supporting the uterus prevents the uterus from being turned inside out. *Vigorous* massage of the uterus (**2**) tires the muscle and results in relaxation of the living ligature and hemorrhage. Firm pressure downward on the uterine fundus (**3**) without supporting the base of the uterus can turn the uterus inside out, even if the fundus is firm. Pressure on a boggy fundus (**4**) can result in turning the uterus inside out. **IMP, APP, 6, PhI, Reduction of risk potential**

16. **(2)** Subinvolution is the delayed return of the uterus to normal tone, size, shape, and position. The uterus is large and flabby, and lacks good tone; there is painless fresh bleeding with hemorrhagic episodes. Management consists of curettage, antibiotics, and oxytocin. The symptoms as given do *not* describe uterine atony (**1**), which would include intermittent uterine relaxation with some "after pains"; uterine tone is achieved with gentle massage. The symptoms also do *not* describe hypofibrinogenemia (**3**), which does not affect uterine tone. Symptoms of hypofibrinogenemia would be emergence of petechiae and bleeding gums; management would include IV infusion of heparin, platelets, and blood. With normal involution (**4**), the uterus *does* contract with gentle massage; lochia gradually changes to serosa and amount decreases. **EV, RE/KN, 6, PhI, Physiological adaptation**

# The Newborn Infant

## Chapter Outline

## 🔑 Key Points

- At term gestation, the newborn's *anatomic* and *physiologic* systems have reached a level of development and functioning that supports a physical existence apart from the mother, and *sensory* capabilities that indicate a state of readiness for social interactions.

- Newborns require a *protective* environment: e.g., correct identification procedures, *safe restraining* techniques (including car seats), measures to *prevent infection*, and *support of physiologic functions*.

- Parents need to learn techniques to *safeguard* their newborns: CPR, maintaining a *patent airway*, knowledge of their *developmental/ behavioral* characteristics, hygiene, *nutrition, cord* and *circumcision* care, and *prevention of infection* (including emphasis on *immunizations* and keeping scheduled medical appointments).

- Parents are entitled to know about newborn *nutrition and feeding*: the benefits of both breastfeeding and formula feeding; the powerful effect the partner's attitude toward breastfeeding has on achieving successful lactation; the need to *avoid* use of honey in home-prepared formulas (can be fatal if newborn
! is infected with botulism).

## Key Words

### (With definitions to facilitate reading of Table 8.2, p. 179–181)

**Acrocyanosis** peripheral cyanosis; blue color of hands and feet in most infants at birth that may persist for 7–10 days.

**Agenesis** *A*: a prefix meaning un, less, lack, not; *genesis*: a combining form denoting origination, development, evolution.

**Caput succedaneum** swelling of the tissue over the presenting part of the fetal head caused by pressure during labor; fluid is serum; swelling *crosses* suture lines.

**Cephalohematoma** extravasation of blood from ruptured vessels between a skull bone and its external covering, the periosteum; fluid is blood; swelling limited by the margins of the cranial bone affected; does *not* cross suture lines.

**Ductus arteriosus** in fetal circulation, an anatomic shunt between the pulmonary artery and arch of the aorta.

**Erythema toxicum** innocuous, pink, papular neonatal rash of unknown cause, appearing within *24–48* hr after birth and resolving spontaneously within a few days.

**Foramen ovale** septal opening between the atria of the fetal heart.

**Imperforate** without the normal opening.

**Lanugo** downy, fine hair characteristic of the fetus between *20 wk* gestation and birth that is most noticeable over the shoulder, forehead, and cheeks but is found on nearly all parts of the body (except the palms of the hands, soles of the feet, and the scalp).

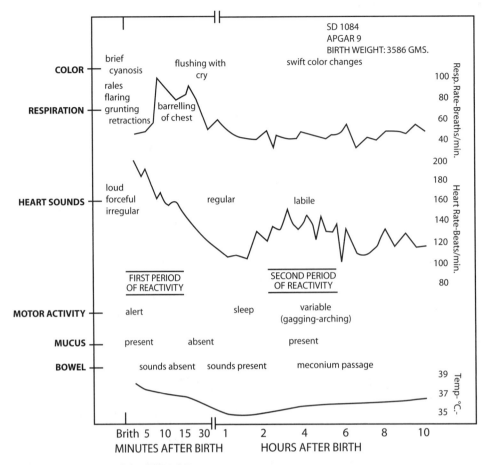

**FIGURE 8.1 NORMAL TRANSITION PERIOD.**
(From M Desmond, A Rudolph, P Phitakspharaiwan. *Pediatr Clin North Am* 13(3):651-68,.)

**Milia** unopened sebaceous glands appearing as tiny, white, pinpoint papules on forehead, nose, cheeks, and chin of a neonate that disappear spontaneously in a *few days* or *weeks*.

**Mongolian spot** bluish-gray or dark, nonelevated pigmented area usually found over the lower back and buttocks; may be present on any part of the newborn; present at birth in some infants, primarily nonwhite.

**Mottling** variability of coloration (with distinct pattern) of newborn skin, secondary to an immature vascular system; a normal variation.

**Periods of reactivity** *first period* (within *30 min* after birth): brief cyanosis, flushing with crying; crackles, nasal flaring, grunting, retractions; heart sounds loud, forceful, irregular; alert; mucus; no bowel sounds; followed by period of sleep. *Second period* (4–8 h after birth): swift color changes; irregular respiratory and heart rates; mucus with gagging; meconium passage; and stabilizing temperature (**Figure 8.1**).

**Phenylketonuria (PKU)** recessive hereditary disease that results in a defect in the metabolism of the amino acid phenylalanine, caused by the lack of an enzyme, *phenylalanine hydroxylase*, that is necessary for the conversion of the amino acid phenylalanine into *tyrosine*. If untreated, brain damage may occur, causing severe mental retardation.

**Physiologic jaundice** hemolysis of excessive fetal RBCs in the early neonatal period; jaundice not apparent during first 24 h.

**Pseudomenstruation** bloody discharge from the newborn girl's vagina in response to maternal hormones during intrauterine life.

**Pulmonary surfactant** a phosphoprotein necessary for normal respiratory function that prevents alveolar collapse (*atelectasis*). (see also **Glossary** section for **lecithin** and **L/S ratio, p. 228, 229**).

**Vernix caseosa** protective gray-white fatty substance of cheesy consistency covering the fetal skin.

**Vitamin K** a necessary component for blood clotting; produced in the GI tract after the introduction of bacteria, starting at about *8 days* after birth.

**Wharton's jelly** white, gelatinous material surrounding the umbilical vessels within the cord.

**Witch's milk** secretion of a whitish fluid for about a *week* after birth from enlarged mammary tissue in the neonate, presumably resulting from maternal hormonal influences.

**! Wry neck (torticollis)** congenital or acquired stiff neck caused by shortening or spasmodic contraction of the neck (sternocleidomastoid) muscles that draws the head to one side with the chin pointing in the other direction.

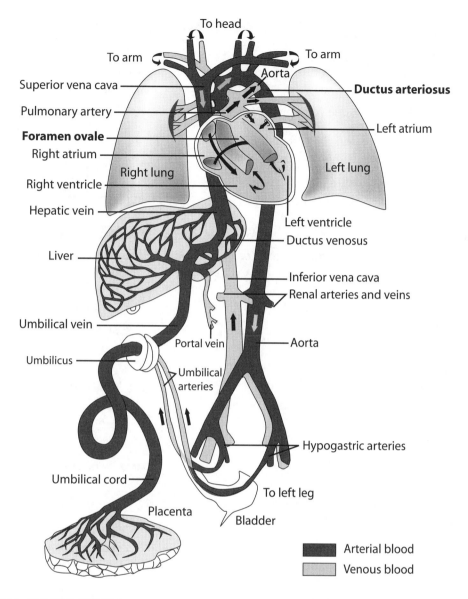

**FIGURE 8.2  FETAL CIRCULATION:** The **foramen ovale** and the **ductus arteriosus** act as bypass channels, allowing a large part of the combined cardiac output to perfuse body tissues without flowing through the lungs. (Courtesy Ross Laboratories, Columbus, OH).

# Biologic Foundations of Neonatal Adaptation—*General Aspects*

**General overview**: Effective nursing care of the newborn infant is based on: (1) knowledge of the conditions present during fetal life; (2) requirements for independent extrauterine life; and (3) alterations needed for successful transition (**Figure 8.1**). *The first 24 hr are the most* ! *hazardous.*

I.   **Fetal anatomy and physiology**

   A. **Fetal circulation**—four intrauterine structures, which differ from extrauterine structures (**Figure 8.2, p. 175**)

      1. *Umbilical vein*—carries oxygen and nutrient-enriched blood from placenta to ductus

venosus and liver. (*Ductus venosus*—connects to inferior vena cava; allows most blood to bypass liver.)

      2. *Foramen ovale*—allows fetal blood to bypass fetal lungs by shunting it from right atrium into left atrium.

      3. *Ductus arteriosus*—allows fetal blood to bypass fetal lungs by shunting it from pulmonary artery into aorta.

      4. *Umbilical arteries* (two)—allow return of deoxygenated blood to the placenta.

   B. **Umbilical cord**—extends from fetus to center of placenta; usually 50 cm (18–22 in.) long and 1–2 cm ( ½–1 in.) in diameter. Contains:

      1. *Wharton's jelly*—protects umbilical vessels from: pressure, cord "kinking," and interference with fetal-placental circulation.

*(continued on p. 177)*

## TABLE 8.1 ESTIMATION OF GESTATIONAL AGE—COMMON CLINICAL PARAMETERS

| Characteristic | Preterm | Term |
| --- | --- | --- |
| **Ankle dorsiflexion** | 90 degrees | 0 degrees |
| **Breast nodules** | 0 mm at 36 wk; 4 mm at 37 wk | 10 mm or more |
| **Cry** | 24 wk: weak; 28 wk: high-pitched; 32 wk: good | Lusty; can persist for some time |
| **Ears**: form, cartilage | Soft, flat, shapeless | Pinna firm; erect from head |
| **Genitalia** | | |
| Boys | Small scrotum, rugae on inferior surface only, and testes undescended | Scrotum pendulous, covered with rugae; testes usually descended |
| Girls | Clitoris large, labia gaping | Labia larger, meet in midline |
| **Hair**: texture, distribution | Fine, fuzzy, or wooly; clumped; appears at 20 wk | Silky; single strands apparent |
| **Head** | Oval—narrow biparietal; large in proportion to body; face looks like "old man"; soft, flat, shapeless | Square-shaped biparietal prominences; ¼ body length |
| **Head lag** | Head lags; arms have little or no flexion | Head follows trunk; strong arm flexion |
| **Heel-to-ear maneuver** | Touches ear easily | 90 degrees |
| **Lanugo** | Apparent at 20 wk; by 33–36 wk, covers shoulders | Minimal or no lanugo |
| **Length** | Under 47 cm (18 ½ in.), usually | 50 cm (20 in.) |
| **Muscle tone** | Hypotonia; extension of arms and legs | Hypertonia; well flexed |
| **Nipples** | No areolae | Formed; raised above skin level |
| **Popliteal angle** | 180 degrees | < 90 degrees |
| **Posture** | Froglike | Attitude of general flexion |
| **Reflexes** | | |
| Grasp | Fair at 28 wk; arm is involved at 32 wk | Strong enough to sustain weight for a few seconds when pulled up; hand, arm, shoulder involved |
| Moro | Apparent at 28 wk; good, but no adduction | Complete reflex with adduction; disappears 4 mo postterm |
| **Scarf sign** | Elbow can extend to opposite axilla | Elbow to midline or less only; infant resists |
| **Skin**: texture, opacity | Visible abdominal veins; thin, shiny | Few indistinct larger veins; thick, dry, cracked, peeling |
| **Sole creases** | Starting at ball of foot, ¹/₃ covered with creases by 36 wk; ²/₃ by 38 wk | Entire sole heavily creased |
| **Square window** | 90 degrees | 0 degrees |
| **Ventral suspension** | Hypotonia; "rag-doll" | Good caudal and cephalic tone |
| **Vernix** | Covers body by 31–33 wk | Small amount or absent at term; *postterm*: dry, wrinkled |
| **Weight** | Under 2500 g (5 lb 5 oz) | 3400 g (7 ½ lb) |

Source: ©Lagerquist, S. *Davis's NCLEX-RN® Success*, Philadelphia.

**(A)**

**(B)**

Vent control puts user in complete command; lets bellows return to its original size, permitting repeated 2 second suctioning cycles.

Anti-reflux valve prevents backflow

Inhaling or applying mechanical suction through mouthpiece causes polyethylene bellows to contract, creating vacuum in rest of unit. Contraction—and suction—terminates within 2 seconds with mechanical suctioning, the maximum recommended time.

Fluid flows through catheter into container that is completely isolated from user's airway or wall unit system

Trap has 2cc gradations, clearly marked and easily readable, to 20cc volume. Overflow reservoir provides additional capacity, also isolated from user or system.

**BEFORE SUCTIONING**
(Bellows expanded.)

**WHILE SUCTIONING**
(Bellows contracted.)

**FIGURE 8.3  SUCTION DEVICES.** (A) Bulb syringe. Compress bulb before inserting. (B) (Isolated) DeLee suction method with catheter and mucus trap. (Courtesy Busse Hospital Disposables, PO Box 011067, Hauppauge, NY 11788-0920.)

2. *Umbilical vein*—carries oxygen and nutrients from placenta to fetus.
3. *Two umbilical arteries*—carry deoxygenated blood and fetal wastes from fetus to placenta. NOTE: Absence of one artery indicates need to rule out intraabdominal anomalies.

**!**

C. **Characteristics of fetal blood**
   1. Fetal hemoglobin (Hb$_f$)
      a. Higher oxygen-carrying capacity than adult hemoglobin.
      b. Releases oxygen easily to fetal tissues.
      c. Ensures high fetal oxygenation.
      d. *Normal range at term: 12–22 g/dL; average: 15–20 g/dL.*
   2. Total blood volume at term: 85 mL/kg body weight; *Hct*: 38–62%, average 53%; *RBC* 3–7 million, average 4.9 million/unit.

II. **Extrauterine adaptation: tasks**
   A. Establish and maintain ventilation, successful gas transfer—requires patent airway and adequate pulmonary surfactant.
   B. Modify circulatory patterns—requires closure of fetal bypass structures.
   C. Absorb and utilize fluids and nutrients.
   D. Excrete body wastes.
   E. Establish and maintain thermal stability.

III. **Nursing care plan/goals**
   A. Facilitate successful transition to independent life.
   B. Protect infant from physiologic stress and environmental hazards.
   C. Encourage development of a strong family unit.

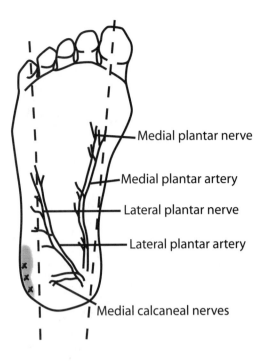

**FIGURE 8.4 ACCEPTABLE INTRAMUSCULAR INJECTION SITE:** Lateral aspect of muscle mass in middle third of distance between greater trochanter and patella. **(A)** preferred injection site in vastus lateralis muscle. **(B)** alternate injection site in rectus femoris muscle.

**FIGURE 8.5 PUNCTURE SITES** (*x*) on infant's foot for heel stick samples of capillary blood. The newborn's foot is wrapped for warmth to increase blood flow to extremity before heel stick.

# Normal Newborn Experience

◄ I. **Assessment of normal, term neonate**
   A. Review antepartum, intrapartum, and recovery period events.
   B. Color and reactivity.
   C. General appearance, symmetry.
   D. Length and weight.
   E. Head and chest circumference.
   F. Vital signs:
      1. Axillary or rectal temperature.
      2. Respirations (check rate, character, rhythm).
      ◄ **Respiratory warning signs:**
         a. **Abnormal rate**
            Bradypnea: respirations ≤ 25/min.
            Tachypnea: respirations ≥ 60/min.
         b. **Abnormal breath sounds:** crackles (rales), wheezes (rhonchi), expiratory grunt.
         c. **Respiratory distress:** nasal flaring, retractions, chin tug, costal breathing, cyanosis.
      3. Apical pulse.
   G. General physical assessment (**Table 8.2, p. 179-181**; see **Key Words** at front of chapter for selected terms and their definitions) and *reflexes* (**Table 8.3, p. 182**).
   H. Estimation of gestational age (**Table 8.1, p. 176**).

◄ II. **Analysis/nursing diagnosis**
   A. *Health maintenance alteration* related to separation from maternal support system.
   B. *Skin integrity impairment* related to umbilical stump; incontinence of urine and meconium stool; skin penetration by scalp electrode, injections, heel stick, scalpel during cesarean birth; abrasion from obstetric forceps or vacuum extractor.
   C. *Airway clearance impairment* related to excessive mucus.
   D. *Pain* related to environmental stimuli and procedures.
   E. *Thermoregulation impairment* related to immature temperature regulation mechanism.

◄ III. **Nursing care plan/implementation**
   A. Goal: *promote effective gas transport.*
      1. Maintain patent airway—to promote effective gas exchange and respiratory function.
      2. *Position: right side lying, head dependent* (gravity drainage of fluid, mucus).
      ☞ 3. Suction for mucus, prn, with bulb syringe or DeLee suction (**Figure 8.3, p. 177**).
   B. Goal: *establish/maintain thermal stability.*
      1. *Avoid* chilling—to prevent metabolic acidosis.
      ☞ 2. Dry, wrap, and apply hat.
      3. Place under radiant warmer.
      4. Monitor vital signs hourly until stable.

*(continued on p. 181)*

## TABLE 8.2 ⋈ PHYSICAL ASSESSMENT OF THE TERM NEONATE[a]

| Criterion | Average Values and Normal Variations | ! Deviations from Normal |
|---|---|---|
| **Vital signs** | | |
| Blood pressure | 80/46; varies with change in activity level | Hypotension: with RDS<br>Hypertension: coarctation of aorta |
| Heart rate | 120–140/min, irregular, especially when crying, and functional murmur | Faint sound—pneumomediastinum; and heart rate < 100 or > 180/min |
| Respiratory rate | 30–60/min with short periods of apnea, irregular; cry—vigorous and loud | Distress—flaring of nares, retractions, tachypnea, grunting, excessive mucus, < 30 or > 60/min; cyanosis |
| Temperature | Stabilizes about 8–10 hr after birth; 36.5°–37° C (97.7°–98.6° F) axillary | Unreliable indicator of infection |
| **Measurements** | | |
| Chest circumference | 2 cm (¾ in.) less than head circumference | If relationship varies, check for reason |
| Head circumference | 33–35 cm (13–14 in.) | Check for microcephalus and hydrocephalus |
| Length | 50 cm (20 in.) | |
| Weight | 3400 g (7 ½ lb) | Birth weight < 2500 g = preterm or SGA infant; > 4000 g = LGA infant; evaluate mother for gestational diabetes |
| **General assessment** | | |
| Abdomen | Dome-shaped, abdominal respirations; soft; may have small umbilical hernia; umbilical cord well formed, containing 3 vessels; dry around base; bowel sounds within 2 hr of birth; voiding; passage of meconium | Scaphoid-shaped, omphalocele, diastasis recti, and distention; umbilical cord containing 2 vessels; redness or drainage around base of cord |
| Anus | Patent, well placed; "wink" reflex | Imperforate, and absence of "wink" (absence of sphincter muscle); fistula |
| Back | Spine straight, easily movable, and flexible; may have small pilonidal dimple at base of spine; may raise head when prone | Fusion of vertebrae; pilonidal dimple with tuft of hair; *spina bifida*, agenesis of part of vertebral bodies; limitation of movement; weak or absent reflexes |
| Chest | Enlarged breasts, "*witch's milk*"; barrel-shaped; both sides move synchronously; nipples symmetrical | Flattened, funnel-chested, asynchronous movement; lack of breast tissue; fracture of clavicle(s); supernumerary or widely spaced nipples; bowel sounds |
| Ears | Well formed, firm; notch of ear should be on straight line with outer canthus | Low placement, clefts; tags; malformed; lack of cartilage |
| Extremeties | Synchronized movements, freely movable through full range of motion; legs appear bowed, and feet appear flat; attitude of general flexion; arms longer than legs; grasp reflex; palmar and sole creases; normal contour | Fractures, *Erb-Duchenne* paralysis (flaccid arm with elbow extended), brachial nerve palsy, *clubbed foot*, phocomelia or amelia, unusual number or webbing of digits, and abnormal palmar creases; poor muscle tone; asymmetry; hypertonicity; unusual hip contour and click sign (*hip dysplasia*); hypermobility of joints |
| Eyes | Edematous eyelids, conjunctival hemorrhage; grayish-blue to grayish-brown in color; *blink reflex*; usually no tears; uncoordinated movements may focus for a few seconds; good placement on face; cornea is bright and shiny; pupillary reflex equal and reactive to light; eyebrows distinct | Epicanthal folds (in non-Asians); discharges; agenesis; opaque lenses; lesions; strabismus; "*doll's eyes*" beyond 10 days; absence of reflexes<br>Gonorrhea: *ophthalmia neonatorum* appears about 3–4 d after birth<br>*Chlamydia trachomatis*: conjunctivitis (congestion and edema) with minimal drainage develops 5 d–2 wk after birth |

*(continued)*

## TABLE 8.2 ◄ PHYSICAL ASSESSMENT OF THE TERM NEONATE[a] (continued)

| Criterion | Average Values and Normal Variations | ! Deviations from Normal |
|---|---|---|
| *Face* | Symmetric movements and contours | Facial palsy (7th cranial nerve); looks "funny" |
| *Genitalia* | | |
|   Girls | Large labia; may have pseudomenstruation, smegma; vaginal orifice open; increased pigmentation; ecchymosis and edema following breech birth; pink-stained urine (uric acid crystals) | Agenesis and imperforate hymen; ambiguous and widely-separated labia, fecal discharge per vagina; *epispadias* or *hypospadias* |
|   Boys | Pendulous scrotum covered with rugae, increased pigmentation; testes usually descended; voids with adequate stream; edema and ecchymosis following breech birth | *Phimosis, epispadias,* or *hypospadias*; ambiguous; scrotum smooth and testes undescended *Hydrocele*: collection of fluid in the sac surrounding the testes |
| *Hair* | Silky, single strands; lies flat; grows toward face and neck | Fine, wooly; unusual swirls, patterns, hair line; coarse |
| *Head* | Molding of fontanels and suture spaces; comprises ¼ of body length | *Cephalohematoma, caput succedaneum,* sunken or bulging fontanels, closed sutures; excessively wide sutures |
| *Mouth* | *Epstein's pearls* on gum ridges; tongue does not protrude and moves freely, symmetrically; uvula in midline; reflexes present: sucking, rooting, gag, extrusion | *Cleft lip or palate*; teeth; cyanosis, circumoral pallor; asymmetric lip movement; excessive saliva; *thrush*; incomplete or absent reflexes |
| *Muscle tone* | Good tone and generalized flexion; full range of motion; spontaneous movement | Flaccid, and persistent tremor or twitching; movement limited; asymmetric |
| *Neck* | Short, freely movable; some head control | Wry neck, webbed neck; restricted movement; masses; distended veins; absence of head control |
| *Nose* | Appears to have no bridge; should have no discharge; preferential nose breathers; sneezes to clear nose | Discharge and *choanal atresia*; malformed; flaring of nares beyond first few moments of life |
| *Skin color* | Mottling, *acrocyanosis,* and physiologic jaundice; petechia (over presenting part), milia, mongolian spotting, lanugo, and vernix caseosa; erythema toxicum ("newborn rash") | Pallor, cyanosis, or jaundice within 24 hr of birth Pethechiae or ecchymoses elsewhere; all rashes, except erythema toxicum; pigmented nevi; hemangioma; and yellow vernix |
| *Stools* | Meconium within first 24 hr; *transitional*—days 2–5; *breastfed*: loose, golden yellow; *bottlefed*: formed, light yellow | Light-colored meconium (dry, hard), or absent with distended abdomen (*cystic fibrosis* or *Hirschsprung's disease*); diarrhetic |
| ∿ **Laboratory values** | | |
| Blood glucose | ≥ 40 mg/dL for *term* > 45 mg/dL for *preterm* | Identify *hypoglycemia* before overt or asymptomatic hypoglycemia—do blood glucose on all at-risk infants (large- or small-for-gestational-age neonates, or neonates of mothers who are diabetic) |
| Hemoglobin (cord) | 13.6–19.6 g/dL | Evaluate for anemia and persistent polycythemia |
| Serum bilirubin | 2–6 mg/dL | Hyperbilirubinemia (*term*: 12 mg or more; *preterm*: 15 mg or more) |

*(continued)*

## TABLE 8.2 ◀ PHYSICAL ASSESSMENT OF THE TERM NEONATE[a] (continued)

| Criterion | Average Values and Normal Variations | ! Deviations from Normal |
|---|---|---|
| Neurologic examination[b] | Specific to gestational age and state of wakefulness | |
| 1. *Behavioral* patterns | | |
|   a. Feeding | Variations in interest, hunger; usually feeds well within 48 hr | Lethargic; poor suck, poor coordination with swallow, choking, cyanosis |
|   b. Social | Crying is lusty, strong, and soon indicative of hunger, pain, attention-seeking; responds to cuddling and voice by quietness and increased alertness | Absent; no focusing on person holding him/her; unconsolable |
|   c. Sleep-wakefulness | Two periods of reactivity: at birth, and 6-8 h later; stabilization, with wakeful periods about every 3-4 hr | Lethargy, drowsiness Disorganized pattern |
|   d. Elimination | Stooling: see *Stools* (p. 180, 182) Urination: *first* few days: 3–4 times qd *end* of first week: 5–6 times qd *later*: 6–10 times qd, with adequate hydration | See *Stools* Diminished number: dehydration |
| 2. *Reflex* response | Bilateral, symmetric response (see **Table 8.3**) | Absent, hyperactive, incomplete, asynchronous |
| 3. *Sensory* capabilities | | |
|   a. Vision | Limited accomodation, with clearest vision within 7-8 in; focuses and follows by 15 min of age; prefers patterns to plain | Absence of these responses may be due to absence of or diminished acuity or to sensory deprivation |
|   b. Hearing | By 2 min of age, can move in direction of sound: responds to high pitch by "freezing," followed by agitation; to low pitch (crooning) by relaxing | Absence of response: deafness |
|   c. Touch | Soothed by massaging, warmth, weightlessness (as in water bath) | Unable to be comforted: possible drug dependence Newborns who are cocaine-addicted avoid eye contact |
|   d. Smell | By 5th day, can distinguish between mother's breasts and those of another woman | |
|   e. Taste | Can distinguish between sweet and sour | |
|   f. Motor | Coordinates body movement to parent's voice and body movement | Absence |

RDS = respiratory distress syndromes; SGA = small for gestational age; LGA = large for gestational age.

[a]See Key Words at front of chapter for definitions of selected terms used in this table.

[b]Based on Brazelton's method.

*Source*: ©Lagerquist, S. *Davis's NCLEX-RN® Success*, Philadelphia.

C. Goal: *reduce possibility of blood loss.*
  1. Check cord clamp for security.
  2. Administer vitamin K injection, as ordered, in anterior or lateral thigh muscle—to stimulate blood coagulability (**Figure 8.4, p. 178**).

D. Goal: *prevent infection.*
  1. Administer *antibiotic* treatment to eyes (if not performed in birth room)—to prevent ophthalmia neonatorum.
  2. Treat cord stump (alcohol), as ordered.
  ▲ 3. Use *standard precautions.*

E. Goal: *promote comfort and cleanliness.* Admission bath when temperature stable.

F. Goal: *promote nutrition, hydration, elimination.*
  1. Encourage breastfeeding immediately after birth.
  2. Check blood sugar (*Dextrostix* or *Chemstrip*) at 30 min, 1, 2, and 4 hr for infants at risk for hypoglycemia (e.g., small for gestational age [SGA], large for gestational age [LGA]), infant of mother who has diabetes. See **Figure 8.5, p. 178** for acceptable puncture sites for heel stick.

## TABLE 8.3 ◄► ASSESSMENT: NORMAL NEWBORN REFLEXES*

| Reflex | Description | ! Implications of Deviations from Normal Pattern |
|---|---|---|
| Babinski | Stroking the sole in an upward fashion elicits *hyperextension* of toes | Same as for **Plantar grasp** |
| Crawling | When placed in prone position, attempts to crawl | Absence may indicate prematurity or depressed infant |
| Moro (startle) | Symmetric *abduction* and *extension* of arms with fingers extended in response to sudden movement or loud noise | Asymmetric reflex may indicate brachial (*Erb's*) palsy or fractured clavicle |
| Palmar grasp | If palm stimulated, fingers *curl*; holds adult finger briefly | Asymmetry may indicate neurologic involvement |
| Plantar grasp | Pressure on sole will elicit *curling* of toes | Absence/asymmetry associated with defects of lower spinal column |
| Rooting and sucking | With stimulus to cheek, turns *toward* stimulus, opens mouth, sucks | Absence of response may indicate prematurity, neurologic problem, or depressed infant (or not hungry) |
| Stepping/dancing | If held in upright position with feet in contact with hard surface, alternately raises feet | Asymmetry may indicate neurologic problem |
| Tonic neck (fencing) | When head turned to one side, arm and leg on *that* side *extends*, and *opposite* arm and leg *flexes* | Asymmetry may indicate cerebral lesion, if persistent |

*NOTE: Reflexes are good indicators of the neurologic system in well infants but not in sick neonates. Infants with infections may not show normal reflexes yet have an intact neurologic system.
*Source*: ©Lagerquist, S. *Davis's NCLEX-RN® Success*, Philadelphia.

## TABLE 8.4 INFANT STOOL CHARACTERISTICS

| Age | Bottle-fed | Breastfed | ! Implications of Abnormal Patterns |
|---|---|---|---|
| 1 day | Meconium | Meconium | Absence may indicate obstruction, atresia |
| 2–5 days (transitional) | Greenish-yellow; loose | Greenish-yellow; loose, frequent | ⚡NOTE: At any time:<br>*Diarrhea*—greenish, mucus or blood-tinged, or forceful expulsion, may indicate infection<br>*Constipation*—dry, hard stools or infrequent or absent stools may indicate obstruction |
| > 5 days | Yellow to brown; firm; 2–4/d; foul odor | Bright golden yellow, loose; 6–10/d | |

*Source*: ©Lagerquist, S. *Davis's NCLEX-RN® Success*, Philadelphia.

🍎 3. First feeding at 1–4 hr of age with formula, if not breastfeeding.

4. Note voiding and/or meconium stool; report
! failure to void or defecate within 24 hr.

G. Goal: *promote bonding.*

1. Encourage parent-infant interaction (holding, touching, eye contact, talking to infant).

2. Encourage breastfeeding within 1 h of birth, if client desires to breastfeed.

3. Encourage parent participation in infant care—to develop confidence and competence in caring for newborn

☞ a. Assist with initial efforts at feeding.

☞ b. Discuss and demonstrate positioning and burping techniques.

☞ c. Demonstrate/assist with basic care procedures, as necessary:

(1) Bath.

(2) Cord care.

(3) Diapering.

(4) Aid parents in distinguishing normal versus abnormal newborn characteristics.

📖 H. Goal: **health teaching.** Provide anticipatory guidance for discharge.

1. Facilitate sibling bonding.

2. Describe/discuss normal newborn behavior

a. *Sleeping*—almost continual (wakes only to feed) or 12–16 h/d.

b. *Feeding*—from every 2–3 h to longer intervals; establish own pattern; babies who are breastfed feed more often.

c. *Weight loss*—5–10% in first few days; regained in 7–14 days.

d. *Stools*—see **Table 8.4, p. 182**.

e. *Physiologic jaundice*—occurs 24–72 h postbirth
   (1) Nonpathologic.
   (2) Need for hydration.
   (3) More common in infants who are breastfed.

3. Demonstrate **cord care**—drops off in 7–10 d.
   a. Keep clean and dry.
   b. Alcohol to stump.

☞ 4. Demonstrate **circumcision care**
   a. Keep clean and dry; heals rapidly.
   b. Watch for bleeding.
   c. Petroleum jelly, gauze, prn, if ordered.
   d. Do *not* remove yellowish exudate.

5. Identify need for newborn screen, biochemical tests for inborn errors of metabolism—see **Figure 8.5**, *heel stick*. (These tests are mandatory in most states; if parents prefer these tests not be done, they need to sign a refusal.)
   a. Phenylketonuria (PKU), after feeding.
   b. Galactosemia.
   c. Thyroxine ($T_4$) for hypothyroidism.
   d. Other tests specific to identified ethnic group, such as sickle cell anemia.

6. Describe suggested sensory *stimulation* modalities (mobiles, color, music).

7. Discuss *safety* precautions:
   a. Infant seat for travel and home safety.
   b. Maintaining contact/control over infant to prevent falls, drowning in bath.
   c. Instruct parents in infant **CPR** (**Figure 8.7, p. 184**)
      • Place mouth over mouth and nose of newborn; repeat word *ho* as you gently puff volume of air from your cheeks into infant; *do not force air*.
      • *Compressions*: using two fingers, on the lower third of the sternum, depress the the third of the anterior-posterior chest diameter at a rate of at least 90 times/min; three compressions in 1 sec or less (3:1 ratio), pausing at end of each compression to allow chest to fall by passive recoil; followed by one breath.
      • *Discontinue*: when infant's spontaneous heart rate reaches or exceeds 80 beats/min.

**FIGURE 8.6   BACK BLOW IN INFANT FOR CLEARING AIRWAY OBSTRUCTION.**

d. Instruct parents in relieving **airway obstruction** for infants of 1 yr of age or younger (**Figure 8.6**) DO NOT USE FOREIGN BODY AIRWAY OBSTRUCTION (HEIMLICH) MANEUVER, AND NO BLIND FINGER SWEEPS.
   Initiate back blows and chest thrusts.
   • *Back blows*: deliver up to five back blows forcefully between infant's shoulder blades with heel of free hand. Turn infant over (while supporting neck and head) and provide up to five quick, downward chest thrusts to same location as chest compressions.
   • *Open airway*: head-tilt/chin lift, and ventilate.
   • *Discontinue*: signs of recovery—palpable peripheral pulses, return of pupils to normal size and responsiveness, and disappearance of mottling and cyanosis.

8. Describe signs of *common health problems*, to be reported promptly:
   a. Diarrhea, constipation.
   b. Colic, vomiting.
   c. Fever.
   d. Signs of inflammation and/or infection at cord stump.
   e. Bleeding at circumcision site.
   f. Rash, jaundice.
   g. Deviation from normal patterns.

**A** Head tilt/chin lift

**B** Mouth-to-mouth and nose seal

**C** Locating and palpating brachial pulse

**D** Locating finger position for chest compressions in infant

**E** When two rescures are present, use your thumbs side by side, placed just below an imaginary line drawn between the two nipples.

## FIGURE 8.7 (A–E) PROCEDURES FOR CARDIOPULMONARY RESUSCITATION.

**IV. Evaluation/outcome criteria**

A. *Infant* demonstrates successful transition to independent life:
1. Breastfeeds well.
2. Normal feeding, sleeping, elimination patterns.
3. No evidence of infection or abnormality.

B. *Mother/family* evidence bonding:
1. Eye contact.
2. Stroking, cuddling.
3. Crooning, calling baby by name, talking to infant.

C. *Mother* demonstrates comfort and skill in basic newborn care.

D. *Mother* verbalizes understanding of subjects discussed:
1. Safety precautions.
2. Health maintenance actions.
3. Signs of normal infant behavior and health.

E. *Evaluate: infant's readiness for hospital discharge:*

■ Term infant (38–42 wk) with birth weight of 2500–4500 g*

■ Normal findings on physical assessment performed by physician*

Normal laboratory data, including negative *Coombs'* test result and hematocrit 40–65%*

■ Stable vital signs*:

*R* < 60 bpm; HR 100–160 bpm;

*T* (axillary) 36.5°C to 37.4°C (97.7°F to 99.3°F)

(Temperature stability*)

■ *Successful feeding* x2 (normal sucking, swallowing, and breathing while feeding)*

Apgar score > 7 at 1 and 5 min

■ Urinated and passed one stool spontaneously.

Screening tests completed.

**General:**

• Hearing screening per hospital protocol

• Initial *hepatitis B vaccine* as indicated by infant's risk status

*Recommendations of American Academy of Pediatrics: Hospital Stay for Healthy Term Newborns *Pediatrics* 113(5) 1434–1436.

# Summary

It is of utmost importance that the newborn nurse be highly skilled in assessment of the neonate—the life and the quality of life of this child can be affected for years to come by the timely identification and treatment of deviations from the norm. The biologic foundations of *neonatal adaptation, fetal anatomy and physiology, extrauterine adaptations*, and nursing goals are presented in this chapter. The nursing process as implemented with the newborn includes guidelines for nurses' hands-on care and teaching the parents about the new member of the family. Teaching topics include *CPR* and relieving *airway obstruction* in the infant of 1 yr of age or less. Guidelines for infant's readiness for hospital discharge are listed.

## Study and Memory Aids

### Newborn—Fluid Maintenance Requirements

| Age | Qty/Feeding | Feedings/24 h |
| --- | --- | --- |
| Birth–3 wk | 2–3 oz (60–90 mL) | 6–10 |
| 3 wk–2 mo | 5 oz (150 mL) | 5–8 |
| 2–3 mo | 5–7 oz (150–210 mL) | 5–6 |

### Newborn —Tests for Inborn Errors of Metabolism

Biotinidase deficiency
Congenital adrenal hyperplasia (CAH)
Congenital hypothyroidism
Galactosemia
Homocystinuria
Maple syrup urine disease
Medium chain acyl-CoA dehydrogenase deficiency (MCAD)
Phenylketonuria (PKU)
Sickle cell anemia

# Questions

1. During a prenatal class for adolescents, the discussion turns to concerns about how the unborn baby breathes "under water." The nurse's reassurance is based on knowledge that during fetal circulation, two fetal structures allow fetal blood to bypass fetal lungs; these are the:
   1. Umbilical vein and ductus venosus.
   2. Foramen ovale and ductus arteriosus.
   3. Umbilical artery and atrial septal shunt.
   4. Ductus venosus and ductus arteriosus.

2. Risk management, a standard for nursing care, requires the nurse to evaluate all assessment findings. The nurse must know that within 3 min of birth, the normal newborn's heart rate may range from:
   1. 100–130.
   2. 110–180.
   3. 120–160.
   4. 130–170.

3. The nurse assesses the Apgar score of a newborn at 1 and 5 min of age based on the following findings: heart rate—118; muscle tone—maintains attitude of general flexion; respirations—lusty cry; reflex response—active at +2; color—pink with some acrocyanosis. What score should the nurse enter on the newborn's records?
   1. 7.
   2. 8.
   3. 9.
   4. 10.

4. The nurse tests the newborn's Babinski reflex by:
   1. Touching the corner of the newborn's mouth or cheek.
   2. Changing the newborn's equilibrium.
   3. Placing a finger in the palm of the newborn's hand.
   4. Stroking the lateral aspect of the sole from the heel upward and across the ball of the foot.

5. To meet the standard of care for risk management, the nurse assessing a newborn must know that asymmetric Moro reflex responses are often associated with:
   1. Injury to the cerebrum or cerebellum.
   2. Injury to cranial nerve VII.
   3. Injury to the brachial plexus, clavicle, or humerus.
   4. Poor muscle tone secondary to a genetic aberration such as Down syndrome.

6. A new mother questions the nurse about the "lump" on her baby's head. She says that the physician told her it was "a collection of blood between a skull bone and its covering" (periosteum). The nurse explains that this is called:
   1. Caput succedaneum.
   2. Molding.
   3. Cephalohematoma.
   4. Subdural hematoma.

7. The home health nurse notices that a newborn has developed purulent conjunctivitis on the sixth day. At this time, the nurse:
   1. Calls the physician for an order to test the infant for allergy.
   2. Assesses the infant for signs of pneumonia.
   3. Demonstrates for the mother how to bathe the infant's eyes with tepid boric acid solution.
   4. Asks the mother if an older sibling has a cold.

8. The nurse must intervene when, after checking the parent's understanding regarding circumcision, the parent states:
   1. "Yellowish crusting (exudate) is normal within 24 hr of the circumcision, so I won't worry if I see any."
   2. "Applying petrolatum gauze wrap will keep the healing wound from sticking to the diaper."
   3. "Brief application of a wrapped ice pack is recommended if bleeding is seen."
   4. "Using cloth diapers will help me see if there is any bleeding."

9. A neonate weighed 7 pounds, 15 oz (3600 g) at birth; at discharge on the second day after birth, the neonate weighs 7 pounds, 8 oz (3402 g). What would be a valid interpretation of the neonate's current condition?
   1. The neonate should show weight gain instead of loss.
   2. The new mother is having trouble breastfeeding.
   3. The weight loss is within normal limits.
   4. The neonate is retaining fluid.

10. When parents question the need for a newborn to receive an injection of vitamin K soon after birth, the nurse's response is based on the knowledge that vitamin K is given to:
    1. Promote hematopoiesis.
    2. Promote synthesis of clotting factors.
    3. Stimulate the formation of platelets.
    4. Stimulate the release of stored iron.

11. Which criteria of gestational age must be assessed within 2 hr of birth for the results to be valid?
    1. Breast tissue.
    2. Posture.
    3. Sole of feet creases.
    4. Scarf sign.

12. A newborn weighed 7 pounds, 8 oz at birth 3 days ago. He now weighs 6 pounds, 12 oz; his mother is concerned. The nurse can assure his mother that her son's weight loss is still within normal limits if he loses up to:
    1. 9 oz.
    2. 12 oz.
    3. 15 oz.
    4. 18 oz.

13. A newborn's head circumference is 34 cm; chest circumference is 32 cm. Which nursing action would be appropriate?
    1. Refer the newborn for evaluation for psychomotor retardation.
    2. Prepare the mother for the probability that the physician will order a head ultrasound.
    3. Measure the occipitofrontal circumference daily.
    4. Record the findings and take no further action.

14. A newborn is admitted to the nursery 15 min after birth. He is moderately cyanotic, has a mottled trunk and active movements of the extremities, and is loosely wrapped in a cotton blanket. The *primary* assessment by the nurse would be to check:
    1. The umbilical stump for bleeding.
    2. The baby's temperature.
    3. For visible abnormalities.
    4. For a patent airway.

15. Suctioning the newborn should follow which procedure?
    1. Suction mouth first, then nose.
    2. Suction nose first, then mouth.
    3. Milk the trachea first, then proceed with suctioning.
    4. Firmly slap the infant's back, then proceed with a bulb syringe or catheter.

16. If bleeding is noted from a newly circumcised penis, the nurse's initial response should be to:
    1. Apply a diaper tightly over the penis to maintain a steady pressure.
    2. Notify the physician immediately.
    3. Apply gentle pressure to the bleeding site with a folded gauze pad.
    4. Wrap the glans penis in a fresh sterile petrolatum gauze and observe for 2 hr.

17. A 5-hr-old newborn boy wakes up in his mother's room, spits up some mucus and has a gagging episode. The nurse's *first* action is to:
    1. Sit him upright and pat his back.
    2. Immediately take him to the nursery for suctioning.
    3. Help his mother hold him face down with his head lower than his buttocks.
    4. Reassure his mother that this is normal at this age, and the baby needs no assistance.

18. The nurse tests a newborn for the rooting reflex by:
    1. Touching the corner of the newborn's mouth or cheek.
    2. Placing a finger in the palm of the newborn's hand.
    3. Stroking the lateral aspect of the sole from the heel upward and across the ball of the foot.
    4. Changing the newborn's equilibrium.

# Answers/Rationale

1. **(2)** The foramen ovale and ductus arteriosus are the two fetal structures that allow fetal blood to bypass the fetal lungs; oxygen is obtained from maternal circulation to placenta to umbilical vein. Because only these structures allow fetal blood to bypass fetal lungs, options **1, 3,** and **4** each contain at least one incorrect structure. **IMP, RE/KN, 5, HPM, Health promotion and maintenance**

2. **(3)** The normal range is 120–160. The rate varies with activity, increasing to 160 while crying and decreasing to 120 when in deep sleep. Bradycardia, rates below 120 (**1** and **2**), and tachycardia, rates above 160 (**2** and **4**), are *not normal* and require further evaluation and intervention. **EV, RE/KN, 5, HPM, Health promotion and maintenance**

3. **(3)** 9 is recorded because the heart rate (> 100), muscle tone, respirations, and reflex response each receive a score of 2, and color pink with acrocyanosis (bluish hands and feet) is scored as 1. Options **1, 2,** and **4** represent *inaccurate* scores. **IMP, APP, 6, HPM, Health promotion and maintenance**

4. **(4)** The Babinski reflex is elicited by stroking the lateral aspect of the sole from the heel upward and across the ball of the foot. A positive test (in neonates) of fanning the toes and dorsiflexing the big toe is an indication of fetal well-being. Touching the corner of the newborn's mouth or cheek (**1**) elicits the *rooting reflex*. Changing the newborn's equilibrium (**2**) elicits the *Moro reflex*. Placing a finger in the palm of the newborn's hand (**3**) elicits the *palmar grasp reflex*. **IMP, RE/KN, 5, HPM, Health promotion and maintenance**

5. **(3)** An asymmetric Moro reflex response is often associated with injury to the brachial plexus, clavicle, or humerus, preventing abductive and adductive movements of the upper extremities. Injuries to the cerebrum or cerebellum (**1**) could result in *symmetric* loss of the reflex. Cranial VII nerve (**2**) is the facial nerve; even if it is paralyzed, there is no effect on the Moro response. Down

---

**Key to Codes**

**Nursing process: AS,** assessment; **AN,** analysis; **PL,** planning; **IMP,** implementation; **EV,** evaluation. (See **Appendix J** for explanation of nursing process steps.)

**Cognitive level: RE/KN,** recall/knowledge; **COM,** comprehension; **APP,** application; **ANL,** analysis; **EVL,** evaluation; **SYN,** synthesis. (See **Appendix J** for explanation.)

**Category of human function: 1,** protective; **2,** sensory-perceptual; **3,** comfort, rest, activity, and mobility; **4,** nutrition; **5,** growth and development; **6,** fluid-gas transport; **7,** psychosocial-cultural; **8,** elimination. (See **Appendix L** for explanation.)

**Client need: SECE,** safe, effective care environment; **HPM,** health promotion and maintenance; **PsI,** psychosocial integrity; **PhI,** physiological integrity. (See **Appendix M** for explanation.)

**Client subneed:** See **Appendix M** for explanation.

syndrome (**4**) is *not* responsible for an asymmetric Moro response. **AN, RE/KN, 3, HPM, Health promotion and maintenance**

6. (**3**) Cephalohematoma is a collection of blood between a skull bone and its covering (periosteum). Caput succedaneum (**1**) is a swelling of the tissue over the presenting part of the fetal head caused by pressure during labor. Molding (**2**) refers to the overlapping of cranial bones or shaping of the fetal head to accommodate and conform to the bony and soft parts of the mother's birth canal during labor. Subdural hematoma (**4**) refers to bleeding between the dural and arachnoid membranes of the brain. **IMP, RE/KN, 5, HPM, Health promotion and maintenance**

7. (**2**) Purulent conjunctivitis that first appears 5 days-2 wk after birth is symptomatic of *Chlamydia trachomatis* infection; this organism causes pneumonia in the untreated child. If untreated, chronic follicular conjunctivitis, with conjunctival scarring and corneal neovascularization, may result. Purulent conjunctivitis is *neither* a sign of allergy (**1**), *nor* related to an older child's cold (**4**). To bathe the eyes with anything (**3**), a physician's order is required. (See treatment note below.)

NOTE: Signs of *pneumonia* include prolonged staccato cough, tachypnea, mild hypoxemia, and eosinophilia. Prevention of *conjunctivitis*: ophthalmic ointment of erythromycin or tetracycline. Treatment of *pneumonia*: oral erythromycin for 2–3 wk, and irrigation of the eye with saline or buffered ophthalmic solution daily. **IMP, APP, 1, SECE, Safety and infection control**

8. (**3**) The nurse *must* intervene if the parent thinks that a wrapped ice pack is to be applied to the healing site if bleeding occurs, because the ice pack can injure the glans penis. Parents should use a sterile *Teflon* gauze (to avoid sticking) to apply gentle intermittent pressure to stem the bleeding. If bleeding continues, the pediatrician should be notified **STAT**. Options **1, 2,** and (**4**) are *correct* regarding circumcision and its care, so *no intervention* is needed. **EV, ANL, 1, SECE, Management of care**

9. (**3**) The weight loss is within normal limits. The normal neonate may lose up to 10% of the birth weight (in this case, 12.7 oz or 360 g). This loss is usually the extra fluid the neonate has at birth until the mother's milk comes in on day 3. Option 1 is the *opposite* of the correct interpretation. Option 2 is incorrect because the mother's milk is not yet in; nature has helped compensate for this by the extra fluid most neonates have at birth. Option 4 is incorrect because the neonate is *losing* (not retaining)fluid, at a rate within normal limits. **EV, ANL, 5, HPM, Health promotion and maintenance**

10. (**2**) Vitamin K's function is to promote synthesis of clotting factors. It is produced in the GI tract by microorganisms, but the newborn's GI tract is sterile; vitamin K is not produced by the newborn until about the eighth day of life. It is given by IM injection, into the vastus lateralis muscle preferably; an alternate injection site is the rectus femoris muscle. Options **1, 3,** and **4** are all unrelated to vitamin $K_1$, since its only purpose is to promote synthesis of clotting factors. **PL, COM, 1, PhI, Pharmacological and parenteral therapies**

11. (**3**) After 2 hr, the edema of tissues present in most newborns begins to resolve and creases appear; these creases do not have the same predictive value as those assessed before resolution of newborn edema. All of the criteria in options **1, 2,** and **4** remain predictive *beyond* the first 2 hr after birth. **AS, COM, 5, HPM, Health promotion and maintenance**

12. (**2**) Normal term newborns whose weight averages from 2500–4000 g (5 lb 8 oz–8 lb 13 oz) can lose about 10% of their birth weight in the first few days of life. This baby can lose 12 oz (7 lb 8 oz = 120 oz x 0.10 = 12 oz) and be within normal limits. This is due to the excretion of fluids through the lungs, urinary bladder, and bowels, and to the small amount of intake during this time. Newborns begin to regain their birth weight by 10–14 days of age. The amounts in options **1, 3,** and **4** are due either to *inaccurate* calculations or to use of the wrong formula. **EV, APP, 5, HPM, Health promotion and maintenance**

13. (**4**) Record the findings and take no further action; this finding is normal. The actions in options **1, 2,** and **3** are *unnecessary* since the finding is within normal limits. **IMP, APP, 5, HPM, Health promotion and maintenance**

14. (**2**) These symptoms reflect a cold body temperature. These symptoms are *not* associated with bleeding from the umbilical stump (**1**), congenital abnormalities (**3**), or respiratory distress (**4**); rather, they *are* the usual symptoms of cold stress (**2**). **AS, ANL, 3, HPM, Health promotion and maintenance**

15. (**1**) The newborn will commence breathing when the nose is stimulated; clearing the mouth first clears oral mucus that might otherwise be aspirated when breathing starts. Stimulating breathing before the mouth is clear (**2**) can lead to aspiration of oral mucus. The trachea should *never* be milked (**3**); this action is ineffective and wastes valuable time. Slapping the infant (**4**) would cause the baby to gasp and aspirate oral and nasopharyngeal contents (and the nurse should *never* hit an infant!). **IMP, ANL, 1, PhI, Reduction of risk potential**

16. **(3)** Gentle pressure to the bleeding site will usually stop the bleeding. Only enough pressure should be exerted to stop the flow of blood; excessive pressure can compromise needed blood flow to the structure. Option **1** is incorrect since bleeding can continue unseen, and too tight a diaper can *obstruct* flow of blood to the diaper area. Option **2** is incorrect because it is *unnecessary at this time*, although it may be necessary if the gentle pressure for a short time does not suffice. Option **4** is incorrect because it does *not* assist with stopping the hemorrhage. **IMP, ANL, 1, PhI, Reduction of risk potential**

17. **(3)** The mother needs to learn what to do when an infant is gagging. The parent(s) should learn how to use a bulb syringe as well. Option **1** is incorrect since this would tend to cause the infant to gasp and *aspirate* mucus. Option **2** is incorrect since this would tell the mother that she is incapable of handling the situation. Option **4** is incorrect since, although this is normal for the second period of reactivity, she needs to know how to manage the situation when she is discharged. **IMP, ANL, 1, HPM, Health promotion and maintenance**

18. **(1)** The rooting reflex is elicited by touching the corner of the newborn's mouth or cheek. Placing a finger in the palm of the newborn's hand (**2**) elicits the *palmar grasp* reflex. Stroking the lateral aspect of the sole from the heel upward and across the ball of the foot (**3**) elicits the *Babinski* reflex. Changing the newborn's equilibrium (**4**) elicits the *Moro* reflex. **IMP, RE/KN, 5, HPM, Health promotion and maintenance**

# Complications During the Neonatal Period: The High-Risk Newborn

## Chapter Outline

---

## Key Points

- To maintain high standards of care, the nurse must identify risk situations caused by **immaturity, alterations in functioning of systems, metabolic imbalances, developmental problems** (*congenital anomalies*), and **acquired problems**, such as *birth injuries, infections*, and *drug dependence*.

- The alert nurse often is the pivotal link between functional and dysfunctional survival for the infant at risk.

- The earliest clinical *signs of neonatal illness* are characterized by a lack of specificity: lethargy, poor feeding, poor weight gain, or irritability.

- The curative and rehabilitative problems of children with some disorders are often complex, requiring a multidisciplinary approach to the care of such a child and the parents.

## Key Words

Bronchopulmonary dysplasia (BPD)
Direct Coombs' test
Erythroblastosis fetalis
Exchange blood transfusion
Fetal alcohol syndrome (FAS)
Hip dysplasia
Hyperbilirubinemia
Iatrogenic (nosocomial)
Kernicterus
Meconium aspiration syndrome
Necrotizing enterocolitis (NEC)
Pilonidal dimple
Retinopathy of prematurity (ROP)
Scaphoid abdomen

# All Infants

**General overview**—successful newborn adaptation to the demands of independent extrauterine life may be complicated by environmental insults during the *prenatal* period (see **Chapter 3**) and/or those arising in the period immediately surrounding birth (see **Chapter 5**). The nursing role focuses on minimizing the effect of present and emerging health problems and on facilitating and supporting a successful transition to extrauterine life. Review **Table 8.2, p. 179-181** for deviations from the norm.

I. **General aspects**—common neonatal risk factors
 A. Gestational age profile (see **Table 8.2, p. 181** and **Table 8.1, p. 176**)
   1. Prematurity.
   2. Dysmaturity.
   3. Postmaturity.
 B. Congenital disorders.
 C. Birth trauma.
 D. Infections.

## Disorders Affecting Protective Function: *Neonatal Infections*

### Oral Thrush (mycotic stomatitis)

I. **Pathophysiology**: local inflammation of oral mucosa due to fungal infection.
II. **Etiology/risk factors:**
 A. Organism—*Candida albicans.*
 B. More common in newborn who is vulnerable (i.e., sick, debilitated, HIV+, those receiving antibiotic therapy).
III. *Mode of transmission*—direct contact with:
 A. Maternal birth canal, nipples, hands, and linens.
 B. Contaminated feeding equipment, staff's hands.
IV. **Assessment**
 A. White patches on oral mucosa, gums, and tongue that bleed when touched.
 B. Occasional difficulty in swallowing.
V. **Analysis/nursing diagnosis**
 A. *Pain* related to irritation of oral mucous membrane secondary to oral moniliasis (candidiasis).
 B. *Nutrition deficit* related to irritability and poor feeding.
VI. **Nursing care plan/implementation:**
 A. Goal: *prevent cross-contamination.*
   1. Aseptic technique; use standard precautions; good handwashing.
   2. Medication, as ordered
    a. *Aqueous gentian violet,* 0.5%: apply to infected area with swab; very messy, stains anything it contacts (rarely used).

b. *Nystatin (Mycostatin)*—instill into mouth with medicine dropper, or apply to lesions with swab, *after* feedings, also apply to nipples.
VII. **Evaluation/outcome criteria**
 A. The newborn's oral mucosa is intact, lesions are healed, with no evidence of infection.
 B. The newborn feeds well; maintains weight or regains weight lost, if any.

### Neonatal Sepsis

I. **Pathophysiology**: generalized infection; may overwhelm infant's immature immune system.
II. **Etiology/risk factors:**
 A. Prolonged rupture of membranes.
 B. Long, difficult labor.
 C. Resuscitation procedures.
 D. Maternal infection (i.e., group ß *beta-hemolytic streptococcus vaginosis*).
 E. Aspiration—amniotic fluid, formula, mucus.
 F. *Iatrogenic* (*nosocomial*)—caused by infected health personnel or equipment.
III. **Assessment**
 A. Respirations—irregular, periods of apnea.
 B. Irritability or lethargy, temperature instability.
IV. **Analysis/nursing diagnosis**
 A. *Fatigue* related to increased oxygen needs.
 B. *Infection risk* related to septic condition.
V. **Nursing care plan/implementation**
 A. Order cultures (spinal, urine, blood).
 B. Check vitals.
 C. Monitor respirations.
VI. **Evaluation/outcome criteria**
 A. The newborn responds to medical/nursing regimen (all assessment findings within normal limits).
 B. Parent(s) verbalize understanding of diagnosis, treatment; demonstrate appropriate techniques in participating in care (as possible).
 C. Parent(s) demonstrate effective coping with situation; express satisfaction with care.

### Hepatitis B and Herpes Simplex Type II Viral Infections

I. **Hepatitis B virus (HBV) infection**
 A. *Mode of transmission*—from the mother to the newborn in about 90% of cases.
 B. HBV is associated with about a 20% increase in preterm birth.
 C. *Medical management*—*infants* who require *hepatitis B immune globulin* (HBIG) should receive 0.5 mL intramuscularly, as soon as possible after birth.
   1. All infants should receive hepatitis B vaccine with the following schedule:
   Dose 1: within the first 12 h of birth.
   Dose 2: at 1 mo.
   Dose 3: at 6 mo.

II. *Herpes* virus infection

⚠ A. *Precautions*—while a mother is awaiting the results of cultures for diagnosis of *herpes virus* infection; both *gown and gloves* should be worn by persons in contact with the infant.

B. *Medical management.*

💊 1. Trifluridine *ophthalmic* solution is administered for prevention of keratoconjunctivitis.

💊 2. Acyclovir 60mg/kg/day divided q 8 hrs, given IV.

3. As long as no suspicious lesions are found on the mother's breasts, breastfeeding is allowed.

4. The infant should be seen by the pediatrician *every week* for the *first month* after birth.

# Disorders Affecting Nutrition:
## Infant of the Mother Who is Diabetic (IDM)

I. **Pathophysiology**: hyperplasia of pancreatic beta cells → increased insulin production → excessive deposition of glycogen in muscles, subcutaneous fat, and tissue growth. Results in fetal:

A. *Macrosomia*—large for gestational age (LGA).

B. *Enlarged internal organs*—common
  1. Cardiomegaly.
  2. Hepatomegaly.
  3. Splenomegaly.

C. Neonatal—inadequate carbohydrate reserve to meet energy needs.

❗ D. *Increased incidence of*:
  1. *Congenital anomalies* (5 times average incidence)—includes cardiac, pelvic, and spinal anomalies.
  2. *Preterm birth*. Respiratory distress syndrome (RDS). Increased insulin needs prenatally → decreased surfactant production.
  3. *Maternal dystocia*—due to cephalopelvic disproportion (CPD).
  4. *Neonatal metabolic problems*:
     a. Hypoglycemia.
     b. Hypocalcemic tetany.
     c. Metabolic acidosis.
     d. Hyperbilirubinemia.

II. **Etiology**: high circulating maternal glucose levels during fetal growth and development; loss of maternal glucose supply following birth; decreased hepatic gluconeogenesis.

▶ III. **Assessment**

A. Characteristics of IDM:
  See **Pathophysiology** above.

📟 B. *Hypoglycemia*—apply *Dextrostix* or *Chemstrip* to heel stick at:
  1. 30 min.
  2. 1, 2, 4, 6, 9, 12, and 24 hr of age.

3. Hypoglycemia laboratory values for *term* infant: ≤ 40 mg/dL.

4. Hypoglycemia laboratory values for *preterm* infant: ≤ 45 mg/dL.

❗ 5. Behavioral signs—tremors, twitching, hypotonia, seizures, lethargy.

C. Gestational age, since macrosomia may mask prematurity.

❗ D. *Hypocalcemia*—usually within first 24 hr:
  1. Irritability.
  2. Coarse tremors, twitching, convulsions.
  3. Lethargy

❗ E. *Birth injuries*:
  1. Fractures: clavicle, humerus, skull.
  2. Brachial palsy, Duchenne-Erb paralysis
  3. Intracranial hemorrhage/signs of *increased intracranial pressure* (ICCP).
     a. Widening of fontanels and sutures.
     b. Bulging fontanels at rest.
     c. High-pitched, whiny cry.
  4. Cephalohematoma.

F. *Respiratory distress in the newborn*:
  1. Nasal flaring.
  2. Sternal and intercostal retraction.
  3. Cyanosis.
  4. Expiratory grunt.

G. *Jaundice.*

▶ IV. **Analysis/nursing diagnosis**

A. *Injury risk* related to CPD, dystocia.

B. *Cardiopulmonary tissue perfusion alteration* related to placental insufficiency, RDS.

C. *Gas exchange impairment* related to RDS.

D. *Nutrition deficit* related to hypoglycemia, hypocalcemia.

E. *Endocrine/metabolic processes alteration* related to hyperbilirubinemia and kernicterus.

▶ V. **Nursing care plan/implementation**

💊 A. *Hypoglycemia*—administer oral or intravenous *glucose*, as ordered (may cause rebound effect).

B. Premature/immature—institute premature care, prn.

💊 C. *Hypocalcemia*—administer oral or intravenous *calcium gluconate*, as ordered.

D. Inform pediatrician **immediately** of signs of:
  1. Jaundice.
  2. Hyperirritability.
  3. Birth injury.
  4. IICP/hemorrhage.

▶ VI. **Evaluation/outcome criteria**: The newborn:

A. Makes successful transition to extrauterine life.

B. Responds to medical/nursing regimen. Experiences minimal or no metabolic disturbances (e.g., hypoglycemia, hypocalcemia, hyperbilirubinemia).

C. Exhibits normal respiratory function and gas exchange.

# Hypoglycemia in the Newborn

I. **Pathophysiology:** low serum-glucose level → altered cellular metabolism → cerebral irritability, cardiopulmonary problems.

II. **Etiology/risk factors:**

A. Loss of maternal glucose supply.

B. Normal physiologic activities of respiration, thermoregulation, and muscular activity *exceed* carbohydrate reserve.

C. *Decreased* hepatic ability to convert amino acids into glucose.

D. More common in:

1. Infants of diabetic mothers (IDM).
2. Preterm, postterm infants.
3. Small for gestational age (SGA).
4. Smaller twin.
5. Infant of mother with pre-eclampsia.
6. Birth asphyxia.

III. **Assessment**

A. Jitteriness, tremors, convulsions; lethargy and hypotonia.

B. Sweating; unstable temperature.

C. Tachypnea; apneic episodes; cyanosis.

D. High-pitched, shrill cry.

E. Difficulty in feeding.

IV. **Analysis/nursing diagnosis**

A. *Tissue perfusion alteration (fetal)* related to placental insufficiency associated with maternal diabetes, pre-eclampsia, renal and/or cardiac disorders; erythroblastosis.

B. *Endocrine/metabolic processes alteration* related to high incidence of morbidity associated with birth asphyxia.

C. *Gas exchange impairment* related to coexisting RDS.

D. *Nutrition deficit* related to hypoglycemia.

E. *Injury risk* related to coexisting infection, metabolic acidosis.

V. **Nursing care plan/implementation:** see **p. 193**, *Infant of the mother who is diabetic.*

VI. **Evaluation/outcome criteria:** see *Infant of the mother who is diabetic*, **p. 193.**

# Disorders Affecting Psychosocial-Cultural Function: *Neonate Who is Drug-Dependent*

I. **General aspects**

A. Maternal drug addiction has been associated with:

1. Prenatal malnutrition and vitamin deficiencies.
2. Increased risk of antepartal infections.
3. Higher incidence of antepartal and intrapartal complications.

B. Infant at risk for:

1. Intrauterine growth restriction (IUGR).
2. Prematurity.
3. Congenital anomalies.
4. Fetal distress.
5. Perinatal death.
6. Child abuse.

II. **Pathophysiology:** withdrawal of accustomed drug levels → physiologic deprivation response.

III. **Etiology:** repeated intrauterine absorption of heroin/cocaine/methadone/methamphetamines from maternal bloodstream → fetal drug dependency.

IV. **Assessment**—degree of newborn drug dependence (withdrawal) depends on type and duration of addiction, and maternal drug levels at birth. Use *neonatal abstinence syndrome (NAS) scoring chart* to determine severity of drug withdrawal, and need for treatment. See **Table 9.1.**

A. Irritability, hyperactivity, hypertonicity, exaggerated reflexes, tremors, high-pitched cry, difficult to comfort

1. *"Step" reflex* (dancing)—infant places both feet on surface; assumes rigid stance—does *not* "step" or dance.
2. *"Head-righting" reflex*—holds head rigid; *fails* to demonstrate head lag.

B. Nasal stuffiness and sneezing; respiratory distress, tachypnea, cyanosis and/or apnea.

C. Exaggerated acrocyanosis and/or mottling in the infant who is warm.

D. Sweating.

E. Hunger—sucks on fists; feeding problems: regurgitation, vomiting, poor feeding; diarrhea and increased mucus production.

F. Convulsions with abnormal eye-rolling and chewing motions.

G. Developmental lags/mental retardation.

V. **Analysis/nursing diagnosis**

A. *Injury risk* related to convulsions secondary to physiologic response to withdrawal, CNS hyperirritability.

B. *Gas exchange* related to respiratory distress secondary to inhibition of reflex clearing of fluid by the lungs.

C. *Nutrition deficit* related to feeding problems secondary to respiratory distress and GI hypermotility.

D. *Skin integrity impairment risk* related to scratching secondary to withdrawal symptoms.

VI. **Nursing care plan/implementation**

A. Goal: *prevent/minimize respiratory distress.*

1. *Position: side lying, head dependent*—to facilitate mucus drainage.
2. Suction, prn, with bulb syringe for excess mucus—to maintain patent airway.
3. Monitor respirations and apical pulse.

## TABLE 9.1   NEONATAL ABSTINENCE SYNDROME (NAS) SCORE

Infants whose mothers have confirmed or suspected drug use during pregnancy and are showing signs of withdrawal should be scored every 4 hours. This scoring system allows personnel to perform a consistent evaluation of symptoms in infants who are drug-exposed.

NOTE: Caution must be exercised before symptoms listed here are solely attributed to drug withdrawal. For example, symptoms such as fever, tachypnea or seizures could be due to sepsis.

| System | Signs and Symptoms | Score |
|---|---|---|
| CNS | High-pitched cry | 2 |
| | Continuous high-pitched cry | 3 |
| | Sleeps <1 hour after feeding | 3 |
| | Sleeps <2 hours after feeding | 2 |
| | Sleeps <3 hours after feeding | 1 |
| | Mild tremors when disturbed | 1 |
| | Mod-severe tremors when disturbed | 2 |
| | Mild tremors when undisturbed | 3 |
| | Mod-severe tremors when undisturbed | 4 |
| | Increased muscle tone | 2 |
| | Excoriation (specify area) | 1 |
| | Mycological jerks | 3 |
| | Generalized convulsions | 5 |
| Metabolic/Vasomotor/Respiratory | Fever (37.3-38.3° C) | 1 |
| | Fever (>38.3° C) | 2 |
| | Frequent yawning (>3-4 times) | 1 |
| | Nasal stuffiness | 1 |
| | Sneezing (>3-4 times) | 1 |
| | Nasal flaring | 2 |
| | Respiratory rate >60/min | 1 |
| | Respiratory rate >60/min + retractions | 2 |
| Gastrointestinal disturbances | Excessive sucking | 1 |
| | Poor feeding | 2 |
| | Regurgitation | 2 |
| | Projectile vomiting | 3 |
| | Loose stools | 2 |
| | Watery stools | 3 |

B. Goal: *minimize possibility of convulsions.*
   1. Decrease environmental stimuli—quiet, touch only when necessary, offer pacifier.
   2. Keep warm, swaddle for comfort.
C. Goal: *maintain nutrition/hydration.*
   1. Food/fluids—oral or IV, as ordered.
   2. I&O.
   3. Daily weight.
D. Goal: *assist in diagnosis of drug and drug level.*
   1. Collect urine during first 24 hr for toxicologic studies.

E. Goal: *maintain/promote skin integrity.*
   1. Mitts over hands—to minimize scratching.
   2. Keep clean and dry.
   3. Medicated ointment/powder, as ordered, every 2–4 hr, to excoriated areas.
   4. Expose excoriated areas to air.
F. Goal: *minimize withdrawal symptoms.*
   1. Administer medications, as ordered.
      a. Morphine sulfate solution 0.4 mg/mL is primary choice for NAS.
      b. *Paregoric elixir—no* longer recommended due to alcohol content and benzoic acid.

c. *Phenobarbital*—to reduce CNS hyperirritability, hyperbilirubinemia.
d. *Methadone*.
G. Goal: *emotional support to mother*.
  1. Encourage verbalization of feelings of guilt, anxiety, fear, concerns.
  2. Refer to social service.

◄ VII. Evaluation/outcome criteria: The newborn:
  A. Responds to medical/nursing regimen
    1. Maintains adequate respirations.
    2. Feeds well, gains weight.
    3. No evidence of CNS hyperirritability, convulsions; demonstrates normal newborn reflexes.
  B. Evidences bonding with parent(s). Responsive to mother's voice.

# Disorders Affecting Psychosocial–Cultural Function: *Fetal Alcohol Syndrome (FAS)*

I. **General aspects:**
  A. Maternal alcohol abuse has been associated with:
    1. Malnutrition, vitamin deficiencies.
    2. Bone marrow suppression.
    3. Liver disease.
    4. Child abuse.

! II. *Infant at risk for*:
  A. Congenital anomalies.
  B. Mental deficiency.
  C. IUGR, (intrauterine growth restriction).

III. **Pathophysiology**: permanent damage to developing embryonic/fetal structures; cardiovascular anomalies (*ventricular septal defects*).

⚡ IV. **Etiology/risk factors**: *high* circulating alcohol levels are lethal to the embryo; *lower* levels cause permanent cell damage.

◄ V. **Assessment**
  A. Characteristic *craniofacial abnormalities*:
    1. Short, palpebral fissure.
    2. Epicanthal folds.
    3. Maxillary hypoplasia.
    4. Micrognathia (abnormal smallness of mandible or chin).
    5. Long, thin upper lip.
  B. Short stature.
  C. Irritable, hyperactive, poor feeding.
  D. High-pitched cry, difficult to comfort.

◄ VI. **Nursing care plan/implementation**
  A. Goal: *reduce irritability*.
    1. Reduce environmental stimuli.
    2. Wrap, cuddle.
    3. Administer *sedatives*, as ordered.
  B. Goal: *maintain nutrition/hydration*.
  C. Goal: *emotional support to mother*.

◄ VII. **Evaluation/outcome criteria**: see *Neonate who is drug-dependent*, **VII.**, p. 196
  A. No respiratory distress.
  B. Infant feeding properly.
  C. Maternal bonding apparent.
  D. Social service—home involvement.

# Classification of Infants by Weight and Gestational Age

I. **Terminology**
  A. *Preterm, or premature*—37 wk gestation or less.
  B. *Term*—38–42 wk gestation.
  C. *Postterm*—over 42 wk.
  D. *Postmature*—gestation greater than 42 wk.
  E. *Appropriate for gestational age (AGA)*—for each week of gestation, there is a normal range of expected weight:
    1. Term infants weighing 2500 g or more are usually mature in physiologic functions.
    2. If respiratory distress occurs, it is usually related to *meconium aspiration syndrome*.
  F. *Small for gestational age (SGA), or dysmature*—weight falls *below* normal range for age.
    1. **Etiology/risk factors**:
      a. Preeclampsia.
      b. Malnutrition.
      c. Smoking.
      d. Placental insufficiency.
      e. Alcohol syndrome.
      f. Rubella.
      g. Syphilis.
      h. Multifetal gestation (twins, etc.).
      i. Genetic.
      j. Cocaine abuse.
  G. *Large for gestational age (LGA)*—above expected weight for age. NOTE: If *preterm*, at risk for *respiratory distress syndrome*. If *postterm*, at risk for meconium aspiration and sudden intrauterine
⚡ death.
    1. **Etiology/risk factors**:
      a. Maternal diabetes or prediabetes.
      b. Maternal weight gain over 35 pounds.
      c. Maternal obesity.
      d. Genetic.
  ! 2. *Associated problems*:
      a. Hypoglycemia.
      b. Hypocalcemia.
      c. Hyperbilirubinemia.
      d. Birth injury, e.g., fractures; conditions secondary to type of birth (scalpel wounds during cesarean; Duchenne-Erb paralysis due to shoulder dystocia during vaginal birth)

II. *Estimation of gestational age*—planning appropriate care for the newborn requires accurate assessment to differentiate between *premature* and *term* infants.

# Preterm/Premature Infant

**Definition:** born at 37 wk gestation or less.

I. **General aspects**

II. **Pathophysiology:** anatomic and physiologic immaturity of body systems compromises ability to adapt to extrauterine environment and independent life:

A. *Interference with* **protective** *functions.*

1. Temperature *regulation*—unstable, due to:
   a. Lack of subcutaneous fat.
   b. Large body surface area in proportion to body weight.
   c. Small muscle mass.
   d. Absent sweat or shiver responses.
   e. Poor capillary response to changes in environmental temperature.

2. *Resistance to infection*—low, due to:
   a. Lack of immune bodies from mother (these cross placenta *late* in pregnancy).
   b. Inability to produce own immune bodies (immature liver).
   c. Poor white blood cell response to infection.

3. *Immature liver.*
   a. Inability to conjugate bilirubin liberated by normal breakdown of red blood cells → increased susceptibility to *hyperbilirubinemia* and *kernicterus*.
   b. Immature production of clotting factors and immune globulins.
   c. Inadequate glucose stores → increased susceptibility to *hypoglycemia*.

B. *Interference with* **elimination:** immature *renal* function → unable to concentrate urine → precarious fluid/electrolyte balance.

C. *Interference with* **sensory-perceptual functions:** central nervous system immaturity → weak or absent reflexes and fluctuating primitive control of vital functions.

D. *Causes of mortality* (in order of frequency):
1. Abnormal pulmonary ventilation.
2. Infection:
   a. Pneumonia.
   b. Septicemia.
   c. Diarrhea.
   d. Meningitis.
3. Intracranial hemorrhage.
4. Congenital defects.

III. **Etiology/risk factors:** (often unknown); preterm labor

A. *Placental factors:*
1. Placenta previa.
2. Abruptio placentae.
3. Placental insufficiency.

B. *Uterine factors:*
1. Incompetent cervix.
2. Overdistention (multifetal gestation, hydramnios).
3. Anomalies (e.g., myomas).

C. *Fetal factors:*
1. Malformations.
2. Infections (e.g., rubella, toxoplasmosis, hepatitis B, human immunodeficiency virus [HIV], AIDS, cytomegalic inclusion disease).
3. Multifetal gestations (e.g., twins, triplets).

D. *Maternal factors:*
1. Severe physical or emotional trauma.
2. Coexisting disorders (e.g., pre-eclampsia, hypertension, heart disease, diabetes, malnutrition).
3. Infections (e.g., strepococcus, syphilis, pyelonephritis, pneumonia, influenza, leukemia).

E. *Miscellaneous factors:*
1. Close frequency of pregnancies.
2. Advanced maternal age.
3. Heavy smoking.
4. High-altitude environment.
5. Cocaine use.

F. *Factors influencing* survival:
1. Gestational age.
2. Lung maturity.
3. Anomalies.
4. Size.

# Disorders Affecting Fluid–Gas Transport:
# ! *Respiratory Distress Syndrome (RDS)*

I. **Pathophysiology:** insufficient pulmonary surfactant (lecithin) and insufficient number/maturity of alveoli predispose to atelectasis; alveolar ducts and terminal bronchi become lined with fibrous, glossy membrane.

II. **Etiology/risk factors:**

A. Primarily associated with prematurity.

! B. Other *predisposing* factors:
1. *Fetal hypoxia*—due to decreased placental perfusion secondary to maternal bleeding (e.g., abruptio) or hypotension.
2. *Birth asphyxia.*
3. *Postnatal hypothermia, metabolic acidosis,* or *hypotension.*

III. Conditions that may enhance production of surfactant and therefore *protect* neonate from RDS:

A. Chronic fetal stress—due to maternal hypertension, pre-eclampsia, or heroin addiction.

B. Premature rupture of membranes (PROM).

C. Maternal steroid ingestion (i.e., *betamethasone*).

D. Low-grade chorioamnionitis.

**IV. Assessment**

A. Usually appears during first or second day after birth.

B. Signs of *respiratory distress*:
  1. Nasal flaring.
  2. Sternal retractions.
  3. Tachypnea (60/min or more).
  4. Cyanosis.
  5. Expiratory grunt.
  6. Increasing number and length of apneic episodes.
  7. Increasing exhaustion.

C. *Respiratory acidosis*—due to hypercapnia and *rising* carbon dioxide level.

D. *Metabolic acidosis*—due to *increased* lactic acid levels and *falling* pH.

**V. Analysis/nursing diagnosis**

A. *Gas exchange impairment* related to lack of pulmonary surfactant secondary to: preterm birth, intrapartal stress and hypoxia, infection, postnatal hypothermia, metabolic acidosis, or hypotension.

B. *Nutrition deficit* related to poor feeding secondary to respiratory distress.

**VI. Nursing care plan/implementation**

A. Goal: *reduce metabolic acidosis, increase oxygenation, support respiratory efforts.*
  1. Ensure warmth (*isolette* at 97.6° F).
  2. Warmed, humidified oxygen (at lowest concentration required to relieve cyanosis), through hood, nasal prongs, or endotracheal tube.
  3. *Monitor continuous positive airway pressure* (CPAP)—oxygen-air mixture administered under pressure during inhalation *and* exhalation to maintain alveolar patency.
  4. *Position: side lying* or *supine* with neck slightly *extended* ("sniffing" position); arms at sides.
  5. Suction, prn, with bulb syringe—for excessive mucus.

B. Goal: *modify care for infant with endotracheal tube.*
  1. Disconnect tubing at adapter.
  2. Inject 0.5 mL sterile normal saline (may not be necessary).
  3. Insert sterile suction tube, start suction, rotate tube, withdraw.
  4. Suction up to 5 sec.
  5. Ventilate with bag and mask during procedure.
  6. Reconnect tubing securely to adapter.
  7. Auscultate for breath sounds and pulse.

C. Goal: *maintain nutrition/hydration.*
  1. Administer: fluids, electrolytes, calories, vitamins, minerals PO or IV, as ordered.
  2. I&O.

D. Goal: *prevent secondary infections.*
  1. Strict aseptic technique.
  2. Handwashing.

E. Goal: *emotional support of infant.*
  1. Gentle touching.
  2. Soft voices.
  3. Eye contact.
  4. Rocking.

F. Goal: *emotional support of parents.*
  1. Keep informed of status and progress.
  2. Encourage contact with infant—to promote bonding, understanding of treatment.

G. Goal: *minimize possibility of iatrogenic disorders associated with oxygen therapy* (see **p. 198**: **Iatrogenic [oxygen toxicity] disorders**: *retinopathy of prematurity*).

**VII. Evaluation/outcome criteria**

A. The infant's respiratory distress is treated successfully; infant breathes without assistance.

B. The infant completes successful transition to extrauterine life.

# Iatrogenic (Oxygen Toxicity) Disorders:
## ! Retinopathy of Prematurity (ROP)

I. **Pathophysiology:** intraretinal hemorrhage → fibrosis → retinal detachment → loss of vision.

II. **Etiology/risk factor:** prolonged exposure to high concentrations of oxygen.

III. **Assessment**
  A. Only perceptible retinal change is vasoconstriction.
  B. NOTE: arterial blood gas ($PaO_2$) readings less than 50 or more than 70 mm Hg.

IV. **Nursing care plan/implementation**
  A. Goal: *prevent disorder.*
    1. Maintain $PaO_2$ of 50–70 mm Hg.

V. **Evaluation/outcome criteria**
  A. The infant demonstrates successful recovery from respiratory distress.
  B. No evidence of disorder.

# Iatrogenic (Oxygen Toxicity) Disorders:
## ! Bronchopulmonary Dysplasia (BPD)

I. **Pathophysiology:** damage to alveolar cells → focal emphysema.

II. **Etiology/risk factors:** positive pressure ventilation (CPAP) and positive end-expiratory pressure (PEEP) and prolonged administration of high concentrations of oxygen.

III. **Assessment**—monitor for signs of:
  A. Tachypnea.
  B. Increased respiratory effort.
  C. Respiratory distress.

IV. **Nursing care plan/implementation**
  A. Goal: *prevent disorder.*
    1. Use of positive pressure devices (CPAP, PEEP).
    2. Maintain oxygen concentration *below* 70%.

3. Supportive care.

☞ 4. Wean off ventilator, as possible.

✖ V. **Evaluation/outcome criteria:** The infant demonstrates:

A. Successful recovery from respiratory distress.

B. No evidence of disorder.

# Intraventricular Hemorrhage

⚡ I. **Pathophysiology:** rupture of thin, fragile capillary walls within ventricles of the brain (more common in preterm).

II. **Etiology/risk factors:**

A. Hypoxia.

B. Respiratory distress.

C. Birth trauma.

D. Birth asphyxia.

E. Hypercapnia.

✖ III. **Assessment**

A. Hypotonia.

B. Lethargy.

C. Hypothermia.

D. Bradycardia.

E. Bulging fontanels.

F. Respiratory distress or apnea.

G. Seizures.

H. Cry: high-pitched whining.

✖ IV. **Nursing care plan/implementation**

A. Goal: *supportive care.*

1. Promote healing.

2. Monitor vital signs.

☞ 3. Maintain thermal stability.

4. Assure adequate oxygenation (may be placed on CPAP).

✖ V. **Evaluation/outcome criteria:** The infant demonstrates:

A. Condition stable, all assessment findings within normal limits.

B. No evidence of residual damage.

# Disorders Affecting Nutrition

I. **Pathophysiology:** underdeveloped feeding abilities, small stomach capacity, immature enzyme system, fat intolerance.

II. **Etiology:** immature body systems associated with preterm birth.

✖ III. **Assessment**

A. Weak suck, swallow, gag reflexes—tendency to aspiration.

B. Signs of malabsorption and fat intolerance (abdominal distention, diarrhea, weight loss, or failure to gain weight).

C. Signs of vitamin E deficiency (edema, anemia).

✖ IV. **Analysis/nursing diagnosis**

A. *Nutrition deficit* related to poor feeding reflexes, reduced stomach capacity, inability to absorb needed nutrients.

B. *Gas exchange impairment* related to aspiration.

✖ V. **Nursing care plan/implementation**

A. Goal: *maintain/increase nutrition.*

1. Frequent, small feedings—to *avoid* exceeding stomach capacity, facilitate digestion.

☞ 2. Frequent "burping" during feeding—to *avoid* regurgitation/aspiration.

⬭ 3. Supplement vitamin E (alpha-tocopherol) intake, as ordered, in infants who are formula-fed (NOTE: intake *adequate* in infants who are breastfed.)

a. *Vitamin E* actions:

(1) Antioxidant.

(2) Maintains structure and function of smooth, skeletal, and cardiac muscle.

(3) Maintains structure and function of vascular tissue, liver, and red blood cell integrity.

(4) Coenzyme in tissue respiration.

(5) Treatment for malnutrition with macrocytic anemia.

4. Encourage parent/family participation.

✖ VI. **Evaluation/outcome criteria:** The infant:

A. Feeds well without regurgitation/aspiration.

B. Maintains/gains weight.

C. Shows no evidence of malabsorption, vitamin deficiency.

# Disorders Affecting Nutrition/Elimination: ⚡ Necrotizing Enterocolitis (NEC)

I. **Pathophysiology:** intestinal thrombosis, infarction, autodigestion of mucosal lining, and necrotic lesions; incidence increased in preterm.

II. **Etiology/risk factors:** intestinal ischemia, due to blood shunt to brain and heart in response to:

A. Fetal distress.

B. Fetal/neonatal asphyxia.

C. Neonatal shock.

D. After birth, may result from:

1. Low cardiac output.

2. Infusion of hyperosmolar solutions.

E. Complicated by action of enteric bacteria on damaged intestine.

✖ III. **Assessment**—early identification is **vital**

A. Abdominal distention and/or erythema.

B. Poor feeding, vomiting.

〰 C. Blood in stool.

D. Systemic signs associated with sepsis that may need temporary colostomy or iliostomy:

1. Lethargy or irritability.

2. Hypothermia.
3. Labored respirations or apnea.
4. Cardiovascular collapse.

E. *Diagnostic tests and procedures*:
1. Lab tests to check for increased gastric residual.
2. X-ray shows ileus, air in bowel wall.

IV. **Analysis/nursing diagnosis**
A. *Nutrition deficit* related to inability to tolerate oral feedings, and gastrointestinal dysfunction secondary to ischemia, thrombosis, and/or necrosis.
B. *Constipation* related to paralytic ileus with stasis; diarrhea related to water loss.
C. *Injury risk* related to infection, thrombosis, metabolic alterations (acidosis, osmotic diuresis, dehydration, hyperglycemia) due to parenteral nutrition.
D. *Parenting alteration* related to physiologic compromise and prolonged hospitalization.
E. *Skin integrity impairment* when colostomy is necessary.

V. **Nursing care plan/implementation**
A. Goal: *supportive care.*
1. Rest GI tract: *no oral intake*—to achieve gastric decompression.
2. IV fluids, as ordered—to maintain hydration.
B. Goal: *prevent infection.*
1. Administer *antibiotics*, as ordered.
C. Goal: *prevent trauma to skin surrounding stoma.*

VI. **Evaluation/outcome criteria**
A. The infant:
1. Tolerates oral feedings.
2. Demonstrates weight gain.
3. Demonstrates normal stool pattern.
B. Parents are accepting and knowledgeable about care of infant.

# Postterm/Postmature Infant

**Definition**: over 42 wk gestation.

I. **General aspects**—labor may be hazardous for mother and fetus.

II. **Pathophysiology**:
A. Large size of infant contributes to maternal dystocia; (diagnosis by *ultrasound*).
B. Placental insufficiency → fetal hypoxia; (diagnosis by: contraction stress test).
C. Meconium passage (common physiologic response) → increased chance of meconium aspiration.

III. **Assessment**
A. If postmature skin: dry, wrinkled—due to metabolism of fat and glycogen reserves to meet in utero energy needs.

B. Long limbs, fingernails, and toenails—due to continued growth in utero.
C. Lanugo and vernix—*absent.*
D. Expression: wide-eyed, alert—probably due to chronic hypoxia (oxygen hunger).
E. Placenta—signs of aging, calcifications.

IV. **Analysis/nursing diagnosis**: *Injury risk* related to high incidence of morbidity and mortality due to dystocia and/or hypoxia.

V. **Nursing care plan/implementation**
A. **During labor:**
1. Goal: *emotional support of mother*—may require cesarean birth due to CPD or fetal distress.
2. Goal: *continuous electronic monitoring of fetal heart rate* (FHR). Report *late* or *variable* decelerations **immediately** (may indicate fetal distress).
B. **After birth:**
1. Goal: *if born vaginally, prompt identification of birth injuries, respiratory distress.* Continual observation.
2. Goal: *early identification/treatment of emerging signs of complications.*
   a. *Hypoglycemia*—Dextrostix readings and behavior.
   b. Administer oral or intravenous glucose, as ordered.

VI. **Evaluation/outcome criterion**: successful transition to extrauterine life (all assessment findings within normal limits).

# Infant with Congenital Disorders

**General overview**: Genetic abnormalities and environmental insults often lead to congenital disorders of the newborn. Successful transition to independent extrauterine life may pose a major challenge to infants compromised by anatomic and/or physiologic disorders. Knowledge regarding the implications of the neonate's structural and/or metabolic problems enables the nurse to identify early signs of health problems and to plan, provide, and evaluate appropriate outcome-directed care to safeguard the status of the infant with a congenital disorder.

## Disorders Affecting Fluid-Gas Transport: *Congenital Heart Disease*

I. **Pathophysiology**: altered hemodynamics, due to persistent fetal circulation or structural abnormalities.
A. *Acyanotic defects*—no mixing of blood in the systemic circulation
1. Patent ductus arteriosus.
2. Atrial septal defect.

3. Ventricular septal defect.

4. Coarctation of the aorta.

B. *Cyanotic defects*—unoxygenated blood enters systemic circulation

1. Tetralogy of Fallot.

2. Transposition of the great vessels.

II. **Etiology**—unknown. **Risk factors:** Associated with maternal:

A. Prenatal viral disease (e.g., rubella, Coxsackie).

B. Malnutrition; alcoholism.

C. Diabetes, poorly controlled.

D. Ingestion of lithium salts.

III. **Assessment**

A. **Patent ductus arteriosus (PDA)**

1. *Characteristic*: machine murmur, mid to upper left sternal border (cardiomegaly); persists throughout systole and most of diastole; associated with a "thrill."

2. Widened pulse pressure.

3. Bounding pulse, tachycardia, "gallop" rhythm.

B. **Atrial septal defect (ASD)**

1. *Characteristic*: crescendo/decrescendo systolic ejection murmur.

2. Fixed $S_2$ splitting.

3. Dyspnea, fatigue on normal activity.

4. *Diagnostic procedures:* cardiac catheterization, echocardiogram, cardiac MRI, ECG, x-ray.

C. **Ventricular septal defect (VSD)**

1. *Characteristic*: loud, harsh, pansystolic murmur; heard best at left lower sternal border; radiates throughout precordium. (NOTE: may be absent—due to high pulmonary vascular resistance $\rightarrow$ equalization of interventricular pressure.)

2. *Diagnostic procedures:* cardiac catheterization, ECG, chest x-ray, echocardiogram.

D. **Coarctation of the aorta**

1. Absent femoral pulse.

2. Late systolic murmur.

3. Decreased blood pressure in *lower* extremities.

4. *Diagnostic procedures*: echocardiogram.

E. **Tetralogy of Fallot** ("blue" baby)

1. Acute hypoxic/cyanotic episodes.

2. Postepisode: limp, sleepy, exhausted; hypotonic extended position.

3. *Diagnostic procedures:* cardiac catheterization, echocardiogram.

F. **Transposition of the great vessels**

1. Cyanotic after crying or feeding.

2. Progressive tachypnea—attempt to compensate for *decreased* $PaO_2$, *metabolic acidosis.*

3. Heart sounds vary, consistent with defect.

4. Signs of heart failure.

5. *Diagnostic procedures*: cardiac catheterization, x-ray, ECG.

IV. **Analysis/nursing diagnosis**

A. *Fluid volume excess* related to persistent fetal circulation, structural abnormalities.

B. *Gas exchange impairment* related to abnormal circulation, secondary to above pathology.

C. *Nutrition deficit* related to exhaustion, dyspnea.

V. **Nursing care plan/implementation**

A. Goal: *minimize cardiac workload.*

1. Minimize crying: snuggle; pacifier—to meet psychological needs.

B. Goal: *maintain thermal stability.*

1. Reduce body need for oxygen.

2. Keep clean and dry.

C. Goal: *prevent infection.*

1. Strict aseptic technique; standard precautions.

2. Handwashing.

D. Goal: *parental emotional support.*

1. Encourage verbalization of anxiety, fears, concerns.

2. Keep informed of status.

E. Goal: **health teaching.** Explain, discuss:

1. Diagnostic procedures.

2. Treatment procedures.

3. Basic care modalities.

F. Goal: *promote bonding.*

1. Encourage to participate in infant care, as possible.

G. *Medical/surgical* management: surgical intervention/repair of congenital cardiac abnormality.

VI. **Evaluation/outcome criteria**

A. The infant experiences no respiratory distress in immediate postnatal period.

B. The infant completes transfer to high-risk center without incident, if applicable.

C. Surgical intervention successful, where applicable.

# Disorders Affecting Fluid-Gas Transport: *Hemolytic Disease of the Newborn*

## Rh Incompatibility

I. **Pathophysiology** and **Etiology**—see *Rh isoimmunization,* **Chapter 3, p. 52-53.**

II. **Assessment**

A. *Prenatal*—maternal Rh titers, amniocentesis.

B. *Intrapartal*—amniotic fluid color:

1. Straw colored: *mild* disease.

2. Golden: *severe* fetal disease.

C. *Postpartal*—**Direct Coombs'** test on cord blood; positive test demonstrates Rh antibodies in fetal blood.

III. **Nursing care plan/implementation—exchange transfusion**

A. Goal: **health teaching.** Explain purpose and process to parents:

1. Removes anti-Rh antibodies and fetal cells that are coated with antibodies.
2. Reduces bilirubin levels—indicated when 20 mg/dL in *term* neonate and 15 mg/dL in *preterm* at ≤ 24 hours of age.
3. Corrects anemia—supplies red blood cells that will not be destroyed by maternal antibodies.
4. ***Rh-negative type O blood*** elicits no reaction; maximum exchange is 500 mL; duration of exchange: 45–60 min.

B. Goal: *minimize transfusion hazards.*

1. Warm blood to room temperature, since cold blood may precipitate cardiac arrest.
2. Use only fresh blood—to reduce possibility of hypocalcemia, tetany, convulsions.
3. Give *calcium gluconate*, as ordered, after each 100 mL of transfusion.

C. Goal: *prepare for transfusion procedure.* Ready necessary equipment—monitor, resuscitation equipment, radiant heater, light.

D. Goal: *assist with exchange transfusion.*

1. Continuous monitoring of vital signs; record baseline, and every 15 min during procedure.
2. Record: time, amount of blood withdrawn; time and amount injected; medications given.
3. *Observe* for: dyspnea, listlessness, bleeding from transfusion site, cyanosis, cardiovascular irregularity or arrest; coolness of lower extremities.

E. Goal: *posttransfusion care.*

1. **Assessment**
   a. Observe for: dyspnea, cyanosis, cardiac arrest or irregularities; jaundice, hypoglycemia; frequent vital signs.
   b. Signs of *sepsis*—fever, tachycardia, dyspnea, chills, tremors.
2. **Nursing care plan/implementation**
   a. Maintain thermal stability—to reduce physiologic stress, possibility of metabolic acidosis.
   b. Give oxygen—to relieve cyanosis.
   c. Keep cord moist—to facilitate repeat transfusion, if necessary.
   d. Maintain nutrition/hydration—feed per schedule.

IV. **Evaluation/outcome criteria**

A. Infant's hemolytic process ceases; bilirubin level drops.
B. Infant makes successful transition to extrauterine life.
C. Infant experiences no complications of therapeutic regimen.
D. Infant demonstrates evidence of bonding.

## ABO Incompatibility

I. **Pathophysiology**: fetal blood carrying antigens A/B enters maternal type O bloodstream → antibody formation → antibodies cross placenta → hemolyze fetal red cells. NOTE: less severe than Rh reaction.

II. **Etiology/risk factors**

A. Type O mother carries anti-A and anti-B antibodies.
B. Even first pregnancy is jeopardized if fetal blood enters maternal system.
C. Reaction possible if fetus is type A, type B, or type AB and mother is type O.

III. **Assessment**

A. Jaundice within first 24 hr.
B. Rising bilirubin levels.
C. Enlarged liver and spleen.

IV. **Nursing care plan/implementation**

A. Goal: *reduce hazard to newborn.*

1. Prepare for possible exchange transfusion with O-negative blood.
2. Provide phototherapy (if bilirubin is ≥ 10 mg/dL, and anemia is mild or absent.)
3. Monitor status closely.
4. Supportive care.

V. **Evaluation/outcome criteria**

A. Infant responds to medical/nursing regimen.
B. Infant's assessment findings within normal limits.

## Hyperbilirubinemia

I. **Pathophysiology**: bilirubin, a breakdown product of hemolyzed red blood cells, appears at increased levels; exceeds 13–15 mg/dL. Bilirubin is safe when bound with albumin and conjugated by user for body excretion; **danger** is when unconjugated and deposits in CNS.

A. **WARNING**: There is no "safe" serum-bilirubin level; *kernicterus* is a function of the bilirubin level *and* neonatal age and condition; poor fluid-and-caloric balance subjects the infant (especially the premature) to kernicterus at low serum-bilirubin levels.

B. **Kernicterus**—high bilirubin levels result in deposition of yellow pigment in basal ganglia of brain → irreversible brain damage.

II. **Etiology/risk factors**

A. Rh or ABO incompatibility, during first 48 hr.
B. Resolution of an enclosed hemorrhage (e.g., cephalohematoma).
C. Infection.
D. Drug-induced—vitamin K injection, maternal ingestion of *sulfisoxazole* (*Gantrisin*).
E. Bile duct blockage.
F. Albumin-binding capacity is exceeded.
G. "Breastfeeding jaundice" (e.g., pregnanediol in milk). Breastfeeding is *not* dangerous and not a cause of physiologic jaundice.

H. Dehydration.

I. Immature liver (interferes with conjugation).

### III. Assessment

A. Jaundice noted after *blanching* skin to suppress hemoglobin color; noted in sclera or mucosa in dark-skinned neonates; make sure light is adequate; spreads from head to toe, with increasing severity.

B. Pallor.

C. Concentrated, dark urine.

D. Blood level determination—hemoglobin or indirect bilirubin (unconjugated, unbound bilirubin deposits in CNS).

E. *Kernicterus*—symptoms similar to intracranial hemorrhage

1. Poor feeding and/or sucking.
2. Regurgitation, vomiting.
3. High-pitched cry.
4. Temperature instability.
5. Hypertonicity/hypotonicity.
6. Progressive lethargy; diminished Moro reflex.
7. Respiratory distress.
8. Cerebral palsy, mental retardation.
9. Death.

### IV. Analysis/nursing diagnosis

A. *Fluid volume (red blood cell) deficit* related to hemolysis secondary to blood incompatibility.

B. *Injury risk* (brain damage) related to kernicterus.

C. *Thought processes alteration* (mental retardation) related to brain damage secondary to kernicterus.

D. *Knowledge deficit (parental)* related to infant condition.

### V. Nursing care plan/implementation

A. *Medical management*

1. *Prenatal*—amniocentesis.
2. *Postnatal*—phototherapy, exchange transfusion.

B. Goal: *assist bilirubin conjugation through phototherapy.*

1. Cover closed eyelids while under light; remove eyepads when not under light (feeding, cuddling, during parental visits)—to protect eyes. Biliblanket—do not need to cover eyes.
2. Expose as much skin as possible—to maximize exposure of circulating blood to light. Remove for only brief time periods.
3. *Change position* every hour—to maximize exposure of circulating blood to light.
4. NOTE: any loose green stools as bile is cleared through gut; watch for skin breakdown on buttocks.
5. Monitor temperature—to identify hyperthermia.
6. *Push fluids* (to 25% more than average) between feedings—to counteract dehydration. Breast milk has natural laxative effects that help clear bile.

C. Goal: **health teaching**. Explain, discuss phototherapy, bilirubin levels, implications.

D. Goal: *emotional support*

1. Encourage verbalization of anxiety, fears, concerns.
2. Encourage contact with infant.
3. Reassure, as possible.

### VI. Evaluation/outcome criteria

A. Infant's hemolytic process ceases; bilirubin level drops.

B. Infant makes successful transition to extrauterine life.

C. Infant experiences no complications of therapeutic regimen.

D. Infant demonstrates evidence of effective bonding.

# Emotional Support of the High-Risk Infant

### I. General aspects

A. The high-risk infant has the same *developmental needs* as the healthy term infant.

1. Social and tactile stimulation.
2. Comfort and removal of discomfort (hunger, soiling).
3. Continuous contact with a consistent, parenting person.

B. Treatment for serious physiologic compromise may result in:

1. Isolation.
2. Sensory deprivation or noxious stimuli.
3. Emotional stress.

### II. Assessment—signs of *neonatal emotional stress*

A. Does not look at person performing care.

B. Does not cry or protest.

C. Poor weight gain; failure to thrive.

### III. Analysis/nursing diagnosis: *sensory/perceptual alterations* related to isolation in Isolette, oxygen hood.

### IV. Nursing care plan/implementation

A. Goal: *provide consistent parenting contact.* Assign same nurses whenever possible.

B. Goal: *emotional support.*

1. Comfort when crying.
2. Provide positive sensory stimulation. Arrange time to:
   a. Stroke skin.
   b. Hold hand.
   c. Hum, sing, talk.
   d. Hold in *en-face* position (nurse looking into infant's eyes).
   e. Hold when feeding, if possible.

C. Goal: *encourage parents to participate in care.*
1. Reduce their psychological stress, anxiety, fear.
2. Promote bonding.
3. Reduce possibility of later child abuse (higher incidence of child abuse against children who have been high-risk infants).

V. **Evaluation/outcome criteria**
A. Infant demonstrates successful resolution of physiologic problems.
B. Parents and infant evidence bonding.
C. Parents express satisfaction with care and result.

# General Aspects: Nursing Care of the High-Risk Infant and Family

I. **General aspects:** The birth of a neonate who is physiologically compromised is psychologically stressful for both infant and family, and physiologically stressful for the neonate. Effective, goal-directed nursing care is focused on:
A. Minimizing physiologic and psychological stress.
B. Facilitating/supporting successful coping and/or adaptation.
C. Encouraging parental attachment/separation/ grieving, as appropriate.

II. **Assessment**—directed toward determining neonate's present and projected status
A. Determine neonate's current physical status.
B. Identify specific status and diagnosis-related problems and needs.
C. Describe family: psychological status, strengths, and coping mechanisms/skills.
D. Determine medical/surgical/nursing approach to problems, and prognosis.

III. **Analysis/nursing diagnosis**
A. *Anxiety/fear* (parental) related to physiologic compromise of neonate.
B. *Self-esteem disturbance* related to feelings of guilt and/or anger.
C. *Individual coping impairment* related to severe psychological stress.
D. *Knowledge deficit* related to diagnosis, treatment, prognosis of infant.
E. *Parenting alteration* related to concern about infant.

IV. **Nursing care plan/implementation**
A. Goal: *preoperative and postoperative care.*
1. Maintain/improve physiologic stability:
   a. Temperature stabilization—keep warm.
   b. Oxygenation
      (1) Position.
      (2) Administer oxygen, as ordered and/ or necessary.
   c. Nutrition/hydration
      (1) Administer/monitor intravenous fluids.
      (2) Provide oral fluids, as ordered.
      (3) Feed, as status permits.
2. Assist with diagnostic testing.
B. Goal: *emotional support of parents.*
1. Encourage exploring and ventilating feelings.
2. Involve parents in decision-making process.
C. Goal: **health teaching.**
1. Determine knowledge/understanding of problem.
2. Explain/simplify/clarify, as needed, physician's discussions with parents.
3. Describe/explain/discuss neonate's present status and any auxiliary equipment; teach CPR to family.
4. Refer, as needed, to hospital/community resources.
D. Goal: *promote bonding.* encourage parental participation in care of the neonate.

V. **Evaluation/outcome criteria**
A. Parents verbalize understanding of relevant information; make informed decisions regarding infant care.
B. Parents demonstrate comfort and increasing participation in care of neonate.
C. Infant maintains/increases adequacy of adaptation to extrauterine life.
D. If relevant, parents demonstrate progress in grieving process.

# Summary

For some neonates, the transition to extrauterine existence is complicated by **high-risk conditions**: *infections*, maternal disorders such as poorly controlled *diabetes mellitus*, and *maternal drug* and *alcohol dependence*. The life and well-being of other infants are threatened by **preterm** or **postterm** births and/or **congenital** disorders. The nurse must have critical care nursing skills, knowledge of the growth and developmental needs of infants, sensitivity to parental needs, and ability to work with an interdisciplinary team of health care providers.

# Study and Memory Aids

## Neonatal Risk Factors: ABC-I

**A**ge (gestational)
**B**irth trauma
**C**ongenital disorders
**I**nfection

## Neonatal Infections—Transmission of HBV

- Serum → serum
- Contact with contaminated: urine, feces, saliva, semen
- Mother → baby: transplacentally or from infected birth canal

## Preterm Infant—Anticipated Problems: TRIES

**T**emperature regulation
**R**esistance to infection
**I**mmature liver
**E**limination
**S**ensory-perceptual functions

## Respiratory Distress Syndrome: Preterm Infant

*Avoid* placing infant on abdomen.

## Prevention of Transmission of Infection (Thrush) and Prevention of Secondary Infections (RDS)

**Handwashing**—for nurse *and* mother—cannot be overemphasized!

## Rh Incompatibility

Rh+ babies receive Rh-, type O blood in exchange transfusion.

# Questions

1. The nurse would not expect to give tetracycline during pregnancy due to:
   1. Its effect on kidney function in the mother.
   2. Its effect on liver function in the mother.
   3. The development of Hutchinson's teeth in the child.
   4. Its stimulation of bone growth in the fetus/newborn.

2. The plan of care developed by nurses for parents of a baby who is drug-dependent includes:
   1. Recommendation for minimal contact between parents and infants.
   2. Ways to encourage parent-infant bonding and any positive parental responses to the baby.
   3. Discouraging attachment between the parent and baby.
   4. Acknowledgement that parents who are drug-dependent are less likely to be interested in their babies.

3. A neonate at 1 min after birth exhibits the following: heart rate, 92; no respiratory effort; muscle tone showing some flexion; grimace in response to slap on sole of foot; pale color. The nurse's first response should be to:
   1. Do nothing because the findings are within normal limits.
   2. Take the neonate to the nursery for further observation.
   3. Administer oxygen by mask until the neonate is pink.
   4. Begin resuscitative actions immediately.

4. Varicella-zoster virus infections are infrequent during pregnancy but can cause serious consequences. Which statement is not relevant to the care of the mother/fetus/newborn?
   1. Transmission occurs through droplet spray (sneeze) or through contact with vesicular fluid and cells from fresh skin lesions.
   2. Infants with varicella embryopathy are highly infectious and should be isolated immediately following birth.
   3. The mother with pneumonia is to be given acyclovir.
   4. Women with chickenpox at the time of birth should not have contact with their newborns until all vesicles have crusted.

5. Health care teaching needs to include information that the most common mode of transmission of *herpes simplex* virus to an infant is:
   1. Across the placenta.
   2. Vertical infection from a vaginal infection.
   3. During passage through an infected birth canal.
   4. From personnel or family who are infected.

6. Congenital syphilis is suspected in a newborn infant. For which specific sign should the nurse assess this neonate?
   1. Tremors, sweating.
   2. Seizure activity.
   3. Anemia.
   4. Snuffles.

7. The home health nurse develops a plan of care for a newborn whose mother was diagnosed with a chlamydial infection during pregnancy. The plan is based on knowledge that *Chlamydia trachomatis* is an intracellular bacterium that causes neonatal conjunctivitis and:
   1. Discolored teeth in baby and adult.
   2. Snuffles and rhagades in the newborn.
   3. Pneumonia.
   4. Central and peripheral hearing defects that progress during infancy.

8. Early signs of neonatal infection are nonspecific. The nurse should be aware that the most accurate predictor of neonatal infection is:
   1. Neutropenia.
   2. Neutrophilia.
   3. Leukopenia.
   4. Leukocytosis.

9. A woman's prenatal record reveals a history of alcohol abuse that continued throughout pregnancy. The nurse's plan of care for this woman's newborn includes assessment of fetal alcohol syndrome (FAS) because of which characteristic?
   1. Saddle nose, red rash on chin, and snuffles.
   2. Neonatal conjunctivitis and pneumonia.
   3. Large for gestational age (LGA).
   4. Facial dysmorphia.

10. Birth injury is a concern during a forceps-assisted or breech birth. Duchenne-Erb paralysis is suspected if the nurse observes:
    1. A flaccid arm with the elbow extended.
    2. Absence of Moro reflex on the unaffected side
    3. Absence of grasp reflex on the affected side.
    4. Torticollis or wry neck.

11. The nurse observes the neonate of the mother whose pregnancy was complicated by the HELLP syndrome for:
    1. High hematocrit.
    2. Hyperglycemia.
    3. Thrombocytopenia.
    4. Cardiomyopathy.

12. What is the most common complication for which the nurse must closely monitor a *preterm* newborn?
    1. Brain damage.
    2. Respiratory distress syndrome.
    3. Meconium aspiration syndrome.
    4. Hemorrhage.

13. The nurse questions the gestational age estimate recorded in the chart if an infant recorded as *preterm* displays:
    1. Absence of lanugo.
    2. Absence of subcutaneous fat.
    3. Parchment-thin skin.
    4. Wrinkled "older person" appearance.

14. The nurse implements cardiopulmonary resuscitation (CPR) on the newborn by maintaining a compression rate of:
    1. 60/min.
    2. 80/min.
    3. 100/min.
    4. 120/min.

15. An important role of the nurse is in risk management. The nurse reviews all assessment findings to determine which, if any, require further investigation/evaluation. Of the following findings on a full-term newborn, which one is *not* a normal result of maternal hormone influence, and needs to be reported?
    1. "Witch's milk."
    2. Vaginal bleeding.
    3. Undescended testes.
    4. *Linea nigra.*

16. When forceps are used for the birth of an infant's head, the nurse should assess the newborn for:
    1. Torticollis.
    2. Facial paralysis.
    3. Fractured clavicle.
    4. Cephalohematoma.

17. A nurse is evaluating a newborn with hospital-specified criteria for discharge. The nurse would determine that the newborn who is *not* a candidate for discharge at < 48 hours is one whose:
    1. Coombs' test is positive, birth weight was 2775 g, and Apgar score was 9, 9.
    2. Hematocrit is 52%; respirations, 40/min; feeding is going well.
    3. Birth weight was 4000 g, gestational age was 38 wk, and temperature is 98.1° F.
    4. Apical heart rate is 122 beats/min, Moro reflex is positive; has passed two meconium stools.

18. The nurse is assessing a newborn on admission to the nursery. In evaluating the findings, the nurse knows that the finding that must be referred for further investigation/evaluation is:
    1. Misshapen head.
    2. Short neck.
    3. Tremors of the extremities.
    4. Flat abdomen (scaphoid).

19. The nurse would closely observe a neonate whose:
    1. Slight heart murmur, heard at 1 hr, is inaudible at 4 hr.
    2. Respiratory rate increased from 30/min to 48/min, then stabilized.
    3. Color became cyanotic during the first feeding.
    4. Heart rate ranged from 122 to 148 within the same hour.

20. Nursing care for a baby treated for jaundice with phototherapy includes:
    1. Discontinuing phototherapy for feedings and parent visits.
    2. Monitoring temperature rectally.
    3. Replacing fluid loss with an additional 2 mL of formula every 2 hr.
    4. Removing eye patches for 5 min every hour.

21. A newborn's record reveals: 42 wk gestation; spontaneous vaginal birth after a 15 hr labor; Apgar scores of 8 and 9; blood glucose of 30 mg/dL. The mother received no sedation, and plans to breastfeed. What is the *priority* nursing action?
    1. Bottle feed with formula, then recheck the blood glucose level.
    2. Start an IV of 10% dextrose in water ($D_{10}W$), then recheck the blood glucose level.
    3. Let the mother breastfeed for 15 min, then recheck the blood glucose level.
    4. Place the baby under a warmer for 15 min, then recheck the blood glucose level.

22. In caring for a preterm infant, the nurse must monitor arterial blood gas readings for oxygen saturation. Following protocol, the nurse discontinues oxygen therapy as soon as possible in order to decrease the possibility of:
    1. Necrotizing enterocolitis.
    2. Retinopathy of prematurity.
    3. Myofibroplasia.
    4. Cerebrospinal dysplasia.

23. Which finding would indicate to the nurse that a newborn has thrush (*candidiasis*)?
    1. Bleeding gums.
    2. Epstein's pearls on roof of mouth.
    3. White patches adherent to mucosa of the mouth.
    4. "Milk blisters" on lips.

24. Which laboratory values in suspected Rh incompatibility will be most relevant in planning nursing care for the infant?
    1. Oxygen concentration.
    2. Direct Coombs' test.
    3. Glucose level.
    4. Hemoglobin $A_{1c}$.

25. For what complication frequently associated with postterm birth must the nurse closely monitor the *postmature* newborn?
    1. Brain damage.
    2. Respiratory distress syndrome.
    3. Meconium aspiration syndrome.
    4. Hemorrhage.

# Answers/Rationale

1. (2) Tetracycline (used for the treatment of syphilis in persons who are allergic to penicillin, and for the treatment of chlamydial infection) is contraindicated in pregnancy because of its effects on liver function in the mother. Tetracycline affects liver, *not* kidney (1), function in the mother. It results in tooth *discoloration*, not Hutchinson's teeth (3), in fetus. (Hutchinson's teeth is a sequel to congenital syphilis.) Tetracycline also results in *decreased* bone growth in the fetus, *not* increased (4). **AN, COM, 1, PhI, Pharmacological and parenteral therapies**

2. (2) Parent-infant bonding and positive parental responses to the baby are encouraged; this may help motivate parents to enter drug rehabilitation. The *opposite* of the other options is true: Contact (1) and attachment (3) between parents and baby are *encouraged*. Parents who are drug-dependent are *not* less likely to be interested in their babies (4). **PL, COM, 7, PsI, Psychosocial integrity**

3. (4) Begin resuscitative actions immediately; the neonate's Apgar score is only 3. The findings *do* require action (1): immediate resuscitation and further investigation. Resuscitation should *not* wait

until the neonate can be taken to the nursery (2). Oxygen (3) will not resuscitate the neonate who is not breathing; resuscitation, preferably by a trained pediatrician (neonatologist), must be initiated **STAT**. **AN, ANL, 6, PhI, Physiological adaptation**

4. (2) Infants with varicella embryopathy are *not* considered infectious and do *not* need to be isolated either in the nursery or at home. The other options *are* relevant: Option **1** correctly describes the mode of transmission of chickenpox. Acyclovir (3) *is* given to women with marked pulmonary involvement. Women with chickenpox at birth *should not* have contact with their newborns until all vesicles have crusted (4).

   ☼ NOTE: There is also a 25% chance that varicella virus will spread vertically from the mother to the fetus or newborn. **PL, APP, 1, SECE, Safety and infection control**

5. (3) The most common mode of transmission of *herpes simplex* virus to an infant is during passage through an infected birth canal. Transplacental transmission (1), vertical infection from a vaginal infection (2), and transmission by infected personnel or family (4) are all possible; however, none of these is *the most common* mode of transmission.

   ☼ NOTE: Thorough handwashing should be practiced by health care providers as well as by family members. Gloves should be worn during contact with lesions or secretions. Family members with oral lesions should be discouraged from kissing the newborn. In general, infants born to mothers who are at risk of transmitting the infection should be isolated. **PL, APP, 1, SECE, Safety and infection control**

---

### Key to Codes

**Nursing process: AS**, assessment; **AN**, analysis; **PL**, planning; **IMP**, implementation; **EV**, evaluation. (See **Appendix J** for explanation of nursing process steps.)

**Cognitive level: RE/KN**, recall/knowledge; **COM**, comprehension; **APP**, application; **ANL**, analysis; **EVL**, evaluation; **SYN**, synthesis. (See **Appendix J** for explanation.)

**Category of human function: 1**, protective; **2**, sensory-perceptual; **3**, comfort, rest, activity, and mobility; **4**, nutrition; **5**, growth and development; **6**, fluid-gas transport; **7**, psychosocial-cultural; **8**, elimination. (See **Appendix L** for explanation.)

**Client need: SECE**, safe, effective care environment; **HPM**, health promotion and maintenance. **PsI**, psychosocial integrity; **PhI**, physiological integrity. (See **Appendix M** for explanation.)

**Client subneed:** See **Appendix M** for explanation.

6. **(4)** Snuffles (rhinitis), rhagades (cracks, fissures around the mouth), hydrocephaly, and corneal opacity are all sequelae to congenital syphilis. Tremors and sweating (**1**), seizure activity (**2**), and anemia (**3**) are *not* sequelae to congenital syphilis. **AS, RE/KN, 1, SECE, Safety and infection control**

7. **(3)** It causes pneumonia. Newborns exhibit prolonged staccato cough, tachypnea, mild hypoxemia, and eosinophilia. Discolored teeth (**1**) are secondary to treatment of the pregnant woman with *tetracycline*. Snuffles and rhagades (**2**) are sequelae to *congenital syphilis. Congenital rubella*, which is not a static disease, results in central and peripheral hearing defects that progress after birth (**4**).

💡 NOTE: *Snuffles* refer to copious, clear, serosanguineous mucous discharge from the obstructed nose. *Rhagades* refer to circumoral radiating scars that result from rough, cracked mucocutaneous lesions of the lips. **AS, COM, 1, HPM, Health promotion and maintenance**

8. **(1)** Neutropenia is the most accurate predictor of neonatal infection. This abnormal *decrease* in neutrophils (circulating white blood cells essential for phagocytosis and proteolysis) is associated with a variety of conditions, including infection. Neutropenia is associated with infection, *not* neutrophilia (**2**), an increase in neutrophils. Leukopenia (**3**) and leukocytosis (**4**) are not accurate predictors of neonatal infection. Leukocytes are of five types; neutrophils are one type of granulocytic leukocytes. **AS, COM, 1, PhI, Reduction of risk potential**

9. **(4)** Facial dysmorphia, growth deficits at birth that do not improve with time, and other neurologic dysfunction are characteristically seen in these children. (Additional problems may include: anomalies of ocular structure and limbs, and a variety of cardiocirculatory defects, especially ventricular septal defects.) Saddle nose, red rash on chin, and snuffles (**1**) are characteristic of *syphilis* (congenital). Neonatal conjunctivitis and pneumonia (**2**) are characteristic of *chlamydial infection*. Newborns with FAS may be preterm and *small* for gestational age (SGA), *not* large (**3**). **AS, COM, 5, PhI, Physiological adaptation**

10. **(1)** The flaccid arm in this paralysis is secondary to damage to spinal nerves C5 and C6. This damage is caused by excessive lateral flexion of the head during birth of the shoulder. The Moro reflex would be absent or lessened on the *affected* side, *not* the unaffected side (**2**). Injury to C5 and C6 does not affect the grasp reflex (**3**); Klumpke's paralysis (paralysis of the hand) results from damage to C8. Torticollis, or wry neck (**4**), is a congenital shortening or spasmodic contraction of the neck (sternocleidomastoid) muscles. **AS, ANL, 3, PhI, Physiological adaptation**

11. **(3)** The neonate of the woman whose pregnancy was complicated with the HELLP syndrome must be observed for thrombocytopenia, a common finding with this disorder. A high hematocrit (**1**), hyperglycemia (**2**), and cardiomyopathy (**4**) are *not* associated with HELLP. **AS, APP, 6, PhI, Reduction of risk potential**

12. **(2)** Respiratory distress syndrome (RDS) is the most common complication in newborns who are preterm, secondary to: a) insufficient surfactant needed to maintain open alveoli on exhalation; b) small, easily collapsible respiratory passages; c) weak respiratory musculature; and d) immature bony thorax. Brain damage (**1**), if present, is diagnosed *later*. (If severe hypoxia occurred during birth, brain damage would be of considerable concern.) Meconium aspiration (**3**) is one of the most common complications of the newborn who is *postterm*. Hemorrhage (**4**) is of concern, but is *not* the *most* common complication seen in the newborn who is preterm. **AS, ANL, 6, PhI, Physiological adaptation**

13. **(1)** Absence of lanugo is characteristic of the newborn who is *full*-term or *postterm*. Absence of subcutaneous fat (**2**), parchment-thin skin (**3**), and wrinkled "old-person" appearance (**4**) due to absence of vernix caseosa *are* all characteristic of the preterm newborn. **AS, COM, 1, HPM, Health promotion and maintenance**

14. **(3)** A compression rate of a minimum of 100/min is required; assist ventilation on the upstroke of every third compression (3:1). The rates in the other options are either *too slow* (**1** and **2**) or *too fast* (**4**). **IMP, RE/KN, 1, PhI, Physiological adaptation**

15. **(3)** Undescended testes are a condition unrelated to maternal hormone influence. Testes begin to descend from the abdominal cavity into the scrotum starting at about 28 wk gestation. Before 36 wk, they should be palpable in the inguinal canal; by 36–38 wk, they should be palpable within the scrotum. "Witch's milk" (**1**) refers to the whitish secretion that comes from the nipples of *some* (boy or girl) newborns who are at term. Vaginal bleeding (**2**), or pseudomenstruation, is seen in *some* full-term newborn girls. *Linea nigra* (**4**) can be seen in *some* full-term (boy or girl) newborns. **EV, ANL, 5, HPM, Health promotion and maintenance**

16. **(2)** Facial paralysis can occur when the forceps blades compress the cranial VII (facial) nerve, anterior to the ears. It is usually mild and temporary, lasting only a few days. Torticollis (**1**), or wry neck, is caused by a shortened sternocleidomastoid muscle on one side of the fetal neck. Fractured clavicle (**3**) is usually caused during birth of the shoulders, when the infant is large, or the mother's pelvic outlet is small. Cephalohematoma (**4**) is *not* caused by properly placed forceps. This bleeding between the periosteum and one or more of the cranial bones (especially the parietal) is *secondary* to *pressure* from the maternal pelvis. **AN, RE/KN, 2, PhI, Reduction of risk potential**

17. **(1)** If a newborn's Coombs' test is positive, further evaluation is needed. If the infant is Coombs positive because of Rh incompatibility, the baby is at risk for anemia and hyperbilirubinemia. (The birth weight of 6 lb 2 oz and the Apgar score of 9, 9 *do* fit the criteria for discharge.) The hematocrit, respirations, and feeding pattern in option **2** *do* fit the criteria for discharge. The birth weight, gestational age, and temperature in option **3** *do* fit the criteria for discharge. The apical heart rate, stooling pattern, and Moro reflex response in option **4** *do* fit the criteria for discharge. **EV, ANL, 6, PhI, Reduction of risk potential**

18. **(4)** A scaphoid abdomen is seen in infants with diaphragmatic hernia, where the abdominal contents have herniated into the thoracic cavity. Within an hour, bowel sounds may be heard in the thoracic cavity and respiratory distress increases markedly. The misshapen head (**1**) is the result of molding (overlapping of cranial bones to accommodate to the dimensions of the maternal pelvis); this is a *normal* finding in infants born vaginally. Normal newborns have very short necks (**2**), but the neck is flexible and moves easily from side to side. Transient tremors of the extremities (**3**) are *normal* in the newborn. **EV, ANL, 8, PhI, Physiological adaptation**

19. **(3)** Cyanosis during feeding may be a sign of a cardiovascular defect. Some cardiovascular defects become apparent as the newborn experiences cold temperatures, handling, feeding, etc. The findings in options **1**, **2**, and **4** are all *normal* in the newborn infant. **EV, ANL, 6, PhI, Physiological adaptation**

20. **(1)** Phototherapy should be discontinued and eye patches removed during feedings and for parent visits to allow for infant stimulation and to allow for bonding/attachment between parent and child. Option **2** is incorrect because taking the temperature rectally is *not* recommended, since this method can result in injury to the rectum. Option **3** is incorrect because the newborn receiving phototherapy needs to have fluid intake increased by 25% to compensate for insensible water loss; since the normal intake requirement is 105 mL/kg/24 hr, this newborn would require an increase of *over* 2 mL *per kg* every 2 hr. Option **4** is incorrect because the newborn under phototherapy lights does *not* need this action; the newborn should be *turned* at least every half hour to expose all areas of the skin and to prevent pressure spots. **IMP, ANL, 5, PhI, Reduction of risk potential**

21. **(1)** Blood glucose for a newborn should be at least 40 mg/dL; this newborn's level is low and requires immediate replacement of glucose; feeding formula or breast milk, if available, provides longer normal glucose levels. Option **2** is incorrect because an *otherwise healthy* newborn should *not* need the *intrusive* procedure of an IV to obtain an adequate glucose level. Use of $D_{10}W$ can result in rebound hypoglycemia (a bolus of glucose stimulates the neonate to produce a large quantity of insulin, which then rapidly uses up the glucose bolus). Options **3** and **4** are incorrect because these do not provide for *immediate* glucose replacement; moreover, breast milk (**3**) is *not available* for about 3 days. **IMP, ANL, 4, PhI, Physiological adaptation**

22. **(2)** Retinopathy of prematurity is caused by the effect of high oxygen concentrations; it results in loss of sight in the infant. The conditions in options **1**, **3** and **4** are not related to the use of high oxygen concentration, but are associated with body damage caused by *other* factors. **IMP, COM, 6, PhI, Reduction of risk potential**

23. **(3)** White patches adherent to mucosa of mouth, gums, and tongue, which tend to bleed when touched, are the lesions of thrush. Bleeding gums (**1**) in the neonate would be an abnormal finding that would necessitate immediate investigation (DIC), but *do not suggest thrush*. Epstein's pearls (**2**), small white blebs found along the gum margins and at the junction of the soft and hard palates, are a *normal* manifestation commonly seen in the newborn (similar to Bohn's nodules). "Milk blisters" (**4**) are *normally* seen in infants (both breast- and bottle fed); they disappear during weaning. **AS, APP, 1, SECE, Safety and infection control**

24. **(2)** Direct Coombs' test is used to determine if maternal Rh-positive antibodies are present in fetal cord blood; a positive test result indicates the presence of antibodies (titer). Oxygen concentration (**1**) does *not* give data relevant to the possible presence of anti-Rh positive antibodies. Glucose level (**3**) does *not* provide data relevant to the possible presence of anti-Rh positive antibodies (however, some of these infants may have low glucose levels, which would require intervention). $Hgb_{Alc}$ (glycosylated hemoglobin) (**4**) determines the status of *glucose* metabolism over the previous 120 days. **AN, RE/KN, 6, PhI, Reduction of risk potential**

25. **(3)** Meconium aspiration is commonly the cause of respiratory distress in the newborn who is *postterm*. It must be suspected if meconium staining is present on the skin, nails, and cord. Brain damage (**1**) if it is present, may be the result of birth trauma, *not* postterm birth. Respiratory distress syndrome (**2**) is seen in infants who are *preterm* and infants of mothers with poorly controlled diabetes mellitus. Hemorrhage (**4**) is not a frequently associated complication. **AS, APP, 6, HPM, Health promotion and maintenance**

# Glossary

Use this list of over **1200 terms** as an additional way to review content.

Key to symbols:

**!**    Alert (awareness of potential problem/condition)

🗠    Diagnostic Test/Procedure

💊    Drugs

⊕    Emergency

☞    Hands-on Care

⚡    Hazard (danger)

▨    Warning (signs/symptoms of impending problems)

**ABC**   Alternative birthing center. Birthing areas in hospitals located away from the traditional obstetric department.

**ABO incompatibility.**   Occurs when the mother's blood type is O and the newborn's is A, B, or AB.

⊕ **Abortion**   The expulsion from the uterus of an embryo or fetus before it is viable and capable of extrauterine existence. See *abortus.*

> **Complete a.**   Abortion in which fetus and all related tissue have been expelled from the uterus.
>
> **Elective a.**   Termination of pregnancy chosen by the woman that is not required for her physical safety.
>
> **Habitual (recurrent) a.**   Loss of three or more successive pregnancies for no known cause.
>
> **Incomplete a.**   Loss of pregnancy in which some but not all the products of conception have been expelled from the uterus.
>
> **Induced a.**   Intentionally produced loss of pregnancy.
>
> **Inevitable a.**   Threatened loss of pregnancy that cannot be prevented or stopped and is imminent.
>
> **Missed a.**   Loss of pregnancy in which the products of conception remain in the uterus after the fetus dies.
>
> **Septic a.**   Loss of pregnancy in which there is an infection of the products of conception and the uterine endometrial lining, usually resulting from attempted termination of early pregnancy.
>
> **Spontaneous a.**   Loss of pregnancy that occurs naturally without interference or known cause.
>
> **Therapeutic a.**   Pregnancy that has been intentionally terminated for medical reasons.
>
> **Threatened a.**   Possible loss of a pregnancy; early symptoms are present (e.g., the cervix begins to dilate).

**Abortus**   An embryo/fetus that is removed or expelled from the uterus at 20 wk gestation or less, or weighing 500 g or less, or measuring 25 cm or less.

⊕ **Abruptio placentae**   Partial or complete premature separation of a normally implanted placenta from the uterine wall, sometimes with massive hemorrhage.

**Abstinence**   Refraining from sexual intercourse periodically or permanently.

**Access to care**   Opportunity to receive health care services.

**Accreta, placenta**   See *placenta accreta.*

▨ **ACHES**   Acronym for possible warning signs secondary to use of oral hormone contraceptives. See *text.*

**Acini cells**   Milk-producing cells in the breast.

**Acrocyanosis**   Peripheral cyanosis; blue color of hands and feet in most infants at birth usually for the first few hours after birth.

**Acromion**   Projection of the spine of the scapula (forming the point of the shoulder); used to explain the presentation of the fetus.

**Acrosome reaction**   Release of proteolytic enzymes from fallopian tubes that enable the sperm to digest the cumulus cells and penetrate the zona pellucida of the ovum.

**Adenomyoma**   Type of tumor affecting glandular and smooth muscle tissue, such as uterine musculature.

**Adnexa**   Adjacent or accessory parts of a structure.

> **Uterine a.**   Ovaries and fallopian tubes.

**!**   **Adult respiratory distress syndrome (ARDS)**   Set of symptoms including decreased compliance of lung tissue, pulmonary edema, and acute hypoxemia. The condition is similar to respiratory distress syndrome (RDS) of the newborn.

**Afibrinogenemia**   Absence or decrease of fibrinogen in the blood such that the blood will not coagulate. In obstetrics, this condition occurs from complications of abruptio placentae or retention of a dead fetus. *See DIC.*

**Afterbirth**   Lay term for the placenta and membranes expelled after the birth of the child.

**Afterpains**   Painful uterine cramps that occur intermittently for approximately 2 or 3 days after birth and that result from contractile efforts of the uterus to return to its normal involuted condition; **afterbirth pains**.

**AGA**   Appropriate (weight) for gestational age.

**Agenesis**   Failure of an organ to develop.

Adapted from IM Bobak, M Jensen. *Maternity and Gynecologic Care—the Nurse and the Family* (5th ed). St. Louis: Mosby; and IM Bobak, DL Lowdermilk, MD Jensen. *Maternity Nursing* (4th ed). St. Louis: Mosby.

**Agonist-antagonist compounds** An agonist is an agent that *activates* something; an antagonist is an agent that *blocks* something.

**Alae nasi** Nostrils.

**Albuminuria** Presence of readily detectable amounts of albumin in the urine; proteinuria.

**Amenorrhea** Absence or suppression of menstruation.

**Amniocentesis** Procedure in which a needle is inserted through the abdominal and uterine walls into the amniotic fluid; used for assessment of fetal health and maturity and for elective or therapeutic abortion.

**Amnioinfusion** Infusion of normal saline or lactated Ringers solution, via an intrauterine catheter into the uterine cavity in an attempt to increase the fluid around the umbilical cord, prevent its compression during uterine contractions, and decrease the viscocity of meconium-stained amniotic fluid.

**Amnion** Inner membrane of two fetal membranes that form the sac and contain the fetus and the fluid that surrounds it in utero.

**Amnionitis** Inflammation of the amnion, occurring most frequently after premature rupture of membranes.

**Amniotic** Pertaining or relating to the amnion.

 **A. fluid** Fluid surrounding fetus derived primarily from maternal serum and fetal urine.

 **A. fluid embolism** Embolism resulting from amniotic fluid entering the maternal bloodstream during labor and birth after rupture of membranes; this is often fatal to the woman due to acute circulatory collapse.

 **A. sac** Thin, transparent sac that holds the fetus suspended in amniotic fluid; popularly called the bag of waters.

**Amniotomy** Artificial rupture of the fetal membranes (AROM).

**Analgesia** Lack of pain without loss of consciousness.

**Analgesic** Any drug or agent that will relieve pain.

**Android pelvis** Male type of pelvis. See *pelvis*.

**Anencephaly** Congenital deformity characterized by the absence of cerebrum, cerebellum, and flat bones of skull.

**Anesthesia** Partial or complete absence of sensation with or without loss of consciousness.

**Aneuploidy** Having an abnormal number of chromosomes.

**Anomaly** Organ or structure that is malformed or in some way abnormal with reference to form, structure, or position.

**Anovular menstrual period** Cyclic uterine bleeding not accompanied by the production and discharge of an ovum. Characteristic of early cycles at menarche and after childbirth.

**Anovulatory** Failure of the ovaries to produce, mature, or release eggs.

**Anoxia** Absence of oxygen.

**Antenatal** Occurring before or formed before birth.

**Antepartal** Before labor and birth.

**Anteroposterior repair** Operation in which the upper and lower walls of the vagina are reconstructed to correct relaxed tissue.

**Anthropoid pelvis** Pelvis in which the anteroposterior diameter is equal to or greater than the transverse diameter. See *pelvis*.

**Anthropometry** Study of human body measurements.

**Antibody** Specific protein substance developed by the body that exerts restrictive or destructive action on specific antigens, such as bacteria, toxins, or Rh factor.

**Anticipatory grief** Grief that predates the loss of a beloved person or object, e.g., anticipated loss of a pregnancy or compromised newborn.

**Antigen** Protein foreign to the body that causes the body to develop antibodies. Examples: bacteria, dust, Rh factor.

**Apgar score** Numeric expression of the condition of a newborn obtained by rapid assessment at 1, 5, and 15 min of age; developed by Dr. Virginia Apgar.

**Apnea** Cessation of respirations for more than 10 sec associated with generalized cyanosis.

**Apt test** Differentiation of maternal and fetal blood when *vaginal bleeding* is present. It is performed as follows: Add 0.5 mL blood to 4.5 mL distilled water. Shake. Add 1 mL 0.25N sodium hydroxide. Fetal and cord blood remain pink for 1 or 2 min. Maternal blood becomes brown in 30 sec. See *Kleihauer-Betke test*.

**Areola** Pigmented ring of tissue surrounding the nipple.

 **Secondary a.**
  During the fifth month of pregnancy, a second faint ring of pigmentation seen around the original areola.

**Artificial insemination** Introduction of semen by instrument injection into the vagina or uterus for impregnation. Preferred term: *therapeutic insemination*.

**Asherman's syndrome** Intrauterine adhesions following inflammation and infection; one cause of impaired fertility.

**Asphyxia** Decreased oxygen and/or excess of carbon dioxide in the body.

 **A. livida** Condition in which the infant's skin is characteristically pale, pulse is weak and slow, and reflexes are depressed or absent; also known as *blue asphyxia*.

 **A. pallida** Condition in which the infant appears pale and limp and suffers from bradycardia (≤ 80 beats/min) and apnea.

**! Fetal a.** Condition occurring in utero, with the following biochemical changes: hypoxemia (lowering of $PO_2$), hypercapnia (increase in $PCO_2$), and respiratory and metabolic acidosis (reduction of blood pH).

**Aspiration pneumonia** Inflammatory condition of the lungs and bronchi caused by the inhalation of vomitus containing acid gastric contents; ARDS may be a sequel.

**Aspiration syndrome** See *meconium aspiration syndrome.*

**Assault** An unlawful act that places another person, without that person's consent, in fear of immediate bodily harm or battery.

**Ataractic** Drug capable of promoting tranquility; a tranquilizer.

**Atelectasis** Pulmonary pathosis involving alveolar collapse.

**Athetosis** Neuromuscular condition characterized by slow, writhing, continuous, and involuntary movement of the extremities, as seen in some forms of cerebral palsy and in motor disorders resulting from lesions in the basal ganglia.

**Atony** Absence of muscle tone.

**Atresia** Absence of a normally present passageway.

**Choanal a.** Complete obstruction of the posterior nares, which open into the nasopharynx, with membranous or bony tissue.

**Esophageal a.** Congenital anomaly in which the esophagus ends in a blind pouch or narrows into a thin cord, thus failing to form a continuous passageway to the stomach.

**Attachment** A feeling of affection or loyalty that binds one person to another, which occurs at critical periods, such as birth or adoption; it is unique, specific, and enduring.

**Augmentation of labor** Artificial stimulation of uterine contractions after labor has started spontaneously but is not progressing satisfactorily.

**Autoimmune disease** Body produces antibodies against itself, causing tissue damage.

**Autoimmunization** Development of antibodies against constituents of one's own tissues (e.g., a man may develop antibodies against his own sperm).

**Autolysis** "Self-digestive" process by which the uterus returns (involutes) to a nonpregnant state following childbirth. The decrease in estrogen and progesterone levels following childbirth results in this destruction of excess and hypertrophied uterine tissue.

**Autosomal inheritance** Characteristics transmitted by genes on the autosomes, not on the sex chromosomes.

**Autosomes** Any of the paired chromosomes other than the sex (X and Y) chromosomes.

**Axis, pelvic** Imaginary curved line that passes through the centers of all the anteroposterior diameters of the pelvis.

**Azoospermia** Absence of sperm in the semen.

**"Baby blues"** See *postpartum blues.*

**Back labor** Uncomfortable labor that occurs when fetus, in occiput posterior position, presses on sacral nerves during contractions.

**Bacteremic shock** Shock that occurs in septicemia when endotoxins are released from certain bacteria in the bloodstream.

**Bag of waters** Lay term for the sac containing amniotic fluid and fetus.

**Ballottement** (1) Movability of a floating object (e.g., fetus). (2) Diagnostic technique using palpation: A floating object, when tapped or pushed, moves away and then returns to touch the examiner's hand.

**Bandl's ring** Abnormally thickened ridge of uterine musculature between the upper and lower segments that follows a mechanically obstructed labor, with the lower segment thinning abnormally.

**Barr body (sex chromatin)** Chromatin mass located against the inner surface of the nucleus in females, possibly representing the inactive X chromosome.

**Bartholin's glands** Two small glands situated on either side of the vaginal orifice that secrete small amounts of mucus during coitus and that are homologous to the bulbourethral glands in the male.

**Basal body temperature (BBT)** Lowest body temperature of a healthy person taken immediately after awakening and before any physical activity.

**Battery** Repeated beating of or use of force on a person without regard to personal rights; may be physical, sexual, psychological, or social.

**Behavioral assessment** Assessment of newborn's activity, feeding and sleeping patterns; responsiveness.

**Bell's palsy** See *palsy, Bell's.*

**Bereavement** The feelings of loss, pain, desolation, and sadness that occur after the death of a loved one.

**Bicornuate uterus** Anomalous uterus that may be either a double or single organ with two horns.

**Bilirubin** Yellow or orange pigment that is a breakdown product of hemoglobin. It is carried by the blood to the liver, where it is chemically changed and excreted in the bile or is conjugated and excreted by the kidneys.

**Billings method** See *ovulation method.*

**Bimanual palpation** Examination of a woman's pelvic organs done by placing one hand on the abdomen and one or two fingers of the other hand in the vagina.

**Biophysical profile (BPP)** Noninvasive assessment of the fetus and its environment using ultrasonography and uterine fetal monitoring; includes fetal breathing movements, gross body movements, fetal muscle tone, reactive fetal heart rate, and amniotic fluid volume.

**Biopsy** Removal of a small piece of tissue for microscopic examination and diagnosis.

**Biparietal diameter** Largest transverse diameter of the fetal head; extends from one parietal bone to the other.

**Birth plan** A tool by which expectant parents can explore their childbirth options and choose those that are most important to them.

**Bishop score** Rating system to evaluate inducibility of the cervix; a higher score increases the rate of successful induction of labor.

**Blastocyst** The stage in development of an embryo following the morula, made of an outer layer of trophoblast and an inner cell mass.

**Blastoderm** Germinal membrane of the ovum.

> **B. vesicle** Stage in the development of a mammalian embryo that consists of an outer layer, or trophoblast, and a hollow sphere of cells enclosing a cavity.

**Blood-brain barrier** Obstruction that prevents passage of certain substances from blood into brain tissue.

**Bloody show** Vaginal discharge that originates in the cervix and consists of blood and mucus; increases as cervix dilates during labor.

**Body image** Person's subjective concept of his or her physical appearance.

**Body mass index (BMI)** Method of evaluating the appropriateness of weight for height; formula: BMI = weight/height$^2$ (weight in kg/height in m).

**Bonding** Describes the initial mutual attraction between people, such as between parent and child, at first meeting. Also see *attachment*.

**Born out of asepsis (BOA)** Pertaining to birth without the use of sterile technique.

**Bradley method** Preparation for parenthood with active participation of father/coach and mother.

**Braxton Hicks contractions** Mild, intermittent, painless uterine contractions that occur more frequently as pregnancy advances but do *not* represent true labor.

**Brazelton assessment** Criteria for assessing the interactional behavior of a newborn.

**Breakthrough bleeding** Escape of blood occurring between menstrual periods; may be noted by women using chemical contraception (birth control pill).

**Breast milk jaundice** See *jaundice, breast milk*.

**Breast self-examination (BSE)** Self-examination of the breasts.

**Breast surgeries for malignant lesions**

> **Lumpectomy (tylectomy)** Excision of tumor and some surrounding normal tissue.

> **Quadrectomy (segmental resection)** Excision of a quadrant of the mammary gland that includes the tumor.

> **Radical mastectomy** Removal of mammary gland, pectoralis major, and axillary lymph nodes.

> **Total (simple) mastectomy** Removal of all of the mammary gland that includes the tumor.

**Breech presentation** Presentation in which buttocks and/or feet are nearest the cervical opening and are born first; occurs in approximately 3% of all births.

> **Complete b.p.** Simultaneous presentation of buttocks, legs, and feet.

> **Footling (incomplete) b.p.** Presentation of one or both feet.

> **Frank b.p.** Presentation of buttocks, with hips flexed so that thighs are against abdomen.

**Bregma** Point of junction of the coronal and sagittal sutures of the skull; the area of the anterior fontanel of the fetus.

**Brim** Edge of the superior strait of the true pelvis; the inlet.

**Bronchopulmonary dysplasia (BPD)** Emphysematous changes caused by oxygen toxicity.

**Brown fat** Source of heat unique to neonates that is capable of greater thermogenic activity than ordinary fat. Deposits are found around the adrenals, kidneys, and neck; between the scapulas; and behind the sternum for several weeks after birth.

**Bruit, uterine** Sound of passage of blood through uterine blood vessels, synchronous with fetal heart rate.

**Calendar method** Method of calculating the fertile days of the *next* menstrual cycle by noting the lengths of the previous 12 cycles; then, subtract 18 from the shortest cycle and 11 from the longest cycle to give the most likely fertile days of the next cycle. *See text.*

*Candida vaginitis* Vaginal, fungal infection; moniliasis.

**Capacitation** Enzymatic process resulting in removal of plasma protein over acrosome of sperm; the process that enables sperm to bind to the egg. (See *Acrosome reaction*.)

**Caput** Occiput of fetal head appearing at the vaginal introitus preceding birth of the head.

> **C. succedaneum** Swelling of the tissue over the presenting part of the fetal head caused by pressure during labor; swelling *does* cross newborn's suture lines.

**Carcinoma** Malignant, often metastatic epithelial neoplasm; cancer.

**Cardiac decompensation** Inability of the heart to maintain a sufficient cardiac output.

**Cardinal movements of labor:** The mechanism of labor in a vertex presentation includes engagement, descent, flexion, internal rotation, extension, external rotation (restitution), and expulsion.

**Carpal tunnel syndrome**   Pressure on the median nerve at the point at which it goes through the carpal tunnel of the wrist. It causes soreness, tenderness, and weakness of the muscles of the thumb.

**Carrier**   Individual who carries a gene that does not exhibit itself in physical or chemical characteristics but that can be transmitted to children (e.g., a female carrying the trait for hemophilia, which is expressed in male offspring).

**Caul**   Hood of fetal membranes covering fetal head during birth.

**Cephalohematoma**   Extravasation of blood from ruptured vessels between a skull bone and its external covering, the periosteum. Swelling is limited by the margins of the cranial bone affected (usually parietals).

**Cephalic**   Pertaining to the head.

> **C. presentation**
> Presentation of any part of the fetal head.

**Cephalocaudal development**   Principle of maturation that development progresses from the head to the feet.

**Cephalopelvic disproportion (CPD)**   Condition in which the infant's head is of such a shape, size, or position that it cannot pass through the mother's pelvis.

**Cerclage**   Use of nonabsorbable suture to keep an incompetent cervix closed; released when pregnancy is at term to allow labor to begin.

**Cervical cap (custom)**   Individually fitted contraceptive covering for the cervix.

**Cervical erosion**   Alteration of the epithelium of the cervix caused by chronic irritation or infection.

**Cervical intraepithelial neoplasm (CIN)**   Uncontrolled and progressive abnormal growth of cervical epithelial cells.

**Cervical mucus method**   See *ovulation method.*

**Cervicitis**   Cervical infection.

**Cervix**   Lowest and narrow end of the uterus; the "neck." The cervix is situated between the external os and the body (corpus) of the uterus, and its lower end extends into the vagina.

**Cesarean birth**   Birth of a fetus by an incision through the abdominal wall and uterus.

**Chadwick's sign**   Violet color of mucous membrane that is visible from about the fourth week of pregnancy; caused by increased vascularity of the vagina.

**Childbed fever**   See *puerperal sepsis.*

**Chloasma**   Increased pigmentation over bridge of nose and cheeks of pregnant women and some women taking oral contraceptives; also known as *mask of pregnancy.*

**Choanal atresia**   See *atresia, choanal.*

**Chorioamnionitis**   Stimulated by organisms in the amniotic fluid, which then become infiltrated with polymorphonuclear leukocytes.

**Chorion**   Fetal membrane closest to the intrauterine wall that gives rise to the placenta and continues as the outer membrane surrounding the amnion.

**Chorionic villi**   See *villi, chorionic.*

**Chorionic villi sampling (CVS)**   Removal of fetal tissue from placenta for genetic diagnostic studies; performed after 10 wk gestation.

**Chromosome**   Element within the cell nucleus carrying genes and composed of DNA and proteins.

**Circumcision**

> **Male**   Excision of the prepuce (foreskin) of the penis, exposing the glans.
> **Female**   Religious or cultural removal of a portion of the clitoris and labia.

**Cleavage**   Cell division following the fertilization of an ovum.

**Cleft lip**   Incomplete closure of the lip; *harelip.*

**Cleft palate**   Incomplete closure of the palate or roof of mouth; a congenital fissure.

**Climacterium**   The period of a woman's life when she is passing from a reproductive to a nonreproductive state, with regression of ovarian function. The cycle of endocrine, physical, and psychosocial changes that occurs during the termination of the reproductive years; also known as perimenopause.

**Clitoris**   Female organ analogous to male penis; a small, ovoid body of erectile tissue situated at the anterior junction of the vulva.

> **Prepuce of the c.**   See *prepuce of the clitoris.*

**Clonus (ankle)**   Spasmodic alternation of muscular contraction and relaxation; deep tendon reflex (DTR) assessed especially in women who are pre-eclamptic.

**Coccyx**   Small bone at the base of the spinal column.

**Coitus**   Penile-vaginal intercourse.

> **C. interruptus**   Intercourse during which penis is withdrawn from vagina before ejaculation.

**Cold stress**   Excessive loss of heat that results in increased respirations and nonshivering thermogenesis to maintain core body temperature. See *heat loss.*

**Colostrum**   Yellow secretion from the breast containing mainly serum and white blood corpuscles preceding the onset of true lactation 2 or 3 days after birth.

**Conception**   Union of the sperm and ovum resulting in fertilization; formation of the one-celled zygote.

**Conceptional age**   In fetal development, the number of completed weeks since the moment of conception. Because the moment of conception is almost impossible to determine, conceptional age is estimated at 2 wk less than gestational age.

**Conceptus**   Embryo or fetus, fetal membranes, amniotic fluid, and the fetal portion of the placenta.

**Condom**  Mechanical barrier worn on the penis for contraception; "rubber"; also provides some protection against transmission of sexually transmitted diseases (STDs).

**Condylomata accuminata**  Wartlike growth on the skin usually seen near the anus or external genitals caused by human papillomavirus (HPV); genital warts. (Must be differentiated from condyloma latum seen in secondary syphilis.)

**Confinement**  *Outdated* term for period of childbirth and early puerperium.

**Congenital**  Present or existing before birth as a result of either hereditary or prenatal environmental factors.

**Conjoined twins**  See *twins, conjoined.*

**Conjugate**

> **Diagonal c.**  Radiographic measurement of distance from i*nferior border* of symphysis pubis (SP) to sacral promontory; may be obtained by vaginal examination; 12.5 to 13 cm (*rarely measured*).

> **True c. (c. vera)**  Radiographic measurement of distance from *upper margin* of SP to sacral promontory; 1.5 to 2 cm less than diagonal conjugate (*rarely measured*).

**Conjunctivitis**  Inflammation of the mucous membrane that lines the eyelids and that is reflected onto the eyeball.

**Conscious relaxation**  Technique used to release the mind and body from tension through conscious effort and practice.

**Contraception**  Prevention of impregnation or conception.

**Contraction stress test (CST)**  Test to stimulate uterine contractions for the purpose of assessing fetal response; a healthy fetus does not demonstrate fetal distress in response to contractions while a compromised fetus demonstrates late decelerations in the fetal heart rate that are indicative of uteroplacental insufficiency.

**Contractions**

> **Acme**  Highest point (e.g., of a contraction).

> **Decrement**  Decrease or stage of decline, as of a contraction.

> **Duration**  The period of time from the beginning of the contraction to the end.

> **Frequency**  How often the contractions occur—the period of time from the beginning of one contraction to the beginning of the next, or number of contractions in a 10 minute time frame.

> **Increment**  An increase, or buildup, as of a contraction.

> **Intensity**  The strength of the contraction at its peak.

> **Interval**  The period of time between uterine contractions—timed from the end of one contraction to the beginning of the next.

> **Resting tone**  The tension in the uterine muscle between contractions.

**Coombs' test**

> **Direct**  Determination of maternal Rh positive antibodies in fetal cord blood. A positive test result indicates the presence of antibodies or titer.

> **Indirect**  Determination of Rh positive antibodies in maternal blood.

**Copulation**  Coitus; sexual intercourse.

**Cordocentesis**  See *Percutaneous umbilical cord sampling.*

**Corpus**  Discrete mass of material; body, e.g., body of uterus.

> **C. luteum**  Yellow body. After rupture of the graafian follicle at ovulation, the follicle develops into a yellow structure that secretes progesterone during the 14 days after ovulation, atrophying about 3 days before sloughing of the endometrium in menstrual flow. If impregnation occurs, this structure continues to produce progesterone until the placenta can take over this function.

**Cotyledon**  One of the 15-28 visible segments of the placenta on the maternal surface, each made up of fetal vessels, chorionic villi, and an intervillous space.

**Couplet care**  One nurse, educated in both mother and infant care, functions as the primary nurse for both mother and infant (also known as mother-baby care or single-room maternity care).

**Couvade**  Custom whereby the man goes through mock labor while the woman is giving birth. Can also refer to men who have pregnancy symptoms.

**Couvelaire uterus**  See *Uterus, Couvelaire.*

**CPAP**  Continuous positive airway pressure.

**Cradle cap**  Common seborrheic dermatitis of infants consisting of thick, yellow, greasy scales on the scalp.

**Craniotabes**  Localized softening of cranial bones.

**Creatinine**  Substance found in blood and muscle; measurement of levels in maternal urine correlates with amount of fetal muscle mass and therefore fetal size.

**Crib death**  Unexpected and sudden death of an apparently normal and healthy infant that occurs during sleep and with no physical or autopsic evidence of disease. Also referred to as *sudden infant death syndrome* (SIDS).

*Cri-du-chat* **syndrome**  Rare congenital disorder recognized at birth by a kittenlike-cry, which may prevail for weeks, then disappear. Other characteristics include: low birth weight, microcephaly, "moon face," wide-set eyes, strabismus, and low-set misshaped ears. Infants are hypotonic; heart defects and mental and physical retardation are common. Also called *cat-cry syndrome.*

**Crisis** Any naturally occurring turning point, such as courtship, marriage, pregnancy, parenthood, or death.

**Developmental crisis** Severe, usually transient, stress that occurs when a person is unable to complete the tasks of a psychosocial stage of development and is therefore unable to move on to the next stage.

**Maturational crisis** Crisis that arises during normal growth and development, e.g., puberty.

**Situational crisis** Crisis that arises suddenly in response to an external event or a conflict concerning a specific circumstance. The symptoms are transient, and the episode is usually brief.

**Crisis intervention** Actions taken by the nurse to help an individual deal with an impending, potentially overwhelming crisis, regain his or her equilibrium, grow from the experience, and improve coping skills.

**Critical path** The exact timing of all key incidents that must occur to achieve the standard outcomes within the diagnosis-related group (DRG)-specific length of stay.

**Crowning** Stage of birth when the top of the fetal head becomes visible at the vaginal opening.

**Cryptorchidism** Failure of one or both of the testicles to descend into the scrotum. Also called *undescended testis*.

**Cul-de-sac of Douglas** Pouch formed by a fold of the peritoneum dipping down between the anterior wall of the rectum and the posterior wall of the uterus; also called *Douglas' cul-de-sac*, pouch of *Douglas*, and rectouterine pouch.

**Culdocentesis** Use of needle puncture or incision to remove intraperitoneal fluid (blood, purulent material) from the posterior cul-de-sac by way of the vagina.

**Culdotomy** Incision or needle puncture of the cul-de-sac of Douglas by way of the vagina.

**!** **Cullen's sign** Faint, irregularly formed, hemorrhagic patches on the skin around the umbilicus. The discolored skin is blue-black and becomes greenish brown or yellow. Cullen's sign may appear 1 to 2 days after the onset of anorexia and the severe, poorly localized abdominal pains characteristic of acute pancreatitis. Cullen's sign is also present in massive upper gastrointestinal hemorrhage, *ruptured ectopic pregnancy*.

**Cultural context** A situation that considers the individual and family's beliefs and practices (culture).

**Curettage** Scraping of the endometrium lining of the uterus with a curet to remove the contents of the uterus (as is done after an inevitable or incomplete abortion) or to obtain specimens for diagnostic purposes.

**Cutis marmorata** Transient vasomotor phenomenon occurring primarily over extremities when the infant is exposed to chilling. It appears as a pink or faint purple capillary outline on the skin. Also called mottling. Occasionally seen in infant in respiratory distress.

**Cycle of violence** Pattern of three phases: period of increasing tension, the abusive episode, and a period of contrition and kindness.

**Cystitis** Inflammatory condition or infection of urinary bladder and ureters.

**Cystocele** Bladder hernia; injury to the vesicovaginal fascia during labor and birth may allow herniation of the bladder into the vagina.

**Daily fetal movement counts (DFMC)** Maternal assessment of fetal activity; the number of fetal movements within a specific time period are counted.

**Death** Cessation of life; mortality.

**Fetal d.** Intrauterine death. Death of a fetus of 20 wk gestation or more.

**Infant d.** Death during the first year of life.

**Maternal d.** Death of a woman during the childbearing cycle.

**Neonatal d.** Death of a newborn within the first 28 days after birth.

**Perinatal d.** Death of a fetus of 20 wk gestation or older or death of a neonate 28 days old or younger.

**Decidua** Mucous membrane, lining of uterus, or endometrium of pregnancy that is shed after giving birth.

**D. basalis** Maternal aspect of the placenta made up of uterine blood vessels, endometrial stroma, and glands. It is shed in lochial discharge after birth.

**D. capsularis** That part of the decidual membranes surrounding the chorionic sac.

**D. vera** Nonplacental decidual lining of the uterus.

**Deep tendon reflexes (DTRs)** Reflex caused by stimulation of tendons, such as elbow, wrist, knee, triceps, and ankle jerk reflexes.

**Deletion** Loss of a piece of a chromosome that has broken off.

**Delivery** Birth of the child with placenta and membranes by the mother or their extraction by the obstetric practitioner.

**Abdominal d.** See *cesarean birth*.

**DOD$_{450}$** (read delta OD$_{450}$) Delta optical density (or absorbance) at 450 nm, obtained by spectral analysis of amniotic fluid. This prenatal test is used to measure the degree of hemolytic activity in the fetus and to evaluate fetal status in women sensitized to Rh(Du).

**Demand feeding** Infant feeds when hungry, not by schedule.

**Deoxyribonucleic acid (DNA)**  Intracellular complex protein that carries genetic information, consisting of two purines (adenine and guanine) and two pyrimidines (thymine and cytosine).

**Depressive reactions**  Depression related to the postpartum period including postpartum blues, postpartum nonpsychotic depression, and postpartum psychosis.

**DES**  Diethylstilbestrol, used in treating menopausal symptoms. Exposure of female fetus predisposes her to reproductive tract malformations and (later) dysplasia.

**Desquamation**  Shedding of epithelial cells of the skin and mucous membranes.

**Diaphragmatic hernia**  Congenital malformation of diaphragm that allows displacement of the abdominal organs into the thoracic cavity.

**Diastasis recti abdominis**  Separation of the two rectus muscles along the median line of the abdominal wall. This is often seen in women with repeated childbirths or with a multifetal gestation (triplets, etc.). In the newborn it is usually due to incomplete development.

**DIC**  Disseminated intravascular coagulation.

**Dick-Read method**  An approach to childbirth developed in the early 20th century based on the premise that fear of pain produces muscular tension, resulting in pain and greater fear. The method includes teaching physiologic processes of labor, exercise to improve muscle tone, and techniques to assist in relaxation and prevent the *fear-tension-pain mechanism.*

**Dilatation and curettage (D and C)**  Vaginal operation in which the cervical canal is stretched enough to admit passage of an instrument called a curet. The endometrium of the uterus is scraped with the curet to empty the uterine contents or to obtain tissue for examination.

**Dilatation and evacuation (D and E)**  A surgical method of pregnancy interruption between weeks 15 and 24; requires extreme cervical dilatation and evacuation of uterine contents using large-bore suction equipment and crushing instruments.

**Dilatation of cervix**  Stretching of the external os from an opening a few millimeters in size to an opening large enough to allow the passage of the infant.

**Diploid number**  Having two sets of chromosomes; found normally in somatic (body) cells; 23 pairs or 46 chromosomes.

**Discordance**  Discrepancy in size (or other indicator) between twins.

**Disparate twins**  See *twins, disparate.*

**Disseminated intravascular coagulation (DIC)**  A pathologic form of coagulation in which clotting factors are consumed to such an extent that generalized bleeding can occur; associated with: abruptio placentae, eclampsia, intrauterine fetal demise, amniotic fluid embolism, and hemorrhage.

**Disseminated lupus erythematosus**  Chronic inflammatory disease affecting many systems of the body. Also called *systemic lupus erythematosus (SLE).*

**Dizygotic**  Related to or proceeding from two zygotes (fertilized ova).

**Dizygotic twins**  See *twins, dizygotic.*

**Döderlein's bacillus**  Gram-positive bacterium occurring in normal vaginal secretions (same as *Lactobacillus acidophilus*).

**Dominant trait**  Gene that is expressed whenever it is present in the heterozygous gene state (e.g., brown eyes are dominant over blue).

**Doppler blood flow analysis**  Device for measuring blood flow noninvasively in the fetus and placenta to detect intrauterine growth retardation.

**Double set-up**  A nursing procedure in which an obstetric operating room is prepared for both vaginal birth or cesarean birth; today, ultrasound has made this *obsolete* in most facilities; used originally to help in diagnosis of vaginal bleeding, to rule out placenta previa.

**Douglas' cul-de-sac**  See *cul-de-sac of Douglas.*

**Doula**  A lay person who provides support during labor.

**Down syndrome**
Abnormality involving the occurrence of a third chromosome (trisomy 21), rather than the normal pair, that characteristically results in a typical picture of mental retardation and altered physical appearance. This condition was *formerly* called *mongolism* or *mongoloid idiocy.*

**Dry labor**  Lay term referring to labor in which amniotic fluid has already escaped. A "dry birth" does not exist.

**Dubowitz assessment**  Estimation of gestational age of a newborn, based on criteria developed for that purpose.

**Ductus arteriosus**  In fetal circulation, an anatomic shunt between the pulmonary artery and arch of the aorta. It is obliterated after birth by a rising $PO_2$ and change in intravascular pressures in the presence of normal pulmonary function. It normally becomes a ligament after birth but in some instances remains patent.

**Ductus venosus**  In fetal circulation, a blood vessel carrying oxygenated blood between the umbilical vein and the inferior vena cava, bypassing the liver. It is obliterated and becomes a ligament after birth.

**Dura (dura mater)**  Outermost, toughest of the three meninges covering the brain and spinal cord.

**Dys-**  Prefix meaning abnormal, difficult, painful, faulty.

**Dysfunctional uterine bleeding**  Abnormal bleeding from the uterus for reasons that are not readily established.

**Dysmaturity**  See *intrauterine growth restriction (IUGR).*

**Dysmenorrhea**  Difficult or painful menstruation.

> **Primary dysmenorrhea**  Painful menstruation beginning 2-6 mo after menarche, related to ovulation.

> **Secondary dysmenorrhea**  Painful menstruation related to organic disease such as endometriosis, pelvic inflammatory disease (PID), uterine neoplasm.

**Dyspareunia**  Painful sexual intercourse.

**Dystocia**  Prolonged, painful, or otherwise difficult birth because of mechanical factors produced by the "6 Ps":
> *Passage*—pelvic structure; full bladder, rectum.

> *Passenger*—fetal size, abnormal presentation/position, anomalies, number.

> *Placenta*—previa, abruptio.

> *Position*—maternal, during labor, birth.

> *Powers*—uterine contractions or maternal bearing-down efforts.

> *Psychological responses*—of mother to labor related to past experiences, preparation, culture and heritage, and support system.

**Ecchymosis**  Bruise; bleeding into tissue caused by direct trauma, serious infection, or bleeding diathesis.

**Eclampsia**  Severe complication of pregnancy of unknown cause and occurring more often in the primigravida; characterized by tonic and clonic convulsions, coma, high blood pressure, albuminuria, and oliguria occurring during pregnancy or shortly after birth.

**Ectoderm**  Outer layer of embryonic tissue giving rise to skin, nails, and hair.

**Ectopic**  Occurring in an abnormal location.

> **E. pregnancy**  Implantation of the fertilized ovum outside of its normal place in the uterine cavity. Locations include the abdomen, fallopian tubes, and ovaries.

**EDD**  Expected date of delivery; "due date."

**EDC**  Expected date of confinement; "due date" (term has been *replaced* by EDD).

**Effacement**  Thinning and shortening or obliteration of the cervix that occurs during late pregnancy or labor or both.

**Effleurage**  Gentle stroking used in massage.

**Ejaculation**  Sudden expulsion of semen from the male urethra.

**ELISA**  *Enzyme*-linked immunosorbent *assay* (uses monoclonal antibodies). Substances detected include hormones, bacterial antigens and antibodies. Laboratory tests: pregnancy, chlamydial infection (Chlamydiazyme), human immunodeficiency virus antibodies.

**Embolus**  Any undissolved matter (solid, liquid, or gaseous) that is carried by the blood to another part of the body and obstructs a blood vessel.

**Embryo**  Conceptus from the second or third wk of development until about the eighth wk after conception, when mineralization (ossification) of the skeleton begins. This period is characterized by cellular differentiation and predominantly hyperplastic growth; embryonic stages are *zygote*, *morula*, and *blastocyst*.

**Emotional lability**  Rapid mood changes.

**Endometriosis**  Tissue closely resembling endometrial tissue but aberrantly located outside the uterus in the pelvic cavity. Symptomatology may include : pelvic pain or pressure, dysmenorrhea, dyspareunia, abnormal bleeding from the uterus or rectum, and sterility.

**Endometritis**  Inflammation of the endometrium.

**Endometrium**  Inner lining of the uterus that undergoes changes caused by hormones during the menstrual cycle and pregnancy; decidua.

**Endorphins**  Endogenous opioids secreted by the pituitary gland that act on the central and peripheral nervous systems to reduce pain.

**En face**  Position in which neonate is held 8 in. (20 cm) away facing the observer to allow for direct eye contact.

**Engagement**  In obstetrics, the entrance of the fetal presenting part into the superior pelvic strait and the beginning of the descent through the pelvic canal.

**Engorgement**  Distention or vascular congestion. In obstetrics, the process of swelling of the breast tissue brought about by an increase in blood and lymph supply to the breast, which precedes true lactation. It lasts about 48 hr and usually reaches a peak between the third and fifth postpartum days.

**Engrossment**  Sustained involvement of a parent with an infant.

**Entoderm**  Inner layer of embryonic tissue giving rise to internal organs such as the intestine.

**Entrainment**  Phenomenon observed in the micro-analysis of sound films in which the speaker moves several parts of the body and the listener responds to the sounds by moving in ways that are coordinated with the rhythm of the sounds. Infants have been observed to move in time to the rhythms of adult speech but not to random noises or disconnected words or vowels. Entrainment is thought to be an essential factor in the process of parental infant bonding.

**Epicanthus**  Fold of skin covering the inner canthus and caruncle that extends from the root of the nose to the median end of the eyebrow; characteristically found in certain races but may occur as a congenital anomaly.

**Epidural anesthesia**  Injection of anesthetic outside the dura mater (anesthetic does not mix with spinal fluid). See *peridural anesthesia*.

**Epidural block**  Type of regional anesthesia produced by injection of a local anesthetic into the epidural (peridural) space.

**Epidural blood patch**  A patch formed by a few milliliters of the mother's blood used to repair a tear or hole in the dura mater around the spinal cord.

**Episiotomy**
Surgical incision of the perineum at the end of the second stage of labor to facilitate birth and to avoid laceration of the perineum.

**Epispadias**  Defect in which the urethral canal terminates on dorsum of penis or above the clitoris (rare).

**Epstein's pearls**  Small, white blebs found along the gum margins and at the junction of the soft and hard palates. They are a normal manifestation and are commonly seen in the newborn. Similar to *Bohn's nodules*.

**Epulis**  Tumorlike benign lesion of the gingiva seen in women who are pregnant.

**Erb-Duchenne paralysis**  Paralysis caused by traumatic injury to the upper brachial plexus, occurring most commonly in childbirth from forcible traction during birth. The signs of Erb's paralysis include: loss of sensation in the arm and paralysis and atrophy of the deltoid, the biceps, and the brachialis muscles. Also called *Erb's palsy*.

**Ergot**  Drug obtained from *Claviceps purpurea*, a fungus, which stimulates the smooth muscles of blood vessels and the uterus, causing vasoconstriction and uterine contractions.

**Erythema toxicum**  Innocuous pink papular neonatal rash of unknown cause, with superimposed vesicles appearing within 24-48 hr after birth and resolving spontaneously within a few days.

**Erythroblastosis fetalis**  Hemolytic disease of the newborn usually caused by isoimmunization resulting from Rh incompatibility or ABO incompatibility.

**Erythropoiesis**  Erythrocyte (RBC) production, which involves the maturation of a nucleated precursor into a hemoglobin-filled, nucleus-free erythrocyte regulated by erythropoietin, a hormone produced by the kidney.

**Estimated date of birth**  Approximate date of birth. Usually determined by calculation using Naegele's rule, also known as EDC (expected date of confinement).

**Estradiol**  An estrogen.

**Estrangement, psychological**  Reaction to the birth of and subsequent separation from an infant who is sick and/or preterm, whereby the mother is diverted from establishing a normal relationship with her baby.

**Estriol**  Major metabolite of estrogen that increases during the second half of pregnancy with an intact fetoplacental unit (normal placenta, normal fetal liver and adrenals) and normal maternal renal function.

**Estrogen**  Female sex hormone produced by the ovaries and placenta.

**Estrogen replacement therapy (ERT)**  Controversial treatment using exogenous estrogen given to women during and after menopause to prevent hot flushes (flashes), mood changes, osteoporosis, and genitourinary symptoms.

**Exchange transfusion**  Replacement of 75-85% of circulating blood by withdrawing the recipient's blood and injecting a donor's blood in equal amounts. The purposes are: to prevent an accumulation of bilirubin in the blood above a dangerous level, to prevent the accumulation of other by-products of hemolysis in hemolytic disease, and to correct anemia and acidosis.

**Expulsive**  Having the tendency to drive out or expel.
    **E. contractions**  Labor contractions that are characteristic of the second stage of labor.

**External cephalic version (ECV)**  Turning the fetus to a vertex position by exerting pressure on the fetus externally through the maternal abdomen.

**Extrauterine**  Occurring outside the uterus.
    **E. pregnancy**  Ectopic pregnancy in which the fertilized ovum implants itself outside the uterus.

**Extrusion reflex**  Infant automatically extends tongue when it is stimulated.

**Facies**  Pertaining to the appearance or expression of the face; certain congenital syndromes typically present with a specific facial appearance.

**FAD**  Fetal activity determination.

**Failure to thrive**  Condition in which neonate's or infant's growth and development patterns are below the norms for age.

**Fallopian tubes**  Two canals or oviducts extending laterally from each side of the uterus through which the ovum travels, after ovulation, to the uterus; uterine tubes.

**False labor**  Uterine contractions that: do *not* result in cervical dilatation, are irregular, are felt more in front, often do *not* last more than 20 sec, and do *not* become longer or stronger.

**False pelvis**  The part of the pelvis superior to a plane passing through the linea terminalis.

**Family dynamics**  The process by which family members assume appropriate social roles.

**Family functions**  Activities carried out within families for the well-being of family members; including: biologic, economic, educational, psychological, and socio-cultural.

**Family types**
    **Blended f.**  Family form that includes stepparents and stepchildren.
    **Communal f.**  Groupings vary from highly formalized structure (Amish) to loosely knit groups; an alternative life-style developed for a variety of ideologic or societal purposes.
    **Extended f.**  Family form that includes the nuclear family and other blood-related persons.

**Homosexual f.** Family form in which parents form a homosexual union. Children may be the offspring of a previous heterosexual union, or may be conceived by one member of a lesbian couple through artificial insemination, or adopted from a surrogate.

**Nuclear f.** Family form consisting of parents and their dependent children.

**Single parent f.** Family with only one parent; may result from loss of a spouse/partner (e.g., death), from out-of-wedlock births, or from adoption.

**Family violence** Interpersonal violence including child, elder, sibling, and spouse/partner.

**Fantasy child** The imagined dream child; the "ideal" unborn child.

**Father—developmental tasks of**

**Announcement phase** The *first* developmental task experienced by expectant fathers. During this phase the expectant father accepts the biologic fact of pregnancy.

**Moratorium phase** The *second* developmental task experienced by expectant fathers. During this phase the expectant father adjusts to the reality of pregnancy.

**Focusing phase** The *third* developmental task experienced by expectant fathers. This phase is characterized by the father's active involvement in both the pregnancy and his relationship with his child.

**Father—expectant, styles of involvement**

**Expressive style** Expectant father's strong *emotional* response to partner's pregnancy.

**Instrumental style** Characteristic style displayed by expectant fathers that emphasizes *tasks* to be accomplished.

**Observer style** Characteristic style displayed by expectant fathers who show a *detached* approach to involvement in their partner's pregnancy.

**Ferguson's reflex** Reflex contractions of the uterus after stimulation of the cervix, e.g., during sexual intercourse or vaginal examination.

**Ferning (arborization) test** The appearance of a fernlike pattern in dried smears of uterine cervical mucus, indicating the presence of estrogen.

**Ovulation f. t.** Test in which cervical mucus, placed on a slide, *dries* in a branching pattern in the presence of high estrogen levels at the time of ovulation.

**Pregnancy f. t.** Test in which cervical mucus, placed on a slide, does *not* dry in a branching pattern because of high levels of progesterone along with estrogen.

**Fertile period** The period before and after ovulation during which the human ovum can be fertilized; usually 3 days before ovulation (life span of sperm in woman's reproductive tract) and 24 hr after ovulation (life span of ovum). Since exact moment of ovulation is unknown, fertile period may extend from before to several days after expected ovulation (see *Calendar method*).

**Fertility** Quality of being able to reproduce.

**Fertility rate** Number of births per 1000 women aged 15 through 44 yr.

**Fertilization** Union of an ovum and a sperm.

**Fetal** Pertaining or relating to the fetus.

**F. asphyxia** See *asphyxia, fetal*.

**F. biophysical profile** Noninvasive dynamic assessment, employing ultrasound and external fetal monitoring, of several parameters: breathing movements, movements, tone, amniotic fluid volume, nonstress test, and often placental grading.

**F. death** See *death, fetal*.

**F. distress** Evidence such as a change in the fetal heartbeat pattern or activity indicating that the fetus is in jeopardy.

**Fetal fibronectin:** A protein produced during pregnancy is the foundation of a screening test for preterm delivery. Fetal fibronectin (fFN) functions as a type of adhesive attaching the fetal amniotic sac to the uterine lining. The presence of fFN during 22–34 weeks of a high-risk pregnancy, along with symptoms of labor, implies that the adhesive is decomposing ahead of schedule and raises the likelihood of a *preterm delivery*. To test fFN, a special cotton swab is used to collect samples of cervico-vaginal secretions using a sterile speculum. A *negative* fFN test result is a highly reliable predictor that delivery will *not occur within the next 2 weeks*. A *positive* fFN test does not guarantee delivery within two weeks, but rather indicates the need for increased surveillance of the *high-risk* pregnancy. *Not* suggested as a *routine* screening tool for all pregnancies.

**Fetal heart rate (FHR)** Beats per minute of the fetal heart. Normal range is 110-160 beats/min.

**Acceleration** Increase in fetal heart rate, usually seen as a reassuring sign; must be a minimum of 15 BPM over the baseline heart rate for 15 seconds.

**Baseline** The average fetal heart rate between uterine contractions.

**Bradycardia** Baseline fetal heart rate below 110 beats/min.

**Prolonged deceleration** Slowing of fetal heart rate lasting longer than 2 min.

**Fetal heart rate deceleration** Slowing of fetal heart rate attributed to a parasympathetic response and described in relation to uterine contractions.

**Early** Onset corresponding to onset of uterine contraction, related to *fetal head compression*.

**Late** Onset after peak of contraction, continuing into interval after contraction; caused by *uteroplacental insufficiency*.

**Variable** Onset anytime unrelated to contraction; caused by *cord compression*.

**Fetal hemoglobin**  Hemoglobin of fetal red blood cells has greater affinity for oxygen than adult hemoglobin A; helps to ensure adequate fetal tissue oxygenation.

**Fetal membranes**
>  **Amnion**  See *amnion*.
>  **Chorion**  See *chorion*.

**Fetal postures**
>  **Attitude**  Relation of fetal parts to each other in the uterus (all parts flexed, except neck is extended, etc.).
>  **Lie**
>  Relation of the fetal spine to the maternal spine; i.e., in *vertical* lie, maternal and fetal spines are parallel and the fetal head or breech presents; in *transverse* lie, fetal spine is perpendicular to the maternal spine and the fetal shoulder presents.
>  **Position**  Relation of an arbitrarily chosen fetal reference point, such as the occiput, sacrum, chin (mentum), or scapula on the presenting part of the fetus to its location in the front, back, or sides of the maternal pelvis.
>  **Presentation**  That part of the fetus that first enters the pelvis and lies over the inlet: may be *cephalic* (also called vertex or head); face, brow; *breech* (sacrum): complete, frank, or footling; and *shoulder* (scapula).

**Fetal syndromes**
>  **Fetal alcohol effects (FAE)**  Set of symptoms that includes prenatal and postnatal growth retardation and CNS malfunctions, including mental retardation; effects may not be evident for several years.
>  **Fetal alcohol syndrome**  Congenital abnormality or anomaly resulting from excessive maternal alcohol intake. It is characterized by: typical craniofacial and limb defects, cardiovascular defects, intrauterine growth retardation, and developmental delay.
>  **Fetal hydantoin syndrome**  Abnormalities such as: microcephaly, mental retardation, developmental delay, intrauterine growth retardation, facial clefts, and nail hypoplasia.

**Fetofetal transfusion**  See *parabiotic syndrome*.

**α-Fetoprotein (AFP)**  Fetal antigen; elevated levels in amniotic fluid associated with neural tube defects.

**Fetotoxic**  Poisonous or destructive to the fetus.

**Fetus**  Child in utero from about the eighth week after conception, until birth.

**Fibroid**  Fibrous benign encapsulated connective tissue tumor, especially of the uterus.

**Fimbria**  Structure resembling a fringe, particularly the fringelike end of the fallopian tube.

**Fissure**  Groove or open crack in tissue.

**Fistula**  Abnormal tubelike passage that forms between two normal cavities, possibly congenital or caused by trauma, abscesses, or inflammatory processes.

**Flaccid**  Having relaxed, flabby, or absent muscle tone.

**Flaring of nostrils**  Widening of nostrils (alae nasi) during inspiration in the presence of air hunger; sign of respiratory distress.

**Flexion**  In obstetrics, resistance to the descent of the baby down the birth canal causes the head to flex, or bend, so that the chin approaches the chest. Thus the smallest diameter (suboccipitobregmatic) of the vertex presents.

**Follicle**  Small secretory cavity or sac.
>  **Graafian f.**  Mature, fully developed ovarian cyst containing the ripe ovum and the epithelial cells that surround it. The follicle secretes estrogens, and after ovulation, the corpus luteum develops within the ruptured graafian follicle and secretes estrogen and progesterone.

**Follicle stimulating hormone (FSH)**  Hormone produced by the anterior pituitary during the first half of the menstrual cycle. Stimulates development of the graafian follicle.

**Fomites**  Nonliving material on which disease-producing organisms may be conveyed (e.g., bed linen).

**Fontanel**  Broad area, or soft spot, consisting of a strong band of connective tissue contiguous with cranial bones and located at the junctions of the bones.
>  **Anterior f.**  Diamond-shaped area between the frontal and two parietal bones just above the baby's forehead at the junction of the coronal and sagittal sutures.
>  **Mastoid f.**  Posterolateral fontanel usually not palpable.
>  **Posterior f.**  Small, triangular area between the occipital and parietal bones at the junction of the lambdoidal and sagittal sutures.
>  **Sagittal f.**  Soft area located in the sagittal suture, halfway between the anterior and posterior fontanels; may be found in normal newborns and in some neonates with Down syndrome.
>  **Sphenoid f.**  Anterolateral fontanel usually not palpable.

**Foramen ovale**  Septal opening between the atria of the fetal heart. The opening normally closes shortly after birth, but if it remains patent, surgical repair usually is necessary.

**Forceps-assisted birth**  Birth in which two curved-bladed instruments are used to assist in birth of the fetal head.

**Foreskin**  Prepuce, or loose fold of skin covering the glans penis.

**Fornix**  Any structure with an arched or vaultlike shape.
>  **F. of the vagina**  Anterior and posterior spaces, formed by the protrusion of the cervix into the vagina, into which the upper vagina is divided.

**Fourth stage of labor**  The initial period of recovery from childbirth. It is usually considered to last for the first 1-2 hr after the expulsion of the placenta.

**Fourth trimester of pregnancy**  Another term for the *puerperium*, the 6-wk interval between the birth of the newborn and the return of the reproductive organs to their nonpregnant state.

**Fowler's position**  Posture assumed by client when head of bed is raised 18 or 20 in. and individual's knees are elevated.

**Freestanding birth center**  A center that provides prenatal care, labor and birth, and postbirth care outside of a hospital setting.

**Frenulum**  Thin ridge of tissue in midline of undersurface of tongue extending from its base to varying distances from the tip of the tongue.

**Friable**  Easily broken. May refer to a fragile condition of the cervix especially during pregnancy that causes the cervix to bleed easily when touched.

**Friedman's curve**  Labor curve; pattern of descent of presenting part and of dilatation of cervix; partogram.

**FSH**  See *follicle stimulating hormone*.

**Fulguration**  Destruction of tissue by means of electricity.

**Fundus**  Dome-shaped upper portion of the uterus between the points of insertion of the fallopian tubes.

**Funic souffle**  See *souffle, funic*.

**Funis**  Cordlike structure, especially the umbilical cord.

**Galacto-, galact-**  Combining form denoting milk.

**Galactorrhea**  Excessive flow or secretion of milk.

**Galactosemia**  Inherited, autosomal recessive disorder of galactose metabolism, characterized by a deficiency of the enzyme galactose-1-phosphate uridyl transferase.

**Gamete**  Mature male or female germ cell; the mature sperm or ovum.

**Gametogenesis**  Development of gametes; ova or sperm.

**Gastroschisis**  Abdominal wall defect at base of umbilical stalk.

**Gastrostomy**  Surgical creation of an artificial opening into the stomach through the abdominal wall, performed to feed a person when oral feeding is not possible.

**Gate control theory**  Proposed in 1965 by Melzack and Wall, this theory explains the neurophysical mechanism underlying the perception of pain.

**Gavage**  Feeding by means of a tube passed to the stomach.

**Gender identity**  The sense or awareness of knowing to which sex one belongs. The process begins in infancy, continues throughout childhood, and is reinforced during adolescence.

**Gene**  Factor on a chromosome responsible for hereditary characteristics of offspring.

**Genetic**  Dependent on the genes. A genetic disorder may or may not be apparent at birth.

**Genetic counseling**  Process of determining the occurrence or risk of occurrence of a genetic disorder within a family and of providing appropriate information and advice about the courses of action that are available, whether care of a child already affected, prenatal diagnosis, termination of a pregnancy, sterilization, or artificial insemination is involved.

**Genitalia**  Organs of reproduction.

**Genotype**  Hereditary combinations in an individual determining physical and chemical characteristics. Some genotypes are not expressed until later in life (e.g., *Huntington's chorea*); some hide recessive genes, which can be expressed in offspring; and others are expressed only under the proper environmental conditions (e.g., diabetes mellitus appearing under the stress of obesity or pregnancy).

**Gestation**  Period of intrauterine fetal development from conception through birth; the period of pregnancy.

**Gestational age**  In fetal development, the number of completed weeks counting from the first day of the last normal menstrual cycle.

**Gestational diabetes**  A carbohydrate intolerance of variable severity that starts or is first recognized during pregnancy.

**GIFT**  Gamete intrafallopian transfer of ova and washed sperm into fallopian tubes.

**Gingivitis**  Inflammation of the gums characterized by redness, swelling, and tendency to bleed.

**Glabella**  Bony prominence above the nose and between the eyebrows.

**Glans penis**  Smooth, round head of the penis, analogous to the female glans clitoris.

**Glucose tolerance test**  A test of the body's ability to utilize carbohydrates; used as a screening measure for gestational diabetes.

**Glycosuria**  Presence of glucose (a sugar) in the urine.

**Glycosylated hemoglobin**  A measurement of glycemic control over time (usually 4-6 wk).

**Gonad**  Gamete-producing, or sex, gland; the ovary or testis.

**Gonadotropic hormone**  Hormone that stimulates the gonads.

**Goodell's sign**  Softening of the cervix, a *probable* sign of pregnancy, occurring during the *second* month.

**Graafian follicle (vesicle)**  See *follicle, graafian*.

**Gravid**  Pregnant.

**Gravidity**  The number of times a woman has been pregnant, regardless of the outcome of the pregnancies.

**Grieving process** A complex of somatic and psychological symptoms associated with some extreme sorrow or loss, specifically the death of a loved one.

**!** **Grunt, expiratory** Sign of respiratory distress (*hyaline membrane disease* [*respiratory distress syndrome* or RDS] or advanced pneumonia) indicative of the body's attempt to hold air in the alveoli for better gaseous exchange.

**Gynecoid pelvis** Pelvis in which the inlet is round instead of oval or blunt. Typical female pelvis.

**Gynecology** Study of the diseases of the female, especially of the genital, urinary, and rectal organs.

**Habitual (recurrent) abortion** See *abortion, habitual.*

**Habituation** An acquired tolerance from repeated exposure to a particular stimulus. Also called negative adaptation; a decline and eventual elimination of a conditioned response by repetition of the conditioned stimulus.

**Habitus** Indications in appearance of tendency or disposition to disease or abnormal conditions.

**!** **Haploid number** Having half the normal number of chromosomes found in somatic (body) cells; 23 chromosomes.

**Harlequin sign** Rare color change of *no* pathologic significance occurring between the longitudinal halves of the neonate's body. When infant is placed on one side, the dependent half is noticeably pinker than the superior half.

**hCG** See *human chorionic gonadotropin.*

**Heat loss, types** See also *cold stress.*
 **Conduction** Heat loss to a cooler surface by direct skin contact.
 **Convection** Heat loss from the warm body surface to cooler air currents.
 **Evaporation** Heat loss incurred when water on the skin surface is converted to a vapor.
 **Radiation** Heat loss incurred when heat transfers to cooler surfaces and objects not in direct contact with the body.

**Hegar's sign** Softening of the lower uterine segment that is classified as a *probable* sign of pregnancy and that may be present during the *second* and *third months* of pregnancy and is palpated during bimanual examination.

**HELLP syndrome** Condition characterized by hemolysis, elevated liver enzymes, and low platelet count (it is *not* disseminated intravascular coagulation); it is a form of severe pre-eclampsia.

**Hematocrit** Volume of red blood cells per deciliter (dL) of circulating blood; packed cell volume (PCV).

**Hematoma** Collection of blood in a tissue; a bruise or blood tumor.

**Hemizygous** Having *only one* of a gene pair that determines a particular genetic trait.

**!** **Hemoconcentration** Increase in the number of red blood cells resulting from either a decrease in plasma volume (as seen in pre-eclampsia/eclampsia) or increased erythropoiesis.

**Hemodilution** An increase in fluid content of blood, resulting in diminution of the proportion of formed elements.

**Hemoglobin** Component of red blood cells consisting of globin, a protein, and hematin, an organic iron compound.

**H. electrophoresis** Test to diagnose sickle cell disease. In newborns, cord blood is used.

**Hemolytic disease of the newborn** Breakdown of fetal red blood cells by maternal antibodies, usually from a mother who is Rh-negative.

**Hemoperitoneum** Blood in the peritoneal cavity.

**Hemorrhagic disease of newborn** Bleeding disorder during first few days of life based on a deficiency of vitamin K (intestinal tract needs bacteria to produce vitamin K).

**Hemorrhagic shock** A clinical condition in which the peripheral blood flow is inadequate to return sufficient blood to the heart for normal function, particularly oxygen transport to the organs/tissue.

**Hereditary** Pertaining to a trait or characteristic transmitted from parent to offspring by way of the genes; used synonymously with *genetic.*

**Hermaphrodite** Person having genital and sexual characteristics of both sexes.

**Heterozygous** Having two dissimilar genes at the same site, or locus, on paired chromosomes (e.g., at the sites for eye color, one chromosome carrying the gene for brown, the other for blue).

**High risk** An increased possibility of suffering harm, damage, loss, or death. See also *risk factors.*

**Hirsutism** Condition characterized by the excessive growth of hair or the growth of hair in unusual places.

**Homan's sign** *Early* sign of phlebothrombosis of the deep veins of the calf in which there are complaints of pain when the leg is in extension and the foot is dorsiflexed. This test has fallen into disfavor because of *risk of precipitating* a pulmonary embolism.

**Home birth** Planned birth of the child at home. Usually under the supervision of a midwife.

**Homoiothermic** Referring to the ability of warm-blooded animals to maintain internal temperature at a specified level regardless of the environmental temperature. This ability is not fully developed in the human neonate.

**Homologous** Similar in structure or origin but not necessarily in function.

**Homologous insemination** Procedure in which a fine catheter is inserted through the cervix and into the uterus to deposit a sperm sample from the woman's mate directly into the uterus. Used in cases of low sperm count or hostile cervical mucus.

**Homozygous**  Having two similar genes at the same locus, or site, on paired chromosomes.

**Hormone**  Chemical substance produced in an organ or gland that is conveyed through the blood to another organ or part of the body, stimulating it to increased functional activity or secretion. See specific hormones.

**Hormone replacement therapy (HRT)**  Controversial therapy in which progestin is added to estrogen replacement therapy to prevent endometrial cancer. See *estrogen replacement therapy (ERT)*.

**Hot flash (flush)**  Transient sensation of warmth experienced by some women during or after menopause, resulting from autonomic vasomotor disturbances that accompany changes in the neurohormonal activity of the ovaries, hypothalamus, and pituitary gland.

**Hourglass uterus**  Uterus in which a segment of circular muscle fibers contracts during labor. The resultant "constriction ring" *dystocia* is characterized by lack of progress in spite of adequate contractions; by pain experienced before palpation of a uterine contraction and persisting after the observer feels the contraction end; and by recession of the presenting part during a contraction, instead of descent of the presenting part.

**Human chorionic gonadotropin (hCG)**  Hormone that is produced by chorionic villi; the biologic marker in pregnancy tests. Two main functions are: prevention of corpus luteum regression and promotion of testosterone production by the fetal testes.

**Hyaline membrane disease (HMD)**  Disease characterized by interference with ventilation at the alveolar level, theoretically caused by the presence of fibrinoid deposits lining alveolar ducts. Membrane formation is related to prematurity (especially with *fetal asphyxia*) and insufficient surfactant production (lecithin-sphingomyelin ratio ≤ 2:1). *Now* known as *respiratory distress syndrome* (RDS).

**Hydatidiform mole**  A mass of abnormal cell growth inside the uterus that produces high levels of human chorionic gonadotropin (hCG), and rapid growth of the uterus with hemorrhage. Signs and symptoms include vaginal bleeding, the discharge containing grapelike vesicles. About 15-20% of molar pregnancies lead to gestational trophoblastic cancer, a highly curable cancer.

**Hydramnios (polyhydramnios)**  Amniotic fluid in excess of 1.5 liters; often indicative of fetal anomaly and frequently seen in pregnant women who have poorly controlled, insulin-dependent diabetes, even if no coexisting fetal anomaly is present.

**Hydrocele**  Collection of fluid in a saclike cavity, especially in the sac that surrounds the testis, causing the scrotum to swell.

**Hydrocephalus**  Accumulation of fluid in the subdural or subarachnoid spaces.

**Hydrops fetalis**  Most severe expression of fetal hemolytic disorder, a possible sequela to maternal Rh isoimmunization; infants exhibit: gross edema (*anasarca*), cardiac decompensation, and profound pallor from anemia, and seldom survive.

**Hymen**  Membranous fold that normally partially covers the entrance to the vagina in the virgin.

**Hymenal caruncles**  Small, irregular bits of tissue that are remnants of the hymen.

**Hymenal tag**  Normally occurring redundant hymenal tissue protruding from the floor of the vagina that disappears spontaneously in a few weeks after birth.

**Hyperbilirubinemia**  Elevation of unconjugated serum bilirubin concentrations.

**Hyperemesis gravidarum**  Abnormal condition of pregnancy characterized by protracted vomiting, weight loss, and fluid and electrolyte imbalance.

**Hyperglycemia**  Excess glucose in the blood.

**Hyperplasia**  Increase in number of cells; formation of new tissue.

**Hyperreflexia**  Overactive or overresponsive reflexes.

**Hyperthyroidism**  Excessive functional activity of the thyroid gland.

**Hypertonic uterine dysfunction**  Uncoordinated, painful, frequent uterine contractions that do not cause dilatation and effacement; primary dysfunctional labor.

**Hypertrophic cardiomyopathy (HCM)**  Enlargement of heart walls and septum impacting on the size of the heart chambers.

**Hypertrophy**  Enlargement, or increase in size, of existing cells.

**Hyperventilation**  Rapid, shallow (or prolonged, deep) respirations resulting in *respiratory alkalosis*: a decrease in H+ concentration and $PCO_2$ and an increase in the blood pH and the ratio of $NaHCO_3$ to $H_2CO_3$. Symptoms may include: faintness, palpitations, and carpopedal (hands and feet) muscular spasms. Relief may result from rebreathing in a paper bag or into one's cupped hands to replace the carbon dioxide "blown off" during hyperventilation.

**Hypofibrinogenemia**  Deficient level of a blood-clotting factor, fibrinogen, in the blood; in obstetrics, it occurs following complications of *abruptio placentae* or retention of a dead fetus. See *disseminated intravascular coagulation (DIC)*.

**Hypogastric arteries**  Branches of the right and left iliac arteries carrying deoxygenated blood from the fetus through the umbilical cord, where they are known as umbilical arteries, to the placenta.

**Hypoglycemia**  Less-than-normal amount of glucose in the blood, usually caused by administration of too much insulin, excessive secretion of insulin by the islet cells of the pancreas, or by dietary deficiency.

**Hypospadias** Anomalous positioning of urinary meatus on undersurface of penis or close to or just inside the vagina.

**Hypothalamus** Portion of the diencephalon of the brain forming the floor and part of the lateral wall of the third ventricle. It activates, controls, and integrates the peripheral autonomic nervous system, endocrine processes, and many somatic functions (e.g. body temperature, sleep, and appetite).

**!** **Hypothyroidism** Deficiency of thyroid gland activity with underproduction of thyroxine.

**!** **Hypotonic uterine dysfunction** Weak, ineffective uterine contractions usually occurring in the active phase of labor; may be related to *cephalopelvic disproportion* (CPD) or malposition of the fetus.

**!** **Hypoxemia** Reduction in arterial $PO_2$ resulting in metabolic acidosis by forcing anaerobic glycolysis, pulmonary vasoconstriction, and direct cellular damage.

**!** **Hypoxia** Insufficient availability of oxygen to meet the metabolic needs of body tissue.

**Hysterectomy** Surgical removal of the uterus.

    **Subtotal h.** Removal of fundus and body of the uterus, but the cervical stump remains.

    **TAH-BSO** Transabdominal hysterectomy and bilateral salpingo-oophorectomy. Removal of uterus, both tubes, and both ovaries.

    **Total h.** Removal of entire uterus, including the cervix, but the ovaries and tubes remain; also called *panhysterectomy.*

    **TVH** Transvaginal hysterectomy.

**Hysterosalpingography** X-ray of the uterus and uterine tubes after filling them with radiopaque material.

**Hysterotomy** Surgical incision into the uterus.

**Iatrogenic** Condition caused by a health care provider's words, actions, or treatment.

**Icterus neonatorum** Jaundice in the newborn.

**Idiopathic peripartum cardiomyopathy** A primary disease of the maternal heart muscle with no apparent cause, occurring during the peripartum period.

**Idiopathic respiratory distress syndrome (hyaline membrane disease)** Severe respiratory condition found almost exclusively in preterm infants and in some infants of mothers who are diabetic regardless of gestational age. See also *hyaline membrane disease (HMD).*

**IDM** Infant of a diabetic mother.

**IgA** Primary immunoglobulin in colostrum.

**IgG** Transplacentally acquired immunoglobulin that confers passive immunity against the infections to which the mother is immune.

**IgM** Immunoglobulin that neonate can manufacture soon after birth.

**Iliopectineal line** Bony ridge on the inner surface of the ilium and pubic bones that divides the true and false pelvis; the brim of the true pelvic cavity; the inlet.

**Immunity**

    **Acquired i.** Protection against microorganisms that develops in response to actual infection or transfer of antibody from an immune donor.

    **Active artificial i.** Immunity acquired by vaccination (e.g., rubella vaccination).

    **Active natural i.** Protection against specific microorganisms that develops in response to actual infection.

    **Natural i.** Nonspecific protection against microorganisms. Natural immunity is the first line of defense and includes skin and phagocytic cells.

    **Passive artificial i.** Immunity acquired by infusion of serum/plasma (e.g., Rh.IG).

    **Passive natural i.** Protection against specific microorganisms that develops in response to the transfer of antibody or lymphocytes from an immune donor (e.g., maternal antibodies in colostrum).

**Immunocompetent** The ability of the immune system to respond appropriately to foreign antigens and to develop antigen-specific antibodies.

**Immunology** The study of the components essential to the recognition and disposal of foreign (nonself or antigenic) material and maintenance of body defenses.

**Impaired fertility** Inability to conceive or carry to live birth at a time a couple chooses to do so.

**Imperforate** Without the normal opening.

**Implantation** Embedding of the fertilized ovum in the uterine mucosa; nidation.

**Impotence** Archaic term designating a man's inability, partial or complete, to perform sexual intercourse or to achieve orgasm; *current* term is *erectile dysfunction.*

**!** **Inborn error of metabolism** Hereditary deficiency of a specific enzyme needed for normal metabolism of specific chemicals (e.g., deficiency of phenylalanine hydroxylase results in *phenylketonuria* ; a deficiency of hexosaminidase results in *Tay-Sachs disease*).

**!** **Incompetent cervix** Cervix that is unable to remain closed until a pregnancy reaches term because of a mechanical defect in the cervix, resulting in painless dilatation and effacement usually during the second or early third trimester of pregnancy.

**Induction** Artificial stimulation or augmentation of labor.

**!** **Inertia** Sluggishness or inactivity; in obstetrics, refers to the absence or weakness of uterine contractions during labor.

**Infant** A child who is under 1 yr of age.

**Infective endocarditis**   Inflammation of the lining membrane of the heart due to invasion of microorganisms.

**Infertility**   Decreased capacity to conceive.

**Inlet**   Passage leading into a cavity.

   **Pelvic i.**   Upper brim of the pelvic cavity.

**Internal os**   Inside mouth or opening.

**Intertuberous diameter**   Distance between ischial tuberosities. Measured to determine dimension of pelvic outlet.

**Intervillous space**   Irregular space in the maternal portion of the placenta, filled with maternal blood and serving as the site of maternal-fetal gas, nutrient, and waste exchange.

**Intimate partner abuse**   Violence between intimate adults.

**Intrapartum**   During labor and birth.

**Intrathecal**   Within the subarachnoid space.

**IUCD**   Abbreviation for intrauterine contraceptive device.

**Intrauterine device (IUD)**   Small copper- or progesterone-containing form used for contraception.

**Intrauterine growth restriction (IUGR)**   The growth of the fetus is abnormally slow due to conditions, such as deficient nutrient supply or intrauterine infection, or associated with congenital malformation.

**Introitus**   Entrance into a canal or cavity such as the vagina.

**Intromission**   Insertion of one part or object into another (e.g., introduction of penis into vagina).

**Intussusception**   Prolapse of one segment of bowel into the lumen of the adjacent segment.

**In utero**   Within or inside the uterus.

**In vitro fertilization (IVF)**   Fertilization in a culture dish or test tube.

**In vitro fertilization with embryo transplant**   Fertilization in a culture dish or tube followed by transplant of embryo into uterus (womb).

**Inversion**   Turning end for end, upside down, or inside out.

   **I. of the uterus**   Condition in which the uterus is turned inside out so that the fundus intrudes into the cervix or vagina; may be caused by a too-vigorous removal of the placenta before it is detached by the natural process of labor.

**Involution**   Integrated processes (contractions and autolysis) by which uterus returns to nonpregnant size, shape, tone, and consistency.

**Isoimmune hemolytic disease**   Breakdown (hemolysis) of fetal/neonatal Rh-positive red blood cells (RBCs) because of Rh antibodies formed by a mother who is Rh-negative and who had been previously exposed to Rh-positive RBCs.

**Isoimmunization**   Development of antibodies in a species of animal with antigens from the same species (e.g., development of anti-Rh antibodies in a person who is Rh-negative).

**ITP**   Abbreviation for idiopathic thrombocytopenic purpura.

**Jaundice**   Yellow discoloration of the body tissues caused by the deposit of bile pigments (unconjugated bilirubin); icterus.

   **Breastfeeding j.**   Appearing about day three, this jaundice is related to the low amount of breast milk available before the mother's milk comes in. Due to relative state of dehydration, the feedings should be ≥ 8 every 24 hr.

   **Breast milk j.**   Yellowing of infant's skin from pregnanediol (in mother's milk) inhibition of enzyme (glucuronyl transferase) necessary for conjugation of bilirubin.

   **Pathologic j.**   Jaundice usually first noticeable within 24 hr after birth; caused by some abnormal condition such as an *Rh* or *ABO incompatibility* and requiring phototherapy treatment.

   **Physiologic j.**   Jaundice usually occurring 48 hr or later after birth, reaching a peak at 5-7 days, gradually disappearing by the seventh to tenth day, and caused by the normal reduction in the number of red blood cells. The infant is otherwise well.

**Jet hydrotherapy**   Use of warm water under pressure to relax muscles and promote comfort.

**Kangaroo care**   Parental skin-to-skin care. An alternative to technology and infant separation. Diaper-clad baby is placed under parent's bare chest.

**Karyotype**   Schematic arrangement of the chromosomes within a cell to demonstrate their numbers and morphology.

**Kegel's exercises**   Exercises to strengthen the pubococcygeal muscles.

**Kehr's sign**   "Referred pain" in the shoulder that indicates intraabdominal bleeding (or rupture of ovarian cyst).

**Kernicterus**   Bilirubin encephalopathy involving the deposit of unconjugated bilirubin in brain cells, resulting in death or impaired intellectual, perceptive, or motor function, and adaptive behavior.

**Kleihauer-Betke test**   Laboratory test that detects the presence of fetal blood cells in the maternal circulation. See *Apt test*.

**Klinefelter's syndrome**   Sex chromosome abnormality; most common deviation in males; trisomy XXY; poorly developed secondary sex characteristics and small testes; infertile; tall; effeminate. Usually, subnormal intelligence.

**!** **Klumpke's palsy** Lower brachial plexus injury, a result of traction on the arm during a difficult birth—results in clawed hand due to paralysis of hand muscles.

**Labia** Lips or liplike structures.

**L. majora** Two folds of skin containing fat and covered with hair that lie on either side of the vaginal opening and from each side of the vulva.

**L. minora** Two thin folds of delicate, hairless skin inside the labia majora.

**Labor** Series of processes by which the fetus is expelled from the uterus; parturition; childbirth.

**Labor-delivery-recovery room (LDR)** Room in which a woman labors, gives birth, and recovers during the fourth stage of labor.

**Labor-delivery-recovery-postpartum room (LDRP)** An LDR in which a woman continues to stay after recovery until discharge home; also called singleroom maternity care.

**Laceration** Irregular tear of wound tissue; in obstetrics, it usually refers to a tear in the perineum, vagina, cervix, or rectum caused by childbirth.

**Lactation** Function of secreting milk, or period during which milk is secreted.

**Lactation amenorrhea** Amenorrhea caused by the act of suckling and the high levels of prolactin, which has an antigonadotrophic effect.

**Lactation suppression** Stopping the production of breast milk through the use of medication and/or nonpharmacologic interventions.

**Lactogenic** Stimulating the production of milk.

**L. hormone** Gonadotropin produced by anterior pituitary and responsible for promoting growth of breast tissue and lactation; *prolactin*; luteotropin.

**Lactose intolerance** Inherited absence of the enzyme lactase.

**Lactosuria** Presence of lactose in the urine during late pregnancy and during lactation. Must be differentiated from glycosuria.

**Lamaze method** Method of psychoprophylaxis for childbirth developed in the 1950s by a French obstetrician, Fernand Lamaze. It requires classes, practice at home, and coaching during labor and birth.

**Lambdoid** Having the shape of the Greek letter lambda ($\lambda$).

**L. suture** Suture line extending across the posterior third of the skull, separating the occipital bone from the two parietal bones, and forming the base of the triangular posterior fontanel.

**Laminaria tent** Cone of dried seaweed or synthetic osmotic dilator that swells as it absorbs moisture. Used to dilate the cervix nontraumatically in preparation for an induced abortion or in preparation for induction of labor.

**Lanugo** Downy, fine hair characteristic of the fetus between 20 wk gestation and birth, that is most noticeable over the shoulder, forehead, and cheeks but is found on nearly all parts of the body except the palms of the hands, soles of the feet, and the scalp.

**Laparoscopy** Examination of the interior of the abdomen by inserting a small telescope through the anterior abdominal wall.

**Large for dates (large for gestational age [LGA])** Exhibiting excessive growth for gestational age > 90% percentile for gestational age.

**Last menstrual period (LMP)** The date of the first day of the last normal menstrual bleeding.

**Learned helplessness** Belief that one is powerless and unable to act independently; the result of socialization.

**Lecithin** A phospholipid that decreases surface tension; surfactant (i.e., surface-active agent).

**Lecithin-sphingomyelin ratio** Ratio of lecithin to sphingomyelin in the amniotic fluid. This is used to assess maturity of the fetal lung.

**Legal terms**

**Abandonment of care** Wrongful cessation of the provision of care to a patient, e.g., leaving a woman in active labor alone. Usually refers to a physician, but can also be the result of a nurse's lack of action.

**Breach** Failure to conform to the standard of care.

**Duty** The standard of care, or external code of behavior or expected performance, for a professional nurse. See *standards of care*.

**Informed consent** Refers to the right of persons to consent to all forms of touching; violation of that right is called **battery**. Includes: information about a procedure, its risks, its anticipated results, and any alternatives to it. The person performing the procedure is usually responsible for obtaining the consent.

**Malpractice** Professional negligence that is the proximate cause of injury or harm to a patient, resulting from a lack of professional knowledge, experience, or skill that can be expected in others in the profession or from a failure to exercise reasonable care or judgment in the application of professional knowledge, experience, or skill.

**Negligence** *Commission* of an act that a prudent person would not have done or the *omission* of a duty that a prudent person would have fulfilled, resulting in injury or harm to another person. In particular, in a malpractice suit a professional person is negligent if harm to a patient results from such an act or such a failure to act, but it must be proven that other prudent persons of the same profession would ordinarily have acted differently under the same circumstances.

**Reasonably prudent nurse**  Nurse who acts with the average degree of skill, care, and diligence as those with similar background, training, and experience. One who acts wisely and judiciously. See *Legal terms, negligence.*

**Reasonably prudent person**  Person who demonstrates the external code of behavior or expected performance (average degree of skill, care, and diligence) exercised by any other person with similar background, training, and experience.

**Tort**  A civil offense.

〰️ **Leopold's maneuver**  Four maneuvers for diagnosing the fetal position by external palpation of the mother's abdomen. See *text.*

**Let-down reflex**  Oxytocin-induced flow of milk from the alveoli of the breasts into the milk ducts.

🕷️ **Leukorrhea**  White or yellowish mucous discharge from the cervical canal or the vagina that may be normal physiologically or caused by pathologic states of the vagina and endocervix (e.g., *Trichomonas vaginalis infections*).

**LH**  See *luteinizing hormone (LH).*

**Libido**  Sexual drive.

**Ligation**  Act of suturing, sewing, or otherwise tying shut.

**Tubal l.**  Abdominal operation in which the fallopian tubes are tied off and a section is removed to interrupt tubal continuity and thus sterilize the woman.

**Lightening**  Sensation of decreased pressure on the diaphragm and stomach produced by fetal descent into the pelvic cavity. It usually occurs 2 wk before the onset of labor in nulliparas.

**Linea nigra**  Line of darker pigmentation seen in some women during the latter part of pregnancy that appears over the midline of the abdomen and extends from the symphysis pubis toward the umbilicus.

**Linea terminalis**  Line dividing the upper (false) pelvis from the lower (true) pelvis.

**Lithotomy position**  Position in which the woman lies on her back with her knees flexed and abducted thighs drawn up toward her chest.

**Live birth**  Birth in which the neonate, regardless of gestational age, manifests any heartbeat, breathes, or displays voluntary movement.

**Living ligature**  In the thick middle myometrial layer of the uterus, the interlaced muscle fibers form a figure-of-eight pattern encircling large blood vessels; contraction of these fibers produces a hemostatic action.

**Local infiltration anesthesia**  Process by which a substance such as a local anesthetic drug is deposited within the tissue to anesthetize a limited region.

**Lochia**  Vaginal discharge during the puerperium, consisting of blood, tissue, and mucus.

**L. rubra**  Red, distinctly blood-tinged vaginal flow that follows birth and lasts 2-4 days.

**L. serosa**  Serous, pinkish brown, watery vaginal discharge that follows lochia rubra until about the *tenth* postpartum day.

**L. alba**  Thin, yellowish to white, vaginal discharge that follows lochia serosa on about the tenth postpartum day and that may *last* from the end of the third *to the sixth* postpartum week.

**Low birth weight (LBW)**  Infant weighing 2500 g or less at birth.  **Extremely low birth weight** ≤ 1000gms at birth

〰️ **L/S ratio (lecithin-sphingomyelin ratio)**  Test for fetal lung maturity (2:1 is desirable).

**Lunar month**  Four wk (28 days).

**Lutein**  Yellow pigment derived from the corpus luteum, egg yolk, and fat cells.

**L. cells**  Ovarian cells involved in the formation of the corpus luteum and that contain a yellow pigment.

**Luteinizing hormone (LH)**  Hormone produced by the anterior pituitary that stimulates ovulation and the development of the corpus luteum.

**Lymphedema**  Collection of excessive fluid in tissue when lymph nodes or vessels have been removed.

**Lysis of adhesions**  Operation to free adhesions (bands of scar tissue) that have caused organs to be abnormally drawn or tied to each other. Intraabdominal adhesions, often sequelae to pelvic inflammatory disease, impair fertility.

**Lysozyme**  Enzyme with antiseptic qualities that destroys foreign organisms and that is found in blood cells of the granulocytic and monocytic series and is also normally present in saliva, sweat, tears, and breast milk.

**Maceration**  (1) Process of softening a solid by soaking it in a fluid. (2) Softening and breaking down of fetal skin from prolonged exposure to amniotic fluid as seen in a dead fetus.

**Macroglossia**  Hypertrophy of tongue or tongue large for oral cavity; seen in some preterm neonates and in neonates with Down syndrome.

**Macrosomia**  Large body size as seen in neonates of mothers who are diabetic or prediabetic; macrosomatia.

〰️ **Magnetic resonance imaging (MRI)**  Noninvasive nuclear procedure for imaging tissues with high fat and water content; use in pregnancy is *limited* because the long-term effects of MRI on fetal development are unknown.

**Mammary gland**  Compound gland of the female breast that is made up of lobes and lobules that secrete milk for nourishment of the young. Rudimentary mammary glands exist in the male.

**Mammography**   X-ray examination technique used to screen for and evaluate breast lesions.

**Manic-depressive psychosis**   Major affective disorder characterized by episodes of mania and depression. One or the other phase may be predominant at any given time; one phase may appear alternately with the other; or elements of both phases may be present simultaneously. Also called *bipolar disorder*.

**Mask of pregnancy**   See *chloasma*.

**Mastalgia**   Breast soreness or tenderness.

**Mastitis**   Inflammation of mammary tissue of the breasts.

**Maternal role-taking**   (Reva Rubin)

**Taking-in phase**   Period after birth characterized by the woman's dependency; *maternal* needs are dominant, talking about the birth is an important task.

**Taking-hold phase**   Period after birth characterized by the woman becoming more independent and more interested in learning *infant care* skills.

**Letting-go phase**   Interdependent phase after birth in which the mother and family move forward as a system with *interacting* members.

**Maturation**   (1) Process of attaining maximum development. (2) In biology, a process of cell division during which the number of chromosomes in the germ cells (sperm or ova) is reduced to one-half the number (haploid) characteristic of the species.

**McDonald's sign**   Easy flexion of the fundus on the cervix.

**Mean arterial pressure (MAP)**   Average of systolic and diastolic blood pressures. A MAP of 90 or more in the second trimester has been used as a predictor of pre-eclampsia in the third trimester. Example: blood pressure: 108/72; pulse pressure: (108 - 72 = 36), 36 ÷ 3 = 12; MAP (diastolic): 72 + 12 = 84.

**Meatus**   Opening from an internal structure to the outside (e.g., urethral meatus).

**Meconium**   First stools of infant: viscid, sticky; dark greenish brown, almost black; sterile; odorless.

**M. aspiration syndrome**   Function of fetal hypoxia: with hypoxia, the anal sphincter relaxes and meconium is released; reflex gasping movements draw meconium and other particulate matter in the amniotic fluid into the infant's bronchial tree, obstructing the air flow after birth.

**M. ileus**   Lower intestinal obstruction by thick, puttylike, inspissated meconium that may be the result of deficiency of trypsin production in the newborn with cystic fibrosis.

**M.-stained fluid**   In response to hypoxia, fetal intestinal activity increases and anal sphincter relaxes, resulting in the passage of meconium, which imparts a greenish coloration.

**Meiosis**   Process by which germ cells divide and decrease their chromosomal number by one-half.

**Melia**   Pertaining to a limb or part of a limb or extremity, as in amelia (absence of a limb) or phocomelia (absence of part of arms or legs).

**Menarche**   Onset, or beginning, of menstrual function.

**Meningomyelocele**   Saclike protrusion of the spinal cord through a congenital defect in the vertebral column.

**Menopause**   From the Greek words *men* (month) and *pausis* (to stop), the actual permanent cessation of menstrual cycles.

**Menorrhagia**   Abnormally profuse or excessive menstrual flow.

**Menses (menstruation)**   Periodic vaginal discharge of bloody fluid from the nonpregnant uterus that occurs from the age of puberty to menopause.

**Mentum**   Chin, a fetal reference point in designating position (e.g., "left mentum anterior" , meaning that the fetal chin is presenting in the left anterior quadrant of the maternal pelvis).

**Mesoderm**   Embryonic middle layer of germ cells giving rise to all types of muscles, connective tissue, bone marrow, blood, lymphoid tissue, and all epithelial tissue.

**Metritis**   Inflammation of the endometrium and myometrium.

**Metrorrhagia**   Abnormal bleeding from the uterus, particularly when it occurs at any time other than the menstrual period.

**Microcephaly**   Congenital anomaly characterized by abnormal smallness of the head in relation to the rest of the body and by underdevelopment of the brain, resulting in some degree of mental retardation.

**Micrognathia**   Abnormal smallness of mandible or chin.

**Midwife**   One who practices the art of helping and aiding a woman to give birth.

**Milia**   Unopened sebaceous glands appearing as tiny, white, pinpoint papules on forehead, nose, cheeks, and chin of a neonate that disappear spontaneously in a few days or weeks.

**Milk ejection**   Milk leaking from the breasts, often before a feeding.

**Milk leg**   See *phlegmasia alba dolens*.

**Miscarriage**   Spontaneous abortion; *lay term* usually referring specifically to the loss of the fetus between the fourth month and viability.

**Misogyny**   Hatred of women.

**Mitosis**   Process of somatic cell division in which a single cell divides, but both of the new cells have the same number of chromosomes as the first.

**Mitral valve prolapse (MVP)**   A disorder in which the cusp(s) of the mitral valve drop into the left atrium during systole characterized by midsystolic click and late systolic murmur.

! **Mitral valve stenosis** Narrowing of the opening of the mitral valve due to stiffening of valve leaflets obstructing free flow from atrium to ventricle.

**Mittelschmerz** Abdominal pain in the region of an ovary during ovulation, which usually occurs midway through the menstrual cycle. Present in many women, mittelschmerz is useful for identifying ovulation, thus pinpointing the fertile period of the cycle.

**Molding** Overlapping of cranial bones or shaping of the fetal head to accommodate and conform to the bony and soft parts of the mother's birth canal during labor.

**Mongolian spot** Bluish-gray or dark, nonelevated pigmented area usually found over the lower back and buttocks present at birth in some infants, primarily nonwhite. The spot usually fades by school age in African-American or Asian infants and within the first year or two of life in other infants.

**Mongolism** See *Down syndrome.*

**Moniliasis** Infection of the skin or mucous membrane by a yeastlike fungus, *Candida albicans; see thrush.*

**Monitrice** One trained in psychoprophylactic methods and in supporting women during labor; also Doula.

**Monosomy** Chromosomal aberration characterized by the absence of one chromosome from the normal diploid complement.

**Monozygotic** Originating or coming from a single fertilized ovum, such as identical twins.

**Mons veneris** Pad of fatty tissue and coarse skin that overlies the symphysis pubis in the woman and that, after puberty, is covered with short curly hair.

**Montgomery's glands, tubercles** Small, nodular prominences (sebaceous glands) on the areolas around the nipples of the breasts that enlarge during pregnancy and lactation.

**Mood disorders** Depression or depression with manic episodes (bipolar disorders).

**Morbidity** (1) Condition of being diseased. (2) Number of cases of disease or sick persons in relationship to a specific population; incidence.

**Morning sickness** Nausea and vomiting that affect some women during the first few months of their pregnancy; may occur at any time of day.

**Moro's reflex** Normal, generalized reflex in a young infant elicited by a sudden loud noise or by striking the table next to the child, resulting in flexion of the legs, an embracing posture of the arms, and usually a brief cry. Also called *startle reflex.*

**Mortality** (1) Quality or state of being subject to death. (2) Number of deaths in relation to a specific population; incidence.

    **Fetal m.** Number of fetal deaths per 1000 births (or per live births).

    **Infant m.** Number of deaths per 1000 children 1 yr of age or younger.

    **Intrauterine m.** Death of a fetus of 20 wk gestation or more.

    **Maternal m.** Number of maternal deaths per 100,000 births during the childbearing cycle.

    **Neonatal m.** Statistical rate of infant death during the first 28 days after live birth, expressed as the number of such deaths per 1000 live births in a specific geographic area or institution in a given period of time.

    **Perinatal m.** Combined fetal and neonatal mortality.

**Morula** Developmental stage of the fertilized ovum in which there is a solid mass of cells resembling a mulberry.

**Mosaicism** Condition in which some somatic cells are normal, whereas others show chromosomal aberrations.

**Mourning** Expressions and behaviors of grief.

**Multigravida** Woman who has been pregnant two or more times.

**Multifetal pregnancy** Pregnancy in which there is more than one fetus in the uterus at the same time; multiple pregnancy.

**Multipara** Woman who has carried two or more pregnancies > 20 weeks gestation, whether they ended in live infants or stillbirths and whether the pregnancy yielded one or more babies.

**Mutation** Change in a gene or chromosome in gametes that may be transmitted to offspring.

**Myoepithelial cells** Contractile cells that surround the mammary alveoli and contract in response to oxytocin, causing milk let-down.

**Naegele's rule** Method for calculating the estimated date of confinement (EDC), estimated date of birth (EDB), EDD (estimated date of delivery) or "due date."

**Narcotic antagonist** A compound such as naloxone (*Narcan*) that promptly reverses the effects of narcotics such as meperidine (*Demerol*).

**Natal** Relating or pertaining to birth.

**Navel** Depression in the center of the abdomen, where the umbilical cord was attached to the fetus; umbilicus.

**Necrotizing enterocolitis (NEC)** Acute inflammatory bowel disorder that occurs primarily in preterm, low-birth-weight, or cocaine-exposed neonates. It is characterized by ischemic necrosis (death) of the gastrointestinal mucosa that may lead to perforation and peritonitis.

! **Neonatal hypovolemic shock** Cardiovascular collapse resulting from a diminished volume of circulating fluid in the cardiovascular system.

**Neoplasia** Growth of new tissue; tumor that serves no physiologic function; may be benign or malignant.

**Neural tube** Tube formed from fusion of the neural folds from which develops the brain and spinal cord.

**N. t. defect** Incomplete development of tube resulting in malformation of brain and/or spinal cord; see (**α**) *fetoprotein* (AFP).

**Neutral temperature range** That grouping of environmental conditions in which the neonate's oxygen consumption is at a minimum and temperature is within normal limits.

**Nevus** Natural blemish or mark; a congenital circumscribed deposit of pigmentation in the skin; mole.

**N. flammeus** Port-wine stain; reddish, usually flat, discoloration of the face or neck.

**N. vasculosus (strawberry hemangioma)** Elevated lesion of immature capillaries and endothelial cells that regresses over a period of years.

**Nidation** Implantation of the fertilized ovum in the endometrium, or lining, of the uterus.

**Nondisjunction** Failure of homologous pairs of chromosomes to separate during the first meiotic division or of the two chromatids of a chromosome to split during anaphase of mitosis or the second meiotic division. The result is an abnormal number of chromosomes in the daughter cells.

**Nonreassuring fetal heart rate pattern** Fetal heart rate pattern that indicates the fetus is not well oxygenated and requires intervention.

**Nonshivering thermogenesis** Infant's method of producing heat by increasing metabolic rate.

**Nonstress test (NST)** Evaluation of fetal response (fetal heart rate) to fetal movement.

**Nosocomial** Pertaining to a hospital or clinic.

**Nuchal cord** Encircling of fetal neck by one or more loops of umbilical cord.

**Nulligravida** Woman who has never been pregnant.

**Nullipara** Woman who has not yet carried a pregnancy ≥ 20 weeks gestation.

**Nurse practitioner** Registered nurse who has additional education to practice nursing in an expanded role.

**Occipitobregmatic** Pertaining to the occiput (the back part of the skull) and the bregma (junction of the coronal and sagittal sutures) or anterior fontanel; the smallest diameter of the fetal head.

**Occiput** Back part of the head or skull.

**Oligohydramnios** Abnormally small amount or absence of amniotic fluid; often indicative of fetal urinary tract defect or maternal dehydration.

**Oliguria** Diminished secretion of urine by the kidneys.

**Omphalic** Concerning or pertaining to the umbilicus.

**Omphalitis** Inflammation of the umbilical stump characterized by redness, edema, and purulent exudate in severe infections.

**Omphalocele** Congenital defect resulting from failure of closure of the abdominal wall or muscles and leading to hernia of abdominal contents through the navel.

**Oogenesis** Formation and development of the ovum.

**Oophorectomy** Excision or removal of an ovary.

**Open glottis** Pushing.

**Operculum** Plug of mucus that fills the cervical canal during pregnancy.

**Ophthalmia neonatorum** Infection in the neonate's eyes, usually resulting from gonorrheal or other infection contracted when the fetus passes through the birth canal (vagina).

**Oral GTT** Test for blood sugar following oral ingestion of a concentrated sugar solution.

**Orchitis** Inflammation of one or both of the testes, characterized by swelling and pain, often caused by mumps, syphilis, or tuberculosis; may result in infertility in males.

**Organogenesis period** Period of embryonic development (between weeks 3-4 and 8) during which all major organ systems are formed. Period of extreme vulnerability to teratogens (e.g., environmental hazards and toxic substances).

**Orifice** Normal mouth, entrance, or opening, to any aperture.

**Os** Mouth, or opening.

**External o.** External opening of the cervical canal.

**Internal o.** Internal opening of the cervical canal.

**O. uteri** Mouth, or opening, of the uterus.

**Ossification** Mineralization of fetal bones.

**Osteoporosis** Deossification of bone tissue resulting in structural weakness.

**-Otomy** Combining form meaning cutting, incision, section.

**Outlet** Opening through which something can exit.

**pelvic o.** Inferior aperture, or opening, of the true pelvis.

**Ovary** One of two glands in the female situated on either side of the pelvic cavity that produce the female reproductive cell, the ovum, and two known hormones, estrogen and progesterone.

**Ovulation** Periodic ripening (maturation) and discharge of the unimpregnated ovum from the ovary, usually 14 days before the onset of menstrual flow.

**O. method** Evaluation of cervical mucus throughout the menstrual cycle; ovulation occurs just after the appearance of the peak mucus sign; Billings method.

**Ovum** Female germ, or reproductive cell, produced by the ovary; egg.

**Oxygen toxicity** Oxygen overdosage that results in pathologic tissue changes (e.g., *retinopathy* of *prematurity, bronchopulmonary dysplasia* in the neonate).

**Oxytocics** Drugs that stimulate uterine contractions, thus accelerating childbirth and preventing postbirth hemorrhage.

**Oxytocin** Hormone produced by the posterior pituitary gland that stimulates uterine contractions and the release of milk in the mammary gland (let-down reflex).

**O. challenge test (OCT)** Evaluation of fetal response (fetal heart rate) to contractile activity of the uterus stimulated by exogenous oxytocin (Pitocin).

**Palmar erythema** Redness on the surface of the palms sometimes seen in pregnancy, caused by estrogen.

**Palsy** Permanent or temporary loss of sensation or ability to move and control movement; paralysis.

**Bell's p.** Peripheral facial paralysis of the facial nerve (cranial nerve VII), causing the muscles of the unaffected side of the face to pull the face into a distorted position.

**Erb's p.** See *Erb-Duchenne paralysis.*

**Papanicolaou (Pap) test** Microscopic examination using scrapings from the cervix, endocervix, or other mucous membranes that will reveal, with a high degree of accuracy, the presence of premalignant or malignant cells.

**Para** Term used to refer to past pregnancies that reached ≥ 20 weeks gestation regardless of whether the infant(s) was dead or alive at birth.

**Parabiotic syndrome** Fetofetal blood transfer caused by placental vascular anastomoses occurring in a small plethoric twin (polycythemia) and one pale twin (anemia) twin-to-twin transfusion syndrome.

**Paracervical block** Type of regional anesthesia produced by injection of a local anesthetic into the lower uterine segment just beneath the mucosa adjacent to the outer rim of the cervix (9 and 3 o'clock positions) after the cervix is more than 5 cm dilated.

**Parity** Number of pregnancies that reached ≥ 20 weeks gestation.

**Parturient** Woman giving birth.

**Parturition** Process or act of giving birth.

**Patent** Open.

**Pathologic hyperbilirubinemia** High (toxic) levels of serum bilirubin resulting from a disease process causing hemolysis (e.g., *Rh incompatibility*); jaundice apparent within first 24 hr. See *jaundice, pathologic.*

**Patulous** Wide spreading or wide open.

**Peak mucus sign** Lubricative, cloudy-to-clear egg white cervical mucus occurring under high estrogen levels close to time of ovulation; ferns; good spinnbarkheit.

**Peau d'orange** "Orange-peel"-like skin seen over edematous breasts found in inflammatory breast cancer.

**Pelvic inflammatory disease (PID)** Infection of internal reproductive structures and adjacent tissues usually secondary to sexually transmitted disease infection.

**Pelvic relaxation** Refers to the lengthening and weakening of the fascial supports of pelvic structures.

**Pelvic tilt (rock)** An exercise used to help relieve low-back discomfort during pregnancy.

**Pelvis** Bony structure formed by the sacrum, coccyx, innominate bones, and symphysis pubis, and the ligaments that unite them. Types:

**Android** Male, heart-shaped.

**Anthropoid** Oval.

**False** Pelvis above the linea terminalis and symphysis pubis.

**Gynecoid** Female, round.

**Platypelloid** Flat.

**True** Pelvis below the linea terminalis.

**Penis** Male organ used for urination and copulation.

**Percutaneous umbilical blood sampling (PUBS)** Procedure during the second or third trimester in which the fetal umbilical vessel is accessed under ultrasound for 1-4 mL blood sampling or for transfusions of severely anemic fetuses. Indications: prenatal diagnosis of inherited organic disorders; fetal infection; fetal acid-base balance assessment and treatment of isoimmunization and thrombocytopenia in women.

**Peridural anesthesia** Injection of anesthetic outside the dura mater (anesthetic does not mix with spinal fluid); epidural anesthesia.

**Perinatal** Of or pertaining to the time and process of giving birth or being born.

**Perinatal period** Period extending from the twentieth week of gestation through the end of the twenty-eighth day after birth.

**Perinatologist** An obstetrician who has a subspecialty in the care of high-risk pregnant women and their fetuses.

**Perineum** Area between the vagina and rectum in the female and between the scrotum and rectum in the male.

**Periodic breathing** Sporadic episodes of cessation of respirations for periods of 10 sec or less not associated with cyanosis; commonly noted in preterm infants.

**Periods of reactivity (newborn infant)** *First period* (within 30 min after birth): brief cyanosis, flushing with crying; crackles (rales), nasal flaring, grunting, retractions; heart sounds loud, forceful, irregular; alert; mucus; no bowel sounds; followed by period of sleep. *Second period* (4-8 hr after birth): swift color changes; irregular respiratory and heart rates; mucus with gagging; meconium passage; and temperature stabilizing.

**Pessary**  Device placed inside the vagina to function as a supportive structure for the uterus or a contraceptive device.

**Petechiae**  Pinpoint hemorrhagic areas caused by numerous disease states involving infection and thrombocytopenia and occasionally found over the face and trunk of the newborn because of increased intravascular pressure in the capillaries during birth.

**pH**  Hydrogen ion concentration.

**Phenotype**  Expression of certain physical or chemical characteristics in an individual, resulting from interaction between genotype and environmental factors.

**Phenylketonuria (PKU)**  Recessive hereditary disease that results in a defect in the metabolism of the amino acid phenylalanine caused by the lack of an enzyme, phenylalanine hydroxylase, that is necessary for the conversion of the amino acid phenylalanine into tyrosine. If PKU is not treated, brain damage may occur, causing severe mental retardation.

**! Phimosis**  Tightness of the prepuce, or foreskin, of the penis.

**! Phlebitis**  Inflammation of a vein with symptoms of pain and tenderness along the course of the vein, inflammatory swelling and acute edema below the obstruction, and discoloration of the skin because of injury or bruise to the vein, possibly occurring in acute or chronic infections or after operations or childbirth.

**Phlebothrombosis**  Formation of a clot or thrombus in the vein; inflammation of the vein with secondary clotting.

**Phlegmasia alba dolens**  Phlebitis of the femoral vein with thrombosis leading to a venous obstruction, causing acute edema of the leg, and occurring occasionally after birth; also called *milk leg*.

**Phocomelia**  Developmental anomaly characterized by the absence of the upper portion of one or more limbs so that the feet or hands or both are attached to the trunk of the body by short, irregularly shaped stumps, resembling the fins of a seal.

**Phosphatidyl glycerol**  A phospholipid, a component of pulmonary surfactant; its presence in amniotic fluid is considered a sign of fetal lung maturity when the pregnancy is complicated by maternal diabetes.

**Phototherapy**  Utilization of specialized lights to reduce serum bilirubin levels by oxidation of bilirubin into water-soluble compounds that are then processed in the liver and excreted in bile and urine.

**Physiologic hyperbilirubinemia**  Hemolysis of excessive fetal red blood cells in the early neonatal period; jaundice not apparent during first 24 hr. Levels generally do not lead to kernicterus. See *jaundice, physiologic.*

**Pica**  Unusual (nonnutritive substance) craving during pregnancy (e.g., for laundry starch, dirt, or red clay).

**PID**  Abbreviation for pelvic inflammatory disease.

**Pinch test**  Determines if nipples are erectile or retractile.

**Pinna**  Ear cartilage.

**Placenta**  Latin, flat cake; afterbirth; specialized vascular disk-shaped organ that permits metabolic interchange between fetus and mother.

  **Abruptio p.**  See *abruptio placentae.*

  **Battledore p.**  Umbilical cord insertion into the margin of the placenta.

  **Circumvallate p.**  Placenta having a raised white ring at its edge.

  **P. accreta**  Invasion of the uterine muscle by the placenta, thus making separation from the muscle difficult if not impossible.

  **P. previa**  Placenta that is abnormally implanted in the thin, lower uterine segment and that is typed according to proximity to cervical os: *total*—completely occludes os; *partial*—does not occlude os completely; and *marginal*—placenta encroaches on margin of internal cervical os.

  **P. succenturiata**  Accessory placenta.

**Placental**  Pertaining or relating to the placenta.

  **P. dysfunction**  Failure of placenta to meet fetal needs and requirements; placental insufficiency.

  **P. dystocia**  See *dystocia, placental.*

  **P. infarct**  Localized, ischemic, hard area on the fetal or maternal side of the placenta.

  **P. souffle**  See *souffle, placental.*

**Platypelloid pelvis**  Broad pelvis with a shortened antero-posterior diameter and a flattened, oval, transverse shape.

**Plethora**  Deep beefy-red coloration ("boiled lobster" hue) of a newborn caused by an increased number of red blood cells (polycythemia) per volume of blood.

**Podalic**  Concerning or pertaining to the feet.

  **P. version**  Shifting of the position of the fetus so as to bring the feet to the outlet during delivery (*rarely performed*).

**! Polycythemia**  Increased number of erythrocytes per volume of blood, which may be caused by large placental transfusion, fetofetal transfusion (in twin pregnancy), or maternal-fetal transfusion, or it may be due to hypovolemia resulting from movement of fluid out of vascular into interstitial compartment.

**Polydactyly**  Excessive number of digits (fingers or toes).

**Polygenic**  Pertaining to the combined action of several different genes.

**Polyhydramnios**  See *hydramnios.*

**Polyuria**  Excessive secretion and discharge of urine by the kidneys.

**Position**  Relationship of an arbitrarily chosen fetal reference point, such as the occiput, sacrum, chin, or scapula, on the presenting part of the fetus to its location in the front, back, or sides of the maternal pelvis.

**Positive sign of pregnancy**  Definite indication of pregnancy (e.g., hearing the fetal heartbeat, visualization and palpation of fetal movement by the examiner, sonographic examination).

**Postmature infant**  Infant born at or after the beginning of week 43 of gestation or later and exhibiting signs of dysmaturity.

**Postnatal**  Happening or occurring after birth (newborn).

**Postpartum**  Happening or occurring after birth (mother).

**Postpartum blues**  A letdown feeling, accompanied by irritability and anxiety, which usually begins 2-3 days after giving birth and disappears within a week or two. Sometimes called the "baby blues."

**Postpartum depression**  Depression occurring within 6 mo of childbirth; lasts longer than postpartum blues and is characterized by a variety of symptoms.

**Postpartum psychosis**  Symptoms begin as postpartum blues or depression but are characterized by a break with reality. Delusions, hallucinations, confusion, delirium, and panic can occur.

**Postterm birth**  Birth of an infant after 42 wk gestation.

**Precipitous labor**  Rapid or sudden labor of less than 3 hr duration beginning from onset of cervical changes to completed birth of neonate.

**Preconception care**  Care designed for health maintenance before pregnancy.

**Pre-eclampsia**  Condition encountered after 20 wk gestation or early in the puerperium; a vasospastic disease process characterized by: increasing hypertension, proteinuria, and hemoconcentration with or without generalized edema; *formerly* called *toxemia, pregnancy-induced hypertention.*

**Pregnancy**  Period between conception through complete delivery of the products of conception. The usual duration of pregnancy in the human is 280 days, 9 calendar mo, or 10 lunar mo.

**Premature infant**  Infant born before completing week 37 of gestation, irrespective of birth weight; preterm infant.

**Premenstrual syndrome (PMS)**  Syndrome of: nervous tension, irritability, weight gain, edema, headache, mastalgia, dysphoria, and lack of coordination occurring during the last few days of the menstrual cycle preceding the onset of menstruation.

**Premonitory**  Serving as an early symptom or warning.

**Prenatal**  Occurring or happening before birth.

**Prepartum**  Before birth; before giving birth.

**Prepuce**  Fold of skin, or foreskin, covering the glans penis of the male.

**P. of the clitoris**  Fold of the labia minora that covers the aroused glans clitoris.

**Presenting part**  That part of the fetus that lies closest to the internal os of the cervix.

**Pressure edema**  Edema of the lower extremities caused by pressure of the heavy pregnant uterus against the large veins; edema of fetal scalp after cephalic presentation (*caput succedaneum*).

**Presumptive signs**  Manifestations that suggest pregnancy but that are not absolutely positive. These include: the cessation of menses, *Chadwick's sign,* morning sickness, and quickening.

**Preterm birth**  Birth occurring before completion of week 37 of gestation; premature birth.

**Preterm infant**  See *premature infant.*

**Primigravida**  Woman who is pregnant for the first time.

**Primipara**  Woman who has carried a pregnancy ≥ 20 weeks gestation without regard to the child's being dead or alive at the time of birth.

**Primordial**  Existing first or existing in the simplest or most primitive form.

**Probable signs**  Manifestations or evidence indicating that there is a definite likelihood of pregnancy. Among the probable signs are: enlargement of abdomen, *Goodell's* sign, *Hegar's* sign, *Braxton-Hicks* sign, and positive hormonal tests for pregnancy.

**Prodromal**  Serving as an early symptom or warning of the approach of a disease or condition (e.g., prodromal labor).

**Progesterone**  Hormone produced by the corpus luteum, adrenal cortex, and placenta whose function is to prepare the endometrium of the uterus for implantation of the fertilized ovum, develop the mammary glands, and maintain the pregnancy.

**Prolactin**  See *lactogenic hormone.*

**Prolapsed cord**  Protrusion of the umbilical cord in advance of the presenting part of the fetus.

**Proliferative phase of menstrual cycle**  Preovulatory, follicular, or estrogen phase of the menstrual cycle.

**PROM**  Rupture of membranes before the onset of labor.

**Preterm rupture of membranes**  Before 38 weeks gestation

**Prolonged rupture of membranes**—Rupture ≥ 24 hours before delivery

**Promontory of the sacrum**  Superior projecting portion of the sacrum at the junction of the sacrum and the L5 vertebra.

**Prophylactic**  Pertaining to prevention or warding off of disease or certain conditions; condom, or "rubber."

**Proscription**  Establish taboos. See *taboo.*

**Prostaglandin (PG)**  Substance present in many body tissues; has a role in many reproductive tract functions.

**Proteinuria**  Excretion of protein into urine.

**Pruritus**  Itching.

**Pruritus gravidarum**  Itching of the skin caused by pregnancy.

**Pseudocyesis (pseudopregnancy)** Condition in which the woman has all the usual signs of pregnancy, such as enlargement of the abdomen, cessation of menses, weight gain, and morning sickness, but is not pregnant; phantom or false pregnancy.

**Pseudomenstruation** Blood-tinged mucus from the vagina in the newborn female infant; caused by withdrawal of maternal hormones that were present during pregnancy.

**Psychoprophylaxis** Mental and physical education of the parents in preparation for childbirth, with the goal of minimizing the fear and perception of pain and promoting positive family relationships.

**Ptyalism** Excessive salivation.

**Puberty** Period in life in which the reproductive organs mature and one becomes functionally capable of reproduction.

**Pubic** Pertaining to the pubis.

**Pubis** Pubic bone forming the front of the pelvis.

**PUBS** See *percutaneous umbilical blood sampling*.

**Pudendal block** Injection of a local anesthetizing drug at the pudendal nerve root in order to produce numbness of the genital and perianal region.

**Pudendum** External genitalia of either sex; Latin, "that of which one should be ashamed."

**Puerperal sepsis** Infection of the pelvic organs during the postbirth period; "childbed fever."

**Puerperium** Time following the third stage of labor and lasting until involution of the uterus takes place, usually about 3-6 wk.

**Pulse oximetry** Noninvasive method of monitoring oxygen levels by detecting the amount of light absorbed by oxygen-carrying hemoglobin.

**Pyrosis** A burning sensation in the epigastric and sternal region from stomach acid; **heartburn**.

**Quickening** Maternal perception of fetal movement; usually occurs between weeks 16 and 20 of gestation.

**Radioimmunoassay** Pregnancy test that tests for the beta subunit of hCG using radioactive labeled markers.

**Rape** Sexual intercourse that is inflicted forcibly on another person, against that person's will; sexual assault.

**Rape trauma syndrome** Characteristic symptoms seen in victims of rape, consisting of several phases; similar to posttraumatic stress syndrome.

**RDS** See *respiratory distress syndrome*.

**Recessive trait** Genetically determined characteristic that is expressed only when present in the homozygotic state (e.g., blue eyes, blond hair).

**Rectocele** Herniation or protrusion of the rectum into the posterior vaginal wall.

**Referred pain** Discomfort originating in a local area such as cervix, vagina, or perineal tissues; the discomfort is felt in the back, flanks, or thighs.

**Reflex** Automatic response built into the nervous system that does not need the intervention of conscious thought (e.g., in the newborn, rooting, gagging, grasp).

**Regional block anesthesia** Anesthesia of an area of the body by injecting a local anesthetic to block a group of sensory nerve fibers.

**Regurgitation** Vomiting or spitting up of solids or fluids.

**Relaxin** Hormone secreted by the corpus luteum, placenta and the lining of the pregnant uterus that causes relaxation of the pelvic ligaments and prepares the uterus for labor.

**Respiratory distress syndrome (RDS)** Condition resulting from decreased pulmonary gas exchange, leading to retention of carbon dioxide (increase in arterial $PCO_2$). Most common neonatal causes are: prematurity, perinatal asphyxia, and maternal diabetes mellitus; hyaline membrane disease (HMD).

**Restitution** In obstetrics, the turning of the fetal head to the left or right after it has completely emerged from the introitus (vaginal opening) as it assumes a normal alignment with the infant's shoulders.

**Retained placenta** Retention of all or part of the placenta in the uterus after birth.

**Retinopathy of prematurity** Associated with hyperoxemia, resulting in eye injury and blindness.

**Retraction** (1) Drawing in or sucking in of soft tissues of chest, indicative of an obstruction at any level of the respiratory tract from the oropharynx to the alveoli. (2) Retraction of uterine muscle fiber. After contracting, the muscle fiber does not return to its original length but remains slightly shortened, a unique attribute of uterine muscle that aids in preventing postbirth hemorrhage and results in involution.

**Retroflexion** Bending backward.

> **R. of the uterus** Condition in which the body of the womb is bent backward at an angle with the cervix.

**Retrolental fibroplasia (RLF)** *Retinopathy of prematurity* associated with hyperoxemia, resulting in eye injury and blindness.

**Retroversion** Turning or a state of being turned back.

> **R. of the uterus** Displacement of the uterus; the body of the uterus is tipped backward with the cervix pointing forward toward the symphysis pubis.

**Retrovirus** A single piece of ribonucleic acid (RNA) surrounded by a protein coat, or envelope. A unique enzyme, reverse transcriptase, allows this RNA retrovirus to go backward, *against the "flow of life."* The RNA becomes a piece of deoxyribonucleic acid (DNA) which infects the cell's DNA nucleus and remains in the cell until its death (e.g., human immunodeficiency virus). (The normal flow of genetic information in life is from DNA to RNA to protein.)

**Rh factor** Inherited antigen present on erythrocytes. The individual with the factor is known as *positive* for the factor.

**Rh immune globulin** Solution of gamma globulin that contains Rh antibodies produced by another person; an example of passive artificial immunity giving a short-term immune response. Intramuscular (IM) administration of Rh immune globulin (trade name RhoGAM) prevents sensitization in Rh-negative women who have been exposed to Rh-positive red blood cells.

**! Rheumatic heart disease** Permanent damage of heart valves secondary to an autoimmune reaction in the heart tissue precipitated by rheumatic heart disease.

**Rhythm method** Contraceptive method in which a woman abstains from sexual intercourse during the ovulatory phase of her menstrual cycle and at least 3 days before and 1 day after the ovulation date.

**Ribonucleic acid (RNA)** Element responsible for transferring genetic information within a cell; a template, or pattern.

**Ring of fire** Burning sensation as vagina stretches and fetal head crowns.

**Risk factors** Factors that cause a person or a group of people to be particularly vulnerable to an unwanted, unpleasant, or unhealthful event.

**Risk management** Actions taken to eliminate or minimize either the chance of injury to a client or the harm that occurs. Requires nurse to be skilled in all steps of the nursing process.

**Risk-taking** Intentional behaviors with uncertain outcomes. Characteristic of adolescence.

**Rite of passage** Significant life event indicating movement from one maturational level to another.

**Ritgen maneuver** Procedure in which the perineum is supported by direct pressure over the coccygeal region.

**Role playing** Psychotherapeutic technique in which a person acts out a real or simulated situation as a means of understanding intrapsychic conflicts.

**Rooming-in unit** Maternity unit designed so that the newborn's crib is at the mother's bedside or in a nursery adjacent to the mother's room.

**Rooting reflex** Normal response in newborns when the cheek is touched or stroked along the side of the mouth to turn the head toward the stimulated side, to open the mouth, and to begin to suck. The reflex disappears by 3-4 mo of age but in some infants may persist until 12 mo.

**Rotation** In obstetrics, the turning of the fetal head as it follows the curves of the birth canal downward.

**Round ligaments** Ligaments that arise from the side of the uterus near the fallopian tube insertion to help the broad ligament keep the uterus in place.

**Rubella vaccine** Live attenuated rubella virus given to women who have not had rubella or who are serologically negative (i.e., titer < 1:3). Exposure to the rubella virus through vaccination causes the woman to form antibodies, producing active artificial immunity. (The person who contracts the infection will develop active *natural* immunity.) Notes:
1. Mothers who are lactating can receive the live attenuated virus.
2. A transient arthralgia or rash may develop, but is benign.
3. Women should not become pregnant for 2-3 mo after vaccination.
4. Women allergic to duck eggs may develop a hypersensitivity reaction.
5. If woman also receives RhoGAM at or around the time of rubella vaccination, the vaccination may not "take"; her titer needs to be retested 3 mo later.

**Rubin, Reva** See *maternal role-taking*.

**Rubin's test** Transuterine insufflation of the fallopian tubes with carbon dioxide to test their patency.

**Rugae** Folds of vaginal mucosa; creases in scrotum.

**Sacroiliac** Of or pertaining to the sacrum and ilium.

**Sacrum** Triangular bone composed of five united vertebrae and situated between L5 and the coccyx; forms the posterior boundary of the true pelvis.

**Saddle block anesthesia** Type of regional anesthesia produced by injection of a local anesthetic solution into the cerebrospinal fluid intrathecal (subarachnoid) space in the spinal canal; "low spinal" anesthesia.

**Safe passage** Normal, uneventful birth process for mother and child.

**Safe period** The days in the menstrual cycle that are not designated as fertile days, i.e., before and after ovulation.

**Sagittal suture** Band of connective tissue separating the parietal bones, extending from the anterior to the posterior fontanel.

**Salpingo-oophorectomy** Removal of a fallopian tube and an ovary.

**Scaphoid abdomen** Abdomen with a sunken interior wall. In newborn, usually indicates a diaphragmatic hernia that allowed abdominal contents to enter the chest cavity during fetal development, thereby compromising development of heart and lungs; a surgical emergency.

**Sclerema** Hardening of skin and subcutaneous tissue that develops in association with such life-threatening disorders as severe cold stress, septicemia, and shock.

**Scrotum** Pouch of skin containing the testes and parts of the spermatic cords.

**Sebaceous glands** Oil-secreting glands found in the skin.

**Secretory phase of menstrual cycle** Postovulatory, luteal, progestational, premenstrual phase of menstrual cycle; 14 days in length.

**Secundines** Fetal membranes and placenta expelled after childbirth; afterbirth.

**Self-care** Patient provides care for self as part of plan of care.

**Self-quieting activity** Infant's ability to use personal resources to quiet and console him or herself.

**Semen** Thick, white, viscid secretion discharged from the urethra of the male at orgasm; the transporting medium of the sperm.

**Semen analysis** Examination of semen specimen to determine: liquefaction, volume, pH, sperm density, and normal morphology.

**Sensitization** Development of antibodies to a specific antigen.

**Sensory behavior** Responses of the five senses; indicate a readiness for social interaction.

**Sepsis** Neonatal bacterial infections of the bloodstream in infants during the first 4 wk of life.

**Sex chromosome** Chromosome associated with determination of gender: the X (female) and Y (male) chromosomes. The normal female has two X chromosomes and the normal male has one X and one Y chromosome.

**Sexual assault** Penetration of any orifice by the penis or object without the victim's consent; achieved through use of actual or implied threats, force, intimidation, or deception.

**Sexual decision making** Selection of choices concerned with intimate and sexual behavior.

**Sexual history** Past and present health conditions, lifestyle behaviors, knowledge, and attitudes related to sex and sexuality.

**Sexual response cycle** The phases of physical changes that occur in response to sexual stimulation and sexual tension release.

**Sexuality** The part of life that has to do with being male or female.

**Sexually transmitted diseases (STDs)** Disease acquired as a result of sexual activity with an infected individual.

**Shake test** Foam stability test for lung maturity of fetus; more rapid than determination of lecithin-sphingomyelin ratio.

**Sibling rivalry** Competition that occurs between brothers and sisters.

**Sickle cell hemoglobinopathy** Abnormal crescent shape red blood corpuscles in the blood.

**Simian line** A single palmar crease frequently found in children with Down syndrome.

**Sims' position** Position in which the person lies on the left side with the right knee and thigh drawn upward toward the chest.

**Single-parent family** Family form characterized by one parent in the household. This may result from loss of spouse by death, divorce, separation, desertion, out-of-wedlock birth of a child, or adoption.

**Singleton** Pregnancy with a single fetus.

**Sitz bath** Application of moist heat to the perineum by sitting in a tub or basin filled with warm water.

**Sleep-wake cycles** Variations in states of newborn consciousness.

**Small for dates (small for gestational age [SGA])** Refers to inadequate growth for gestational age.

**Smegma** Whitish secretion around labia minora; also under the foreskin in uncircumcised penis.

**Somatic** Pertaining to the body, not reproductive, cells.

**Souffle** Soft, blowing sound or murmur heard by auscultation.

    **Funic s.** Soft, muffled, blowing sound produced by blood rushing through the umbilical vessels and synchronous with the fetal heart sounds.

    **Placental s.** Soft, blowing murmur caused by the blood current in the placenta and synchronous with the maternal pulse.

    **Uterine s.** Soft, blowing sound made by the blood in the arteries of the pregnant uterus and synchronous with the maternal pulse.

**Sperm** Male sex cell. Also called spermatozoon.

**Spermatogenesis** Process by which mature spermatozoa are formed, during which the diploid chromosome number (46) is reduced by half (haploid, 23).

**Spermicide** Chemical substance (usually nonoxynol-9) that kills sperm by reducing their surface tension, causing the cell wall to break down by a bactericidal effect or by creating a highly acidic environment.

**Spina bifida occulta** Congenital malformation of the spine in which the posterior portion of laminas of the vertebrae fails to close but there is no herniation or protrusion of the spinal cord or meninges through the defect. The newborn may have a dimple in the skin or growth of hair over the malformed vertebrae.

**Spinal block anesthesia** See *saddle block anesthesia*.

**Spinnbarkheit** Formation of a stretchable thread of cervical mucus under estrogen influence at time of ovulation.

**Splanchnic engorgement** Excessive filling or pooling of blood within the visceral vasculature that occurs following the removal of pressure from the abdomen, e.g., birth of a child, removal of an excess of urine from bladder (≥ 1000 mL), removal of large tumor.

**Square window** Angle of wrist between hypothenar prominence and forearm; one criterion for estimating gestational age of neonate.

**Standard body weight** An appropriate weight for height, a body mass index (BMI) within the normal range.

**Standards of care** Actions that a reasonably prudent person would have performed or omitted under specific conditions; conduct against which the defendant's actions are judged in a malpractice/ negligence case.

**State-related behavior** Behavioral responses dependent on current state of infant.

**Station** Relationship of the presenting fetal part to an imaginary line drawn between the ischial spines of the pelvis.

**Sterility** (1) State of being free from living microorganisms. (2) Complete inability to reproduce offspring.

**Sterilization** Process or act that renders a person unable to produce children, e.g., fallopian tube occlusion or ligation; vasectomy or occlusion of vas deferens.

**Stillbirth** The birth of a baby after 20 wk gestation who does not show any signs of life.

**Stork bites** See *telangiectatic nevi*.

**Striae gravidarum ("stretch marks")** Shining reddish lines caused by stretching of the skin, often found on the abdomen, thighs, and breasts during pregnancy. These streaks turn to a fine pinkish white or silver tone in time in fair-skinned women and brownish in darker-skinned women.

! **Subinvolution** Failure of a part (e.g., the uterus) to reduce to its nonpregnant size and condition after enlargement from functional activity (i.e., pregnancy).

**Suboccipitobregmatic diameter** Smallest diameter of the fetal head--follows a line drawn from the middle of the anterior fontanel to the under surface of the occipital bone.

**Succedaneum** See *caput succedaneum*.

**Supine hypotension** Fall in blood pressure caused by impaired venous return when gravid uterus presses on ascending vena cava, when woman is lying flat on her back; *vena caval syndrome*.

**Support systems** Network from which people receive help in times of crisis.

**Surfactant** Phosphoprotein necessary for normal respiratory function that prevents the alveolar collapse (*atelectasis*). See also *lecithin and lecithin-sphingomyelin ratio*.

**Suture** (1) Junction of the adjoining bones of the skull. (2) Operation uniting parts by sewing them together.

**Symphysis pubis** Fibrocartilaginous union of the bodies of the pubic bones in the midline.

**Syndactyly** Malformation of digits, commonly seen as a fusion of two or more fingers or toes to form one structure.

**Synostosis** Articulation by osseous tissue of adjacent bones; union of separate bones by osseous tissue.

**Systemic analgesia** Analgesics, either intramuscular (IM) or intravenous (IV), that cross the blood-brain barrier and provide central analgesic effects.

**Systemic lupus erythematosus** A chronic, autoimmune disorder that can affect any organ of the body. Characterized by periods of illness, flares and periods of wellness.

**Taboo** Proscribed (forbidden) by society as improper and unacceptable.

**Tachypnea** Excessively rapid respiratory rate (e.g., in neonates, respiratory rate of 60 breaths/min or more).

**Talipes equinovarus** Deformity in which the foot is extended and the person walks on the toes.

**Telangiectasia** Permanent dilatation of groups of superficial capillaries and venules.

**Telangiectatic nevi ("stork bites")** Clusters of small, red, localized areas of capillary dilatation commonly seen in neonates at the nape of the neck or lower occiput, upper eyelids, and nasal bridge that can be blanched with pressure of a finger.

**Teratogenic agent** Any drug, virus, or irradiation, the exposure to which can cause malformation of the fetus.

**Teratogens** Nongenetic factors that cause embryonic/ fetal malformations and disease syndromes in utero; examples: rubella, thalidomide, x-ray.

**Teratoma** Tumor composed of different kinds of tissue, none of which normally occur together or at the site of the tumor.

**Term infant** Infant born between weeks 38 and 42 of completed gestation.

**Testis** One of the two glands contained in the male scrotum that produce the male reproductive cell, or sperm, and the male hormone testosterone; testicle.

! **Tetany, uterine** Extremely prolonged uterine contractions.

! **Tetralogy of Fallot** Congenital cardiac malformation consisting of pulmonary stenosis, intraventricular septal defect, dextroposed aorta that receives blood from both ventricles, and hypertrophy of the right ventricle.

! **Thalassemia anemia** Affecting Mediterranean and Southeast Asian populations in which there is an insufficient amount of globin produced to fill the red blood cells.

**Therapeutic intrauterine insemination** See *artificial insemination*.

**Therapeutic rest** Administration of analgesics to decrease pain and induce rest for management of hypertonic uterine dysfunction.

**Thermoneutral environment** Environment that enables the neonate to maintain a body temperature of 36.5°C (97.7°F) with minimum use of oxygen and energy.

**!** **Thrombocytopenia** Abnormal hematologic condition in which the number of platelets is reduced, usually by destruction of erythroid tissue in bone marrow owing to certain neoplastic diseases or to an immune response to a drug.

**⚡** **Thrombocytopenic purpura** Hematologic disorder characterized by: prolonged bleeding time, decreased number of platelets, increased cell fragility, and purpura, which result in hemorrhages into the skin, mucous membranes, organs, and other tissue.

**⚡** **Thromboembolism** Obstruction of a blood vessel by a clot that has become detached from its site of formation.

**⚡** **Thrombophlebitis** Inflammation of a vein with secondary clot formation.

**⚡** **Thrombus** Blood clot obstructing a blood vessel that remains at the place it was formed.

**※** **Thrush** Fungal infection of the mouth or throat characterized by the formation of white patches on a red, moist, inflamed mucous membrane and caused by *Candida albicans*.

**Toco- (toko-)** Combining form that means childbirth or labor.

**▭** **Tocolytic drug** Drug used to suppress preterm labor, e.g., ritodrine (*Yutopar*), terbutaline (*Brethine*), magnesium sulfate.

**〰** **Tocotransducer** Electronic device for measuring uterine contractions.

**Tongue-tie** Congenital shortening of the frenulum, which, if severe, may interfere with sucking and articulation; a rare condition.

**※** **TORCH organisms** Organisms that damage the embryo or fetus; acronym for **t**oxoplasmosis, **o**ther (e.g., syphilis), **r**ubella, **c**ytomegalovirus, and **h**erpes simplex.

**!** **Torticollis** Congenital or acquired stiff neck caused by shortening or spasmodic contraction of the neck (sternocleidomastoid) muscles that draws the head to one side with the chin pointing in the other direction; wryneck.

**Toxemia** Term *previously* used for hypertensive states of pregnancy.

**⚡** **Tracheoesophageal fistula** Congenital malformation in which there is an abnormal tubelike passage between the trachea and esophagus.

**Trait** A distinguishing feature or characteristic.

**Transition—labor** Last phase of first stage of labor; 8-10 cm cervical dilatation.

**Transition period—newborn** Period from birth to 4-6 hr later; infant passes through period of reactivity, sleep, and second period of reactivity.

**Translocation** Condition in which a chromosome breaks and all or part of that chromosome is transferred to a different part of the same chromosome or to another chromosome.

**Trauma** Physical or psychic injury.

**Trial of labor (TOL)** Period of observation to determine if a laboring woman is likely to be successful in progressing to a vaginal birth.

**!** **Trichomonas vaginitis** Inflammation of the vagina caused by *Trichomonas vaginalis*, a parasitic protozoan and characterized by persistent burning and itching of the vulvar tissue and a profuse, frothy, white discharge.

**Trimester** Period of 3 mo.

**Trisomy** Condition in which any given chromosome exists in triplicate instead of the normal duplicate pattern.

**Trophoblast** Outer layer of cells of the developing blastodermic vesicle that develops the trophoderm or feeding layer which will establish the nutrient relationships with the uterine endometrium.

**!** **Trophoblastic disease, gestational (GTD)** A condition in which trophoblastic cells covering the chorionic villi proliferate and undergo cystic changes that may be malignant. See *hydatidiform mole*.

**⚡** **TSS** Toxic shock syndrome.

**Tubercles of Montgomery** Small papillae on surface of nipples and areolae that secrete a fatty substance that lubricates the nipples.

**Turner's syndrome** Most common sex chromosome abnormality; monosomy X; juvenile external genitalia with undeveloped ovaries; short stature; webbed neck.

**Twins** Two neonates from the same impregnation developed within the same uterus at the same time.

   **Conjoined t.** Twins who are physically united; Siamese twins.

   **Disparate t.** Twins who are different (e.g., in weight) and distinct from one another.

   **Dizygotic t.** Twins developed from two separate ova fertilized by two separate sperm at the same time; fraternal twins.

   **Fraternal twins** Nonidentical twins who come from two separate fertilized ova. Dizygotic.

   **Identical twins** Come from one fertilized ovum that then divides; same sex; same genotype. Monozygotic.

   **Monozygotic twins** Twins developed from a single fertilized ovum; identical twins.

**〰** **Ultrasonography** Using high-frequency sound waves to construct an image of a body organ or fetus.

**〰** **Ultrasound transducer** External signal source for monitoring fetal heart rate electronically.

**Umbilical cord (funis)** Structure connecting the placenta and fetus and containing two arteries and one vein encased in a tissue called *Wharton's jelly*. The cord is ligated at birth and severed; the stump falls off in 4-10 days.

**Umbilicus** Navel, or depressed point in the middle of the abdomen that marks the attachment of the umbilical cord during fetal life.

☞ **Universal precautions**  Universal blood and body-fluid precautions, recommended by the Centers for Disease Control (CDC); infection control measures to protect care providers and to prevent nosocomial infection of clients.

**Urachus**  Epithelial tube connecting the apex of the urinary bladder with the allantois. Its connective tissue forms the median umbilical ligament.

! **U. persistent**  Urachus does not close; urine can be seen oozing from the umbilical cord.

**Urethra**  Small tubular structure that drains urine from the bladder.

**Urinary frequency**  Need to void often or at close intervals.

**Urinary meatus**  Opening, or mouth, of the urethra.

**Uterine**  Referring or pertaining to the uterus.

**U. adnexa**  See *adnexa, uterine.*

**U. bruit**  Abnormal sound or murmur heard while auscultating the uterus.

! **U. ischemia**  Decreased blood supply to the uterus.

! **U. prolapse**  Falling, sinking, or sliding of the uterus from its normal location in the body.

**U. souffle**  See *souffle, uterine.*

⚡ **Uteroplacental insufficiency**  Decline in placental function—exchange of gases, nutrients, and wastes—leading to *fetal hypoxia* and *acidosis;* evidenced by late fetal heart rate decelerations in response to uterine contractions.

**Uterus**  Hollow muscular organ in the female designed for the implantation, containment, and nourishment of the fetus during its development until birth.

⚡ **Couvelaire u.**  Interstitial myometrial hemorrhage following premature separation (abruptio) of placenta. A purplish-bluish discoloration of the uterus and boardlike rigidity of the uterus are noted.

**Vaccination**  Intentional injection of antigenic material given to stimulate antibody production in the recipient.

**Vacuum curettage**  Uterine aspiration method of early abortion.

**Vacuum extraction**  Birth involving attachment of vacuum cup to fetal head and using negative pressure to assist in birth of the fetus.

**Vagina**  Normally collapsed musculomembranous tube that forms the passageway between the uterus and the entrance to the vagina.

**Vaginal birth after cesarean (VBAC)**  Giving birth vaginally after having had a previous cesarean birth.

**Valsalva maneuver**  The process of making a forceful attempt at expulsion while holding one's breath and tightening the abdominal muscles; *not recommended* as a method for pushing during the second stage.

**Variability**  Normal irregularity of fetal cardiac rhythm; short term—beat-to-beat changes; (internal scalp electrode) long term—rhythmic changes (waves) from the baseline, usually 3-5 beats/min.

**Varices (varicose veins)**  Swollen, distended, and twisted veins that may develop in almost any part of the body but are most commonly seen in the legs, caused by pregnancy, obesity, congenitally defective venous valves, and occupations that require much standing.

**Varicocele**  Enlargement of veins of the spermatic cord.

**Varicosity**  See *Varices (varicose veins).*

**Vascular spiders**  See *telangiectasia.*

**Vasectomy**  Ligation or removal of a segment of the vas deferens, usually done bilaterally to produce sterility in the male.

**VBAC**  Vaginal birth after cesarean.

〰 **VDRL test**  Abbreviation for Venereal Disease Research Laboratory test, a serologic flocculation test for syphilis.

〰 **Velocimetry**  See *Doppler blood flow analysis.*

**Vernix caseosa**  Protective gray-white fatty substance of cheesy consistency covering the fetal skin.

**Version**  Act of turning the fetus in the uterus to change the presenting part and facilitate birth (*rarely performed*).

**Podalic v.**  Shifting of the fetus' position so as to bring the feet to the outlet during birth (*rarely performed*).

**Vertex**  Crown or top of the head.

**V. presentation**  Presentation in which the fetal skull is nearest the cervical opening and born first.

**Very low birth weight (VLBW)**  Infant weighing 1500 g or less at birth.

**Viable**  Capable of living, such as a fetus that has reached a stage of development, usually 22 menstrual (20 wk gestation), which will permit it to live outside the uterus.

**Villi**  Short, vascular processes or protrusions growing on certain membranous surfaces.

**Chorionic v.**  Tiny vascular protrusions on the chorionic surface that project into the maternal blood sinuses of the uterus and that help to form the placenta and secrete hCG.

**Visceral pain**  Discomfort from cervical changes and uterine ischemia located over the lower portion of the abdomen; radiates to the lumbar area of the back and down the thighs.

**Voluntary abortion**  See *abortion, elective.*

**Vulva**  External genitalia of the female that consist of the labia majora, labia minora, clitoris, urinary meatus, and vaginal introitus.

**Vulvar self-examination (VSE)**  Systematic examination of the vulva by the woman herself.

**Weaning**  Process of changing from breastfeeding or bottle feeding to drinking from a cup.

**Wharton's jelly**  White, gelatinous material surrounding the umbilical vessels within the cord.

**Witch's milk**  Secretion of a whitish fluid for about a week after birth from enlarged mammary tissue in the neonate, presumably resulting from maternal hormonal influences.

**Womb**  See *uterus*.

**X chromosomes**  Sex chromosome in humans existing in duplicate in the normal female and singly in the normal male.

**X linkage**  Genes located on the X chromosome.

**X-linked inheritance**  Characteristics transmitted by genes on the X chromosome.

**Y chromosome**  Sex chromosome in the human male necessary for the development of the male gonads.

**Zona pellucida**  A thin layer of proteins and polysaccharides that surrounds the oocyte and provides protection during transport in the female genital tract.

**Zona reaction**  After one sperm has entered an egg, other sperm cannot; this process causes destruction of sperm receptors and hardening of the zona pellucida.

**Zygote**  Cell formed by the union of two reproductive cells or gametes; the fertilized ovum resulting from the union of a sperm and an ovum.

# Common Acronyms and Abbreviations

This list provides a review of over **350 need-to-know acronyms and abbreviations** used in charting, verbal communication, directives, and study guides.

| | |
|---|---|
| a | Before (*ante*) |
| Ab | Antibody/Abortion |
| ABC | Alternative birthing center |
| Abd | Abdomen/Abdominal |
| ABG | Arterial blood gas |
| ABO | Blood typing system |
| ac | Before meals (*ante cibum*) |
| ACHES | Acronym for possible warning signs secondary to use of oral hormone contraceptives |
| ADH | Antidiuretic hormone |
| ad lib | As much as desired (*ad libitum*) |
| ADLs | Activities of daily living |
| AFB | Acid-fast bacillus |
| Afib | Atrial fibrillation |
| Aflutter | Atrial flutter |
| AFP | Alpha-fetoprotein |
| AG | Antigen |
| AGA | Average (weight) for gestational age |
| AIDS | Acquired immunodeficiency syndrome |
| A-K (or AKA) | Above-the-knee (amputation) |
| ALL | Acute lymphocytic (lymphoblastic) leukemia |
| ALT | Alanine aminotransferase (*formerly* SGPT) |
| AMA | Against medical advice |
| A&O X 3 | Alert, oriented to person, place, time |
| AP | Anteroposterior/Alkaline phosphatase |
| ARC | AIDS-related complex |
| ARDS | Adult respiratory distress syndrome |
| ARF | Acute renal failure |
| aPPT | Activated partial thromboplastin time |
| ASA | Acetylsalicylic acid (aspirin) |
| ASAP | As soon as possible |
| ASD | Atrial septal defect |
| AST | Aspartate aminotransferase (*formerly* SGOT) |
| AV | Atrioventricular/Arteriovenous/Aortic valve |
| AVB | Atrioventricular block |
| AVM | Arteriovenous malformation |
| | |
| BBT | Basal body temperature |
| bid | Twice daily (*bis in die*) |
| BKA | Below-the-knee (amputation) |
| BM | Bowel movement/Bone marrow |
| BMI | Body mass index |
| BMR | Basal metabolic rate |
| BOA | Born out of asepsis |
| BP | Blood pressure |
| BPH | Benign prostatic hyperplasia |
| BPD | Biparietal diameter/Bronchopulmonary dysplasia |
| BPM | Beats per minute |

| | |
|---|---|
| BPP | Biophysical profile |
| BSE | Breast self-examination |
| BSST | Breast stimulation stress test |
| BUN | Blood urea nitrogen |
| Bx | Biopsy |
| | |
| c̄ | With (*cum*) |
| CA | Carcinoma/Cancer |
| CABG | Coronary artery bypass graft operation (X 1,2,3,4 = number of grafts) |
| CAD | Coronary artery disease |
| CBC | Complete blood count |
| CCU | Cardiac (intensive) care unit |
| CDC | Centers for Disease Control |
| CF | Cystic fibrosis |
| CHD | Congenital heart disease |
| CIN | Cervical intraepithelial neoplasm |
| CK | Creatine kinase |
| CMV | Cytomegalovirus |
| CNS | Central nervous system/Coagulase-negative staphylococcus |
| C/O | Complains of |
| CO₂ | Carbon dioxide |
| COPD | Chronic obstructive pulmonary disease |
| CPAP | Continuous positive airway pressure |
| CPD | Cephalopelvic disproportion |
| CPK | Creatine phosphokinase (*now* creatine kinase) |
| CPR | Cardiopulmonary resuscitation |
| CRF | Chronic renal failure/Cardiac risk factors |
| CRP | C-reactive protein |
| CSF | Cerebrospinal fluid |
| CSM | Circulation, sensation, motion checks |
| CST | Contraction stress test |
| CT | Computed tomography |
| CVA | Costovertebral angle |
| CVP | Central venous pressure |
| CVS | Chorionic villi sampling |
| Cx | Cervix |
| Δ | Change (Greek letter delta) |
| | |
| D&C | Dilatation and curettage |
| D&E | Dilatation and evacuation |
| DBM | Diabetes mellitus |
| DES | Diethylstilbestrol |
| DFMC | Daily fetal movement counts |
| DI | Diabetes insipidus |
| DIC | Disseminated intravascular coagulation |
| Dig | Digitalis |
| DM | Diabetes mellitus (also called DBM) |
| DNA | Deoxyribonucleic acid |
| DNR | Do not resuscitate |
| DOA | Dead on arrival |
| DOB | Date of birth |

Adapted from: M. Delong: *Medical Acronyms, Eponyms & Abbreviations* (4th edition) Los Angeles: Practice Management Information Corporation.

| | |
|---|---|
| DOE | Dyspnea on exertion |
| DPT | Diphtheria, pertussis, and tetanus |
| DRG | Diagnosis-related group |
| DTs | Delirium tremens |
| DTR | Deep tendon reflex |
| DVT | Deep-venous thrombosis |
| $D_5W$ | 5% dextrose in water |
| Dx | Diagnosis |
| | |
| ECG | Electrocardiogram (purist's version) |
| Echo | Echocardiogram |
| ECT | Electroconvulsive therapy |
| EDB | Estimated date of birth |
| EDC | Estimated date of "confinement" (old term) |
| EDD | Estimated date of delivery |
| EEG | Electroencephalogram |
| EKG | Electrocardiogram (common version) |
| ELISA | Enzyme-linked immunosorbent assay |
| EMG | Electromyogram |
| EMT | Emergency medical technician |
| ENT | Ear, nose, and throat |
| ER | Emergency room (now called emergency department) |
| ERT | Estrogen replacement therapy |
| ESR | Erythrocyte sedimentation rate |
| ETOH | Alcohol (ethanol) |
| | |
| FAS | Fetal alcohol syndrome |
| FBS | Fasting blood sugar |
| FSBS | Fingerstick blood sugar |
| $FEV_1$ | Forced expiratory volume in 1 sec |
| FHR | Fetal heart rate |
| FM | Fetal movement |
| FRC | Functional residual capacity |
| FSH | Follicle stimulating hormone |
| FTT | Failure to thrive |
| FUO | Fever of unknown origin |
| FVC | Forced vital capacity |
| Fx | Fracture |
| | |
| g | Gram |
| G | Gravida |
| GB | Gallbladder |
| GC | Gonococcus/Gonorrhea |
| GDM | Gestational diabetes meuitus |
| GFR | Glomerular filtration rate |
| G-6-P-D | Glucose-6-phosphate dehydrogenase |
| GI | Gastrointestinal |
| GIFT | Gamete intrafallopian transfer |
| GT | Gastric tube |
| GTD | Gestational trophoblastic disease |
| GTT | Glucose tolerance test |
| gtt(s) | Drop(s) (guttae) |
| GU | Genitourinary |
| GYN | Gynecologic |
| | |
| HbsAg | Hepatitis B surface antigen |
| HBV | Hepatitis B virus |
| hCG | Human chorionic gonadotropin |
| Hct | Hematocrit |

| | |
|---|---|
| HDL | High-density lipoprotein |
| HEENT | Head, eyes, ears, nose, and throat |
| HELLP | Hemolysis, elevated liver enzymes, low platelets |
| HF | Heart failure |
| Hgb | Hemoglobin |
| $Hgb_{A1c}$ | Glycosylated hemoglobin |
| HIV | Human immunodeficiency virus |
| HMO | Health maintenance organization |
| HOB | Head of bed |
| HR | Heart rate |
| HRT | Hormone replacement therapy |
| hs | Bedtime (hora somni) |
| HSV | Herpes simplex virus |
| HTN | Hypertension |
| Hx | History |
| | |
| ICN | Intensive care nursery |
| ICP | Intracranial pressure |
| ICU | Intensive care unit |
| I&D | Incision and drainage |
| IDDM | Insulin-dependent diabetes mellitus |
| IDM | Infant of a diabetic mother |
| Ig | Immunoglobulin |
| IM | Intramuscular |
| INH | Isoniazid |
| I&O | Intake and output |
| IPPB | Intermittent positive-pressure breathing |
| ITP | Idiopathic thrombocytopenic purpura |
| IUD | Intrauterine device |
| IUGR | Intrauterine growth restriction |
| IV | Intravenous |
| IVC | Inferior vena cava |
| IVF | In vitro fertilization |
| IVP | Intravenous pyelogram/Intravenous push |
| IZ | Immunization |
| | |
| JRA | Juvenile rheumatoid arthritis |
| JVD | Jugular venous distention |
| | |
| KUB | Kidneys, ureters, and bladder (flat/upright abdominal x-ray) |
| KVO | Keep vein open |
| | |
| LDR | Labor-delivery-recovery room |
| LDRP | Labor-delivery-recovery-postpartum room |
| LGA | Large for gestational age |
| LH | Luteinizing hormone |
| LLL | Left lower (lung) lobe |
| LLQ | Left lower quadrant |
| LMP | Last menstrual period |
| LNMP | Last normal menstrual period |
| LOC | Loss of consciousness/Level of consciousness |
| LPN | Licensed practical nurse |
| L/S | Lecithin-sphingomyelin ratio |
| LUL | Left upper (lung) lobe |
| LUQ | Left upper quadrant |
| LVN | Licensed vocational nurse |
| | |
| MAP | Mean arterial pressure |

| | |
|---|---|
| MCL | Midclavicular line |
| **Med** | Medication |
| MI | Myocardial infarction |
| MMR | Measles, mumps, and rubella |
| MODS | Multiple organ dysfunction syndrome |
| MOM | Milk of magnesia |
| **Mono** | Mononucleosis |
| MR | Mitral regurgitation/Mental retardation |
| MRI | Magnetic resonance imaging |
| MRSA | Methicillin- resistant *Staphylococcus aureus* |
| MS | Mental status/Mitral stenosis/Multiple sclerosis/Morphine sulfate |
| MVP | Mitral valve prolapse |
| MVR | Mitral valve replacement |
| | |
| NA | Not applicable |
| NEC | Necrotizing enterocolitis |
| NG | Nasogastric |
| NIDDM | Non-insulin-dependent diabetes mellitus |
| NL | Normal |
| NOC | Night (nocturnal) |
| NPH | Neutral-protamine-Hagedorn (intermediate-acting insulin) |
| NPO | Nothing by mouth (*nil per os*) |
| NS | Normal saline |
| NSAID | Nonsteroidal anti-inflammatory drug |
| NSR | Normal sinus rhythm |
| NST | Nonstress test |
| NTG | Nitroglycerin |
| N/V | Nausea, vomiting |
| NVD | Nausea, vomiting, and diarrhea |
| | |
| $O_2$ | Oxygen |
| OB | Obstetrics |
| OCT | Oxytocin stress test (oxytocin challenge test) |
| OD | Overdose |
| OOB | Out of bed/Out of breath |
| O&P | Ova and parasites |
| OR | Operating room |
| OS | Left eye (*oculus sinister*)/Opening snap |
| OT | Occupational therapy |
| OU | Both eyes (*oculo utro*) |
| | |
| P | Para/Pulse |
| p̄ | Post (after) |
| PA | Posterior-anterior/Physician's assistant/Pulmonary artery |
| PAINS | Acronym for possible warning signs of problems related to use of the intrauterine device |
| $PAO_2$ | Alveolar oxygen pressure |
| $PaO_2$ | Arterial partial pressure of oxygen |
| Pap | Papanicolaou test |
| PAS | Para-aminosalicylic acid |
| PAT | Paroxysmal atrial tachycardia |
| pc | After meals (*post cibum*) |
| PCA | Patient-controlled analgesia (pump) |
| PCP | *Pneumocystis carinii* pneumonia/Phencyclidine |
| PCV | Packed-cell volume |

| | |
|---|---|
| PDA | Patent ductus arteriosus |
| PEEP | Positive end-expiratory pressure |
| PERRL(A) | Pupils equally round and reactive to light (and accommodation) |
| PG | Prostaglandin |
| pH | Hydrogen ion concentration |
| PID | Pelvic inflammatory disease |
| PIH | Pregnancy-induced hypertension (*old term*) |
| PKU | Phenylketonuria |
| PMI | Point of maximum impulse |
| PMS | Premenstrual syndrome |
| PND | Paroxysmal nocturnal dyspnea |
| PO | By mouth (*per os*) |
| PPD | Purified protein derivative (tuberculosis skin test |
| PPO | Preferred provider organization |
| prn | When necessary (*pro re nata*) |
| PROM | Premature (prolonged) preterm rupture of membranes |
| PSA | Prostate-specific antigen |
| Pt | Patient |
| PT | Prothrombin time/Physical therapy |
| PTA | Prior to admission |
| PTCA | Percutaneous transluminal coronary angioplasty |
| PTT | Partial thromboplastin time |
| PUBS | Percutaneous umbilical blood sampling |
| PUD | Peptic ulcer disease |
| PVC | Premature ventricular contraction |
| | |
| q | Each, every (*quaque*) |
| qid | Four times a day (*quarter in die*) |
| | |
| R | Respirations |
| RA | Rheumatoid arthritis/Right atrium |
| RBC | Red blood cell |
| RDS | Respiratory distress syndrome |
| REEDA | Acronym for warning signs of problems related to episiotomy |
| RHD | Rheumatic heart disease |
| RLL | Right lower (lung) lobe |
| RLQ | Right lower quadrant |
| RML | Right middle (lung) lobe |
| RNA | Ribonucleic acid |
| R/O | Rule out |
| ROM | Range of motion/Rupture of membranes |
| ROP | Retinopathy of prematurity |
| ROS | Review of systems |
| RUL | Right upper (lung) lobe |
| RUQ | Right upper quadrant |
| Rx | Prescription/Therapy/Treatment |
| | |
| s̄ | Without (*sine*) |
| $S_1$ | First heart sound |
| $S_2$ | Second heart sound |
| $S_3$ | Third heart sound |
| $S_4$ | Fourth heart sound |
| SBE | Subacute bacterial endocarditis |
| SGA | Small for gestational age |

| | |
|---|---|
| SIADH | Syndrome of inappropriate antidiuretic hormone |
| SICU | Surgical intensive care unit |
| SIDS | Sudden infant death syndrome |
| SIRS | Sudden inflammatory response syndrome |
| SL | Sublingually |
| SLE | Systemic lupus erythematosus |
| SOB | Short(ness) of breath |
| SR | Sinus rhythm |
| S/S | Signs, symptoms |
| Stat | Immediately (*statim*) |
| STD | Sexually transmitted disease |
| SVD | Spontaneous vaginal delivery |
| SVT | Supraventricular tachycardia |
| Sx | Symptoms |
| | |
| T | Temperature |
| T&A | Tonsillectomy and adenoidectomy |
| TAH-BSO | Transabdominal hysterectomy and bilateral salpingo-oophorectomy |
| TB | Tuberculosis |
| TIA | Transient ischemic attack |
| tid | Three times a day (*ter in die*) |
| TKO | To keep open |
| TLC | Total lung capacity/Tender loving care |
| Toco-(Toko-) | Combining form meaning childbirth or labor |
| TOL | Trial of labor |
| TPN | Total parenteral nutrition |
| TPR | Temperature, pulse, and respirations |
| TSH | Thyroid-stimulating hormone |

| | |
|---|---|
| TSS | Toxic shock syndrome |
| TURP | Transurethral resection of prostate |
| TV | Total volume/Tidal volume |
| TVH | Transvaginal hysterectomy |
| Tx | Treatment |
| | |
| UA | Urinalysis |
| UGI | Upper gastrointestinal |
| UOQ | Upper outer quadrant |
| UQ | Upper quadrant |
| URI | Upper respiratory infection |
| UTI | Urinary tract infection |
| UV | Ultraviolet |
| | |
| VBAC | Vaginal birth after cesarean |
| VC | Vital capacity |
| VDRL | Venereal Disease Research Laboratory test |
| Vfib (VF) | Ventricular fibrillation |
| VLBW | Very low birth weight |
| VS | Vital signs |
| VSD | Ventricular septal defect |
| VTx | Vertex |
| | |
| WBC | White blood count/White blood cells |
| WNL | Within normal limits |
| w/o | Without |

# Quick Guide to Common Clinical Signs

Many clinical signs have been named for the physicians who first described them, or the phenomena they resemble. Following is a list of **28 of the most common clinical signs**, for use as a quick reference as you review.

**Babinski reflex**    Dorsiflexion of the big toe after stimulation of the lateral sole; normal response in newborn, but associated with *corticospinal tract lesions in the adult*

**Blumberg's sign**    Transient pain in the abdomen after approximated fingers pressed gently into abdominal wall are suddenly withdrawn—rebound tenderness; associated with *peritoneal inflammation*

**Braxton Hicks sign**    Mild, intermittent, painless uterine contractions that occur more frequently as pregnancy advances, but do *not* represent *true* labor

**Brudzinski's sign**    Flexion of the hip and knee induced by flexion of the neck; associated with *meningeal irritation*

**Chadwick's sign**    Cyanosis of vaginal and cervical mucosa; associated with *pregnancy*

**Cheyne-Stokes respiration**    Rhythmic cycles of deep and shallow respiration, often with apneic periods; associated with *central nervous system respiratory center dysfunction*

**Chvostek's sign**    Facial muscle spasm induced by tapping on the facial nerve branches; associated with *hypocalcemia*

**Coppernail's sign**    Ecchymoses on the perineum, scrotum, or labia; associated with *fracture* of the *pelvis*

**Cullen's sign**    Bluish discoloration of the umbilicus; associated with acute *pancreatitis* or *hemoperitoneum*, especially *rupture of fallopian tube* in ectopic pregnancy

**Doll's eye sign**    Dissociation between the movements of the head and eyes: as the head is raised, the eyes are lowered; and as the head is lowered, the eyes are raised; associated with global-diffuse disorders of the *cerebrum*

**Fluid wave**    Transmission across the abdomen of a wave induced by snapping the abdomen, associated with *ascites*

**Goldstein's sign**    Wide distance between the great toe and the adjoining toe; associated with *cretinism and trisomy 21*

**Goodell's sign**    Softening of the cervix, a *probable* sign of pregnancy, occurring during the second month

**Harlequin sign**    In the newborn infant, reddening of the lower half of the laterally recumbent body and blanching of the upper half, due to a *temporary vasomotor disturbance*

**Hegar's sign**    Softening of the isthmus of the uterus; associated with the *first trimester of pregnancy*

**Homan's sign**    Pain behind the knee, induced by dorsiflexion of the foot; associated with peripheral vascular disease, especially *venous thrombosis* in the calf (**not recommended** due to risk of pulmonary embolism)

**Kehr's sign**    Severe pain in the left upper quadrant, radiating to the top of the shoulder; associated with *splenic rupture*

**Kernig's sign**    Inability to extend leg when sitting or lying with the thigh flexed on the abdomen; associated with *meningeal irritation*

**Knie's sign**    Unequal dilatation of the pupils; associated with *Graves'* disease

**Kussmaul's respiration**    Paroxysmal air hunger; associated with acidosis, especially *diabetic ketoacidosis*

**McBurney's sign**    Tenderness at McBurney's point (located two-thirds of the distance from the umbilicus to the anterior-superior iliac spine); associated with *appendicitis*

**Ortolani's (click) sign**    "Click" sound sometimes heard if hip *dysplasia* is present; on assessment, head of femur can be felt (or heard as a click) to slip forward in acetabulum and slip back when pressure is released and legs are returned to their original position

**Osler's sign**    Small painful erythematous swellings in the skin of the hands and feet; associated with *bacterial endocarditis*

**Psoas sign**    Pain induced by hyperextension of the right thigh while lying on the left side; associated with *appendicitis*

**Setting-sun sign**    Downward deviation of the eyes so that each iris appears to "set" beneath the lower lid, with white sclera exposed between it and the upper lid; associated with *increased intracranial pressure* or irritation of the *brain stem*

**Tinel's sign**    Tingling sensation felt from light percussion on the radial side of the palmaris longus tendon; associated with *carpal tunnel syndrome*

**Trousseau's sign**    Carpopedal spasm that develops when BP cuff is inflated above systolic pressure for 3 minutes; associated with *hypocalcemia*

**Williamson's sign**    Markedly diminished blood pressure in the leg as compared with that in the arm on the same side; associated with *pneumothorax* and *pleural effusions*

Adapted from: E. Braunwald (ed.) et al. *Harrison's Principles of Internal Medicine*, 15th Edition, New York: McGraw Hill Professional.

For a quick review, use this index to locate over **75 diagnostic tests and procedures** covered in this book as they relate to specific maternal-newborn conditions. Also *see* **Glossary** for ⊞.

**Miscellaneous tests**

# ➤⌾⭠ Index to: Maternal–Newborn Emergencies

For a quick review, use this index to locate content on over **35 maternal-newborn emergencies** covered in this book.

# 🍎 Index to: Diets

For a quick review, use this index to locate over **36 special dietary considerations** covered in this book as they relate to specific conditions/situations in pregnancy.

# ☞ Index to: Positioning the Client

For a quick reference as you study or review, use this index to locate **18 positions** of choice (or contraindicated) for various conditions related to pregnancy.

# ☞ Index to: Nursing Treatments (Essential "Hands-on" Care, Skills, Activities and Nursing Procedures)

Use this index as a quick checklist of over **58 skills and procedures** to locate pages where they are mentioned in this book that nurses need to know about or be able to perform in giving client care.

# ☀ Index to: Memory Aids (Mnemonics and Acronyms)

| Condition | Memory Aid | Page(s) |
|---|---|---|
| Blood vessels in cord | AVA | 120 |
| Dystocia: etiology | 6 P's | 131-132, 137 |
| Episiotomy: assessment | REEDA | 118, 121 |
| Gestational diabetes: assessment | 3 P's | 83 |
| Infections during pregnancy | TORCH | 63, 64, 83 |
| IUDs: signs of potential problems | PAINS | 9 |
| Neonatal risk factors | ABC.I | 205 |
| Newborn assessment components | APGAR | 112, 120 |
| Oral contraceptives: signs of potential problems | ACHES | 9 |
| Preterm infant: anticipated problems | TRIES | 205 |
| Recording gravidity/parity | GT PAL | 33, 42 |
| Severe pre-eclampsia (HELLP Syndrome) | HELLP | 77, 84 |
| Validation of pregnancy | 3 P's | 42 |

# NANDA-Approved Nursing Diagnoses

(with modifications)

This list represents modifications of some of the North American Nursing Diagnosis Association (NANDA) approved nursing diagnoses for clinical use.

## PATTERN 1: EXCHANGING

Airway clearance impairment
Aspiration risk
Autonomic dysreflexia
Blood pressure alteration
Bowel elimination alteration
Bowel incontinence
Breathing pattern impairment
Cardiac alteration
Cardiovascular alteration
Colonic constipation
Constipation, perceived
Constipation, unspecified
Contraceptive risk
Delivery risk
Diarrhea
Disuse syndrome
Endocrine alteration
Failure to thrive
Fecal impaction
Fertility risk
Fluid volume alteration
Fluid volume deficit
Fluid volume deficit risk
Fluid volume excess
Gas exchange impairment
Hyperthermia
Hypothermia
Immunologic alteration
Infection risk
Infertility risk
Injury risk
Intracranial adaptive capacity impairment
Kinesthetic alteration
Labor risk
Latex allergy response
Medication risk
Nutrition alteration
Nutrition deficit (less than body requirements)
Nutrition excess (more than body requirements)
Oral mucus membrane impairment
Perinatal risk
Perioperative injury risk
Poisoning risk
Polypharmacy
Postpartum risk

Pregnancy risk
Protection alteration
Reflex urinary incontinence
Reproductive risk
Respiration alteration
Skin integrity impairment
Skin integrity impairment risk
Stress urinary incontinence
Suffocation risk
Surgical recovery delay
Thermoregulation impairment
Tissue integrity alteration
Tissue perfusion alteration (specify type)
     (Renal, cerebral, cardiopulmonary, gastrointestinal, peripheral)
Tobacco use
Trauma risk
Urinary elimination alteration
Urinary incontinence, functional
Urinary incontinence, total
Urinary retention
Urinary urge incontinence
Ventilatory weaning impairment

## PATTERN 2: COMMUNICATING

Communication impairment
Verbal impairment

## PATTERN 3: RELATING

Adolescent behavior alteration
Adult behavior alteration
Alcohol abuse
Caregiver role strain
Drug abuse
Family process alteration
Older adult behavior alteration
Parental role conflict
Parenting alteration
Role performance alteration
Sexual dysfunction
Sexuality patterns alteration
Social interaction alteration
Social isolation
Socialization alteration
Substance abuse

Adapted from: NANDA. *Nursing Diagnosis: Definitions and Classification*, Philadelphia: North American Nursing Diagnosis Association

# PATTERN 4: VALUING

Meaningfulness alteration
Spiritual distress
Spiritual state alteration
Suicide risk

# PATTERN 5: CHOOSING

Adjustment impairment
Community coping impairment
Coping, defensive
Decisional conflict (specify)
Denial
Family coping, compromised
Family coping, disabled
Family coping impairment
Health-seeking behavior alteration (specify)
Individual coping impairment
Noncompliance (specify)
     (Diagnostic test, dietary regimen,
       medication regime, safety precautions,
       therapeutic regime)

# PATTERN 6: MOVING

Activities of daily living (ADLs) alteration:
     Bathing/hygiene self-care deficit
     Dressing/grooming self-care deficit
     Feeding self-care deficit
     Toileting self-care deficit
Activity alteration
Activity intolerance
Breastfeeding impairment
Child behavior alteration
Diversional activity deficit
Fatigue
Growth and development alteration
Health maintenance alteration
Home maintenance alteration
Infant behavior alteration
Infant feeding pattern impairment
Musculoskeletal alteration
Newborn behavior alteration
Perioperative positioning injury
Peripheral alteration
Physical mobility impairment
Relocation stress syndrome
Sleep deprivation
Sleep pattern disturbance
Swallowing impairment

# PATTERN 7: PERCEIVING

Body image disturbance
Chronic low self-esteem disturbance
Hopelessness
Personal identity disturbance
Powerlessness
Self-concept alteration
Sensory/perceptual alteration (specify)
     (Visual, auditory, kinesthetic, gustatory, tactile,
       olfactory)
Situational self-esteem disturbance
Unilateral neglect

# PATTERN 8: KNOWING

Confusion
Knowledge deficit (specify)
     (Diagnostic test, dietary regime, disease process,
       medication regime, safety precautions, therapeutic
       regime)
Memory impairment
Thought processes alteration

# PATTERN 9: FEELING

Anxiety
Comfort alteration
Dying process
Fear
Grieving
Grieving, anticipatory
Grieving, dysfunctional
Nausea
Pain, acute
Pain, chronic
Pain, unspecified
Post-trauma response
Rape-trauma syndrome
Self-mutilation risk
Violence risk (self-directed or directed at others)

# NCLEX-RN® Test Plan:
# ⋈ Nursing Process/Cognitive Level: Definitions/Descriptions

The phases of the nursing process include the following:

## I. DATA COLLECTION

⋈ **A. Assessment: establishing a database**

   1. *Gather objective and subjective information relative to the client:*

     **a.** Collect information from the client, significant others, and/or health care team members; current and prior health records; and other pertinent resources.

     **b.** Utilize assessment skills appropriate to client's condition.

     **c.** Recognize *symptoms* and significant findings.

     **d.** Determine client's ability to assume care of daily health needs (self-care).

     **e.** Determine health team member's ability to provide care.

     **f.** Assess *environment* of client.

     **g.** Identify own or staff reactions to client, significant others, and/or health care team members.

   2. *Confirm data:*

     **a.** *Verify* observation or perception by obtaining additional information.

     **b.** *Question* prescriptions and decisions by other health care team members when indicated.

     **c.** *Observe* condition of client directly when indicated.

     **d.** *Validate* that an appropriate client assessment has been made.

   3. *Communicate information gained in assessment:*

     **a.** Document assessment findings thoroughly and accurately.

     **b.** Report assessment findings to relevant members of the health care team.

⋈ **B. Analysis: identifying actual or potential health care needs and/or problems based on assessment**

   1. *Interpret data:*

     **a.** Validate data.

     **b.** Organize related data.

     **c.** Determine need for *additional* data.

     **d.** Determine client's unique needs and/or problems.

   2. *Formulate client's nursing diagnoses:*

     **a.** Determine significant relationship between data and client needs and/or problems.

     **b.** Utilize *standard taxonomy* for formulating nursing diagnoses.

   3. *Communicate results of analysis:*

     **a.** Document client's *nursing diagnoses.*

     **b.** Report results of analysis to relevant members of the health care team.

⋈ **II. Planning: setting goals for meeting client's needs and designing strategies to achieve these goals**

   A. *Prioritize nursing diagnoses:*

     1. Involve client, significant others, and/or health care team members when establishing nursing diagnoses.

     2. Establish *priorities* among nursing diagnoses.

     3. Anticipate needs and/or problems on the basis of established priorities.

   B. *Determine goals of care:*

     1. Involve client, significant others, and/or health care team members in setting goals.

     2. Establish *priorities among goals.*

     3. Anticipate needs and/or problems on the basis of established priorities.

   C. *Formulate outcome criteria for goals of care:*

     1. Involve client, significant others, and/or health care team members in formulating outcome criteria for goals of care.

     2. Establish *priorities* among outcome *criteria* **for goals of care.**

     3. Anticipate needs and/or problems on the basis of established priorities.

   D. *Develop plan of care and modify as necessary:*

     1. Involve the client, significant others, and/or health care team members in designing strategies.

     2. *Individualize* the plan of care based on such information as *age, gender, culture, ethnicity, and religion.*

     3. Plan for client's *safety,* comfort, and maintenance of optimal functioning.

     4. Select nursing interventions for delivery of client's care.

     5. Select *appropriate* teaching approaches.

   E. *Collaborate with other health care team members when planning delivery of client's care:*

     1. Identify health or social resources available to the client and/or significant others.

     2. *Select appropriate health care team members* when planning assignments.

     3. Coordinate care provided by health care team members.

*Source* Adapted from: National Council of State Boards of Nursing, Inc. most current *NCLEX-RN® Test Plan.*

F. *Communicate plan of care:*
1. Document plan of care thoroughly and accurately.
2. Report plan of care to relevant members of the health care team.
3. Review plan of care with client.

▶ III. **Implementation: initiating and completing actions necessary to accomplish the defined goals**
A. *Organize and manage client's care:*
1. Implement a plan of care.
2. Arrange for a client care conference.
B. *Counsel and teach client, significant others, and/or health care team members:*
1. Assist client, significant others, and/or health care team members to recognize and manage stress.
2. Facilitate client relationships with significant others and health care team members.
3. *Teach* correct principles, procedures, and techniques for maintenance and promotion of health.
4. Provide client with health status information.
5. Refer client, significant others, and/or health care team members to appropriate *resources.*
C. *Provide care to achieve established goals of care:*
1. Use *safe* and *appropriate techniques* when administering client care.
2. Use precautionary and *preventive* interventions in providing care to client.
3. *Prepare client for surgery, delivery,* or other *procedures.*
4. Institute *interventions* to compensate for adverse responses.
5. Initiate *life-saving interventions* for emergency situations.
6. Provide an *environment* conducive to attainment of goals of care.
7. Adjust care in accord with client's expressed or implied needs, problems, and/or preferences.
8. Stimulate and motivate client to achieve *self-care* and independence.
9. Encourage client to follow a treatment regime.
10. Assist client to maintain optimal functioning.
D. *Supervise and coordinate the delivery of client's care provided by nursing personnel:*
1. *Delegate* nursing interventions to appropriate nursing personnel.
2. *Monitor* and follow up on delegated interventions.
3. Manage health care team members' *reactions* to factors influencing therapeutic relationships with clients.

E. *Communicate nursing interventions:*
1. Record actual client responses, nursing interventions, and other information relevant to implementation of care.
2. Provide complete, accurate reports on assigned client(s) to relevant members of the health care team.

▶ IV. **Evaluation: determining the extent to which goals have been achieved and interventions have been successful**
A. *Compare actual outcomes with expected outcomes of care:*
1. Evaluate responses (*expected and unexpected*) in order to determine the degree of success of nursing interventions.
2. Determine impact of therapeutic interventions on the client and significant others.
3. Determine need for modifying the plan of care.
4. Identify factors that may interfere with the client's ability to implement the plan of care.
B. *Evaluate the client's ability to implement self-care:*
1. Verify that *tests or measurements are performed correctly* by the client and/or other caregivers.
2. Ascertain client's, and/or others' *understanding* of information given.
C. *Evaluate health care team members' ability to implement client care:*
1. Determine *impact of teaching* on health care team members.
2. Identify factors that might alter health care team members' response to teaching.
D. *Communicate evaluation findings:*
1. Document client's response to therapy, care, and/or teaching.
2. Report client's response to therapy, care, and/or teaching to relevant members of the health care team.
3. Report and document others' responses to teaching.
4. Document other caregivers' responses to teaching.

Notes:

1. Throughout the outline in this book, the stages of the nursing process are referred to as: assessment, analysis/nursing diagnosis, nursing care plan/implementation, evaluation/outcome criteria.

2. The practice questions in this book are coded as to the phase of the nursing process being tested; the codes are found following the answer/rationale for each question. *Key to Nursing Process Codes:*

AS  Assessment
AN  Analysis  > Data Collection
PL  Planning
IMP  Implementation
EV  Evaluation

For an **index to questions relating to each phase of the nursing process**, see **Appendix K**.

---

**The phases of the cognitive level** include:

A. **Recall/Knowledge**: Rote remembering of significant facts or terms; to *define*, to name and to *list*.

B. **Comprehension**: To understand; to restate; to reorganize; to translate; to find an *illustration* or *example*; to *interpret by explanation* or *summary*; to determine *implications, consequences* and effects.

C. **Application**: The *use of abstractions in particular* or *concrete* situations. They may be in the form of general ideas, *rules, procedures,* or *general methods*. The abstractions may also be technical *principles, ideas,* and *theories* that need to be remembered and applied, *using a concept or principle in a new situation.*

D. **Analysis**: The breakdown of the whole into constituent *parts* or elements so that a rank *priority* of ideas can emerge and *relationships* between ideas can be made clear.

E. **Synthesis**: Putting ideas together to form a *new* whole.

F. **Evaluation**: *Judging* material using specific criteria.

*Key to cognitive level codes:*

RE/KN    Recall/Knowledge
COM      Comprehension
APP      Application
ANL      Analysis
SYN      Synthesis
EVL      Evaluation

For an **index to questions relating to each phase of the cognitive level**, see **Appendix K**.

# ⋈ Index to: Questions Related to Nursing Process/Cognitive Level

Use this index to locate *practice questions* throughout the book in each of the phases of the nursing process and cognitive level.

Please refer to the following pages for the complete table.

# Appendix K

| Chapter | Nursing Process | | | | | Cognitive Level | | | | | |
|---|---|---|---|---|---|---|---|---|---|---|---|
| | Assessment (AS) Question #: | Analysis (AN) Question #: | Planning (PL) Question #: | Implementation (IMP) Question #: | Evaluation (EV) Question #: | Recall/Know. (RE/KN) Question #: | Comprehension (COM) Question #: | Application (APP) Question #: | Analysis (ANL) Question #: | Evaluation (EVL) Question #: | Synthesis (SYN) Question #: |
| 1—Growth and Development | 14, 19 | 5, 6, 20, 24, 26 | 1, 11, 16 | 3, 4, 7, 8, 9, 12, 13, 15, 18, 23, 25 | 2, 10, 17, 21, 22 | 3, 4, 8, 12, 13, 14, 15, 18, 20, 23, 24, 25, 26 | 1 | 5, 6, 7, 9 | 11, 16, 19, 22 | 2, 10, 17, 21 | |
| 2—Normal Pregnancy | 1 | 6, 7, 9, 16, 20, 21, 27 | 2, 15, 17, 29 | 4, 8, 10, 12, 13, 14, 18, 23, 24, 25, 26, 28, 32 | 3, 5, 11, 19, 22, 30, 31 | 1, 4, 6, 7, 8, 9, 10, 12, 29 | 2, 5, 13, 14, 17, 28 | 16, 18, 20, 23, 25, 26, 32 | 3, 15, 21, 24, 27, 30 | 11, 19, 22, 31 | |
| 3—High-Risk Conditions & Complications During Pregnancy | 11, 20, 28, 38, 40, 44, 52 | 1, 10, 14, 26, 27, 42, 43, 48, 51 | 5, 8, 16, 17, 18, 19, 21, 24, 33, 36, 37 | 2, 6, 12, 15, 23, 32, 34, 35, 39, 41, 45, 46, 47, 50, 53, 54, 55, 56 | 3, 4, 7, 9, 13, 22, 25, 29, 30, 31, 49 | 1, 3, 14, 20, 21, 23, 32, 34, 35, 42, 47, 50, 51, 53, 55 | 6, 16, 33, 38, 43, 44, 46, 48 | 2, 8, 10, 12, 15, 17, 18, 19, 24, 26, 37, 41, 52, 54, 56 | 4, 5, 7, 9, 11, 22, 25, 27, 28, 29, 30, 31, 36, 39, 40, 45, 49 | 13 | |
| 4—The Intrapartal Experience | 1, 21, 24, 26 | 2, 8, 9, 11, 23, 27, 28 | 4, 16, 22, 25 | 3, 5, 12, 14, 15, 17, 18, 20 | 6, 7, 10, 13, 19, 29, 30, 31 | 5, 8, 9, 10, 13, 15, 16, 17, 19, 22 | 1, 2, 4, 6, 7, 14, 20, 24 | 11, 25, 28, 31 | 3, 12, 18, 21, 26, 27 | | 23, 29, 30 |
| 5—Complications During the Intrapartal Period | 17 | 4, 5 | 2, 16 | 3, 7, 8, 9, 12, 14, 18, 19 | 1, 6, 10, 11, 13, 15 | 1, 2, 4, 5, 6, 7, 9, 17 | 8 | 3, 10 | 11, 12, 13, 14, 15, 16, 18, 19 | | |
| 6—The Postpartal Period | 13, 15, 23 | 9, 16, 20, 21 | 4, 6, 18, 19 | 1, 2, 5, 8, 10, 11, 12, 14, 22, 25, 26 | 3, 7, 17, 24, 27 | 2, 9, 13, 15, 24, 26 | 4, 10, 11, 16, 20, 23, 25 | 3, 6, 7, 8, 14 | 1, 5, 12, 17, 18, 19, 21, 22 | 27 | |
| 7—Complications During the Postpartal Period | | 6, 8, 13, 14 | 2, 3, 9 | 4, 5, 10, 11, 12, 15 | 1, 7, 16 | 4, 9, 16 | 1, 2, 3, 7 | 5, 8, 11, 12, 15 | 6, 10, 13, 14 | | |
| 8—The Newborn Infant | 11, 14 | 5 | 10 | 1, 3, 4, 6, 7, 13, 15, 16, 17, 18 | 2, 8, 9, 12 | 1, 2, 4, 5, 6, 18 | 10, 11 | 3, 7, 12, 13 | 8, 9, 14, 15, 16, 17 | | |

*(continued)*

## Nursing Process

| Chapter | Assessment (AS) Question #: | Analysis (AN) Question #: | Planning (PL) Question #: | Implementation (IMP) Question #: | Evaluation (EV) Question #: |
|---|---|---|---|---|---|
| 9—Complications During the Neonatal Period: The High-Risk Newborn | 6, 7, 8, 9, 10, 11, 12, 13, 23, 25 | 1, 3, 16, 24 | 2, 4, 5 | 14, 20, 21, 22 | 15, 17, 18, 19 |

## Cognitive Level

| Recall/Know. (RE/KN) Question #: | Comprehension (COM) Question #: | Application (APP) Question #: | Analysis (ANL) Question #: | Evaluation (EVL) Question #: | Synthesis (SYN) Question #: |
|---|---|---|---|---|---|
| 6, 14, 16, 24 | 1, 2, 7, 8, 9, 13, 22 | 4, 5, 11, 23, 25 | 3, 10, 12, 15, 17, 18, 19, 20, 21 | | |

# Index to: Definitions and Questions Related to Categories of Human Functions

This index lists practice questions for you to use in reviewing categories of human functions (which are detailed examples of what subtopics are covered by the four broad client needs categories).

The eight categories of human functions include:

**Protective Functions** client's ability to maintain defenses and prevent physical and chemical trauma, injury, and threats to health status (e.g., communicable diseases, abuse, safety hazards, poisoning, skin disorders, and pre- and post-operative complications).

**Sensory-Perceptual Functions** client's ability to perceive, interpret, and respond to sensory and cognitive stimuli (e.g., auditory, visual, verbal impairments, brain tumors, aphasia, sensory deprivation or overload, body image, reality orientation, learning disabilities).

**Comfort, Rest, Activity, and Mobility Functions** client's ability to maintain mobility, desirable level of activity, adequate sleep, rest, and comfort (e.g., pain, sleep disturbances, joint impairment).

**Nutrition** client's ability to maintain the intake and processing of essential nutrients (e.g., obesity, gastric and metabolic disorders that primarily affect the nutritional status).

**Growth and Development** client's ability to maintain maturational processes throughout the life span (e.g., child bearing, child rearing, maturational crisis, changes in aging, psychosocial development).

**Fluid-Gas Transport Functions** client's ability to maintain fluid-gas transport (e.g., fluid volume deficit/overload, acid-base balance, CPR, anemias, cardiopulmonary diseases).

**Psychosocial-Cultural Functions** client's ability to function in intrapersonal/interpersonal relationships (e.g., grieving, death/dying, psychotic behaviors, self concept, therapeutic communication, ethical-legal aspects, community resources, situational crises, substance abuse).

**Elimination Functions** client's ability to maintain functions related to relieving the body of waste products (e.g., conditions of GI and/or GU systems).

# Appendix L

| Chapter | Protective Functions (1) Question #: | Sensory–Perceptual Functions (2) Question #: | Comfort, Rest, Activity, and Mobility Functions (3) Question #: | Nutrition (4) Question #: | Growth and Development (5) Question #: | Fluid–Gas Transport Functions (6) Question #: | Psychosocial–Cultural Functions (7) Question #: | Eliminations Functions (8) Question #: |
|---|---|---|---|---|---|---|---|---|
| 1—Growth and Development | 3, 4, 16, 17, 18, 19, 21 | | 1, 22 | 2 | 5, 6, 7, 8, 9, 10, 12, 13, 14, 15, 23, 24, 25, 26, 27 | 11, 20 | | |
| 2—Normal Pregnancy | 12 | 19 | 13, 22, 23 | 1, 2, 3, 4, 18, 24, 25, 26, 31, 32 | 5, 6, 9, 10, 15, 16, 17, 20, 21, 27, 29 | 7, 8, 11, 30 | 14, 28 | |
| 3—High-Risk Conditions & Complications During Pregnancy | 2, 3, 12, 20, 22, 30, 33, 34, 39, 43, 44, 47, 50, 51, 52, 53, 55 | 9, 25, 27, 28, 49 | 24, 37 | 8, 17, 18 | 15, 21, 31, 38, 42, 54, 56 | 4, 5, 6, 7, 10, 11, 13, 14, 16, 19, 23, 26, 32, 35, 36, 40, 41, 44, 45, 46, 48 | 1 | 29 |
| 4—The Intrapartal Experience | 25 | | 6, 8, 9, 14, 20 | | 1, 2, 3, 5, 7, 10, 11, 15, 16, 17, 19, 22, 23, 24, 26, 27, 28, 29, 30, 31 | 4, 12, 13, 21 | 18 | |
| 5—Complications During the Intrapartal Period | 7, 13, 14, 15, 18 | | 3, 12 | | 2, 4, 5, 10 | 1, 6, 8, 9, 11, 16, 17, 19 | | |
| 6—The Postpartal Period | 14, 16, 24 | | 4, 5, 8, 11 | 9, 25, 27 | 2, 3, 10, 12, 13, 26 | 1, 18, 19, 20, 21, 22, 23 | 6, 7 | 15, 17 |
| 7—Complications During the Postpartal Period | 1, 2, 7, 12, 13 | | | 4, 5 | | 3, 6, 8, 9, 10, 11, 14, 15, 16 | | |
| 8—The Newborn Infant | 7, 8, 10, 15, 16, 17 | | 5, 14 | | 1, 2, 4, 6, 9, 11, 12, 13, 18 | 3 | | |
| 9—Complications During the Neonatal Period: The High-Risk Newborn | 1, 4, 5, 6, 7, 8, 13, 14, 23 | 16 | 10 | 21 | 9, 15, 20 | 3, 11, 12, 17, 19, 22, 24, 25 | 2 | 18 |

To *practice questions* in each of the 4 categories of **client needs** and *6 client subneeds* that are tested on NCLEX-RN®, refer to the questions listed on the following pages.

## CLIENT NEEDS/*Client Subneeds:*

**1. SAFE, EFFECTIVE CARE ENVIRONMENT**
*Management of Care*
*Safety and Infection Control*

**2. HEALTH PROMOTION AND MAINTENANCE—has no** *client subneeds.*

**3. PSYCHOSOCIAL INTEGRITY— has no** *client subneeds.*

**4. PHYSIOLOGICAL INTEGRITY**
*Basic Care and Comfort*
*Pharmacological and Parenteral Therapies*
*Reduction of Risk Potential*
*Physiological Adaptation*

---

The four broad categories of **CLIENT NEEDS** include:

**SAFE, EFFECTIVE CARE ENVIRONMENT**—coordinated care, environmental safety, safe and effective treatment and procedures (e.g., client rights, confidentiality, principles of teaching/learning, control of infectious agents).

**HEALTH PROMOTION AND MAINTENANCE**—normal growth and development from birth to death, self-care and support systems, prevention and early treatment of disease (e.g., newborn care, normal perinatal care, family planning, human sexuality, parenting, end-of-life process, lifestyle choices, immunity).

**PSYCHOSOCIAL INTEGRITY**—psychosocial adaptation, coping (e.g., behavioral norms, chemical dependency, communication skills, family systems, mental health concepts, psychodynamics of behavior, psychopathology, treatment modalities).

**PHYSIOLOGICAL INTEGRITY**—physiological adaptation, reduction of risk potential, provision of basic care (e.g., drug administration, emergencies, nutritional therapies).

---

The six categories of *client subneeds* include:

1. *Management of Care*—staff development, collaboration, supervision of multidisciplinary health team; delegation; client rights; prioritization, ethical and legal responsibilities; referrals.

2. *Safety and Infection Control*—protecting clients, family/significant others and health care personnel from health and environmental hazards; e.g., disaster planning, home safety, medical and surgical asepsis, use of restraint/safety devices, safe use of equipment, standard precautions.

3. *Basic Care and Comfort*—performing routine nursing activities of daily living.

4. *Pharmacological and Parenteral Therapies*—expected and unexpected effects, chemotherapy; blood products; pain management; calculations; TPN, IV; central venous access devices.

5. *Reduction of Risk Potential*—monitoring, and reducing likelihood of complications related to existing conditions, treatments or procedures.

6. *Physiological Adaptation*—meeting acute, chronic or life-threatening physical health conditions.

## Appendix M

| Chapter | SECE: Management of Care | SECE: Safety/Infection Control | HPM: Question # | PsI: Question # | PhI: Basic Care/Comfort | PhI: Pharmacological/Parenteral Therapies | PhI: Reduction of Risk Potential | PhI: Physiological Adaptation |
|---|---|---|---|---|---|---|---|---|
| 1—Growth and Development | | | 1, 4, 6, 7, 8, 10, 12, 13, 14, 15, 18, 19, 21, 24, 25, 26 | 9, 17 | 2 | 5, 22, 23 | 3, 16 | 11, 20 |
| 2—Normal Pregnancy | 16 | | 5, 6, 7, 8, 9, 10, 11, 12, 13, 15, 17, 19, 20, 22, 23, 24, 27, 31 | 14, 28, 29 | 1, 2, 3, 4, 18, 25, 26, 32 | | 21, 30 | |
| 3—High-Risk Conditions and Complications During Pregnancy | | 2, 3, 12, 33, 44, 50, 52, 53, 55 | 10, 20, 21, 31, 42, 43, 51, 54 | 1 | 8, 24 | 16, 28, 38, 45, 46, 49 | 7, 15, 17, 19, 22, 23, 27, 34, 35, 36, 37, 39, 41, 47, 56 | 4, 5, 6, 9, 11, 13, 14, 18, 25, 26, 29, 30, 32, 40, 48 |
| 4—The Intrapartal Experience | | | 1, 2, 3, 4, 5, 6, 7, 8, 9, 11, 14, 15, 17, 19, 22, 23, 24, 26, 28, 29, 31 | 16, 18 | | 10, 13, 21 | 12, 20, 25, 27, 30 | |
| 5—Complications During the Intrapartal Period | 12, 14, 19 | | 10, 15 | | 4, 5, 11, 14 | 1, 2, 6, 7, 8 | 4, 5, 16, 17, 18 | 3, 9, 11, 13 |
| 6—The Postpartal Period | 16 | 24 | 1, 2, 3, 8, 9, 10, 12, 13, 17, 18, 21, 25, 26, 27 | 6, 7 | | 23 | 15 | 19, 20, 22 |
| 7—Complications During the Postpartal Period | | 5 | 1, 4, 8 | | | 2, 3, 11, 13, 14 | 7, 15 | 6, 9, 10, 12, 16 |
| 8—The Newborn Infant | 8 | 7 | 1, 2, 3, 4, 5, 6, 9, 11, 12, 13, 14, 17, 18 | | | 10 | 15, 16 | |

*(continued)*

| | CLIENT NEED: SAFE, EFFECTIVE CARE ENVIRONMENT (SECE) | | CLIENT NEED: HEALTH PROMOTION/ MAINTENANCE (HPM) | CLIENT NEED: PSYCHOSOCIAL INTEGRITY (PsI) | CLIENT NEED: PHYSIOLOGICAL INTEGRITY (PhI) | | | |
|---|---|---|---|---|---|---|---|---|
| **Chapter** | Client Subneed: Management of Care Question #: | Client Subneed: Safety/Infection Control Question #: | Question #: | Question #: | Client Subneed: Basic Care/ Comfort Question #: | Client Subneed: Pharmacological/ Parenteral Therapies Question #: | Client Subneed: Reduction of Risk Potential Question #: | Client Subneed: Physiological Adaptation Question #: |
| 9—Complications During the Neonatal Period: The High-Risk Newborn | | 4, 5, 6, 23 | 7, 13, 15, 25 | 2 | | 1 | 8, 11, 16, 17, 20, 22, 24 | 3, 9, 10, 12, 14, 18, 19, 21 |

# Resources

Selected sources of information and services. (Every effort has been made to provide current names and addresses; however, addresses do change frequently.)

## Health and Welfare Agencies/Associations

**American Cancer Society**
1599 Clifton Rd. NE
Atlanta, GA 30329
800-ACS-2345
*www.cancer.org*

**American Diabetes Association**
National Center
1701 North Beauregard St.
Alexandria, VA 22311
800-342-2383
*www.diabetes.org*

**Centers for Disease Control**
Department of Health and Human Services
U.S. Public Health Service
Atlanta, GA 30333
800-311-3435
*www.cdc.gov*

**Endometriosis Association**
8585 N. 76th Place
Milwaukee, WI 53223
414-355-2200
*www. endometriosis.assn.org*

**HELP (Herpes Resource Center)**
PO Box 100
Palo Alto, CA 94302
*www.herpes.org*

**La Leche League International**
1400 N. Meacham Rd.
Schaumburg, IL 60173-4808
847-519-7730
*www.lalecheleague.org*

**Maternity Center Association, Inc.**
281 Park Ave South, 5th Floor
New York, NY 10010
212-777-5000
*www.maternitywise.org*

**National Coalition Against Domestic Violence**
P.O. Box 18749
Denver, CO 80218
1-800-799-SAFE (24-hr line)
*www.ncadv.org*

**National Coalition Against Sexual Assault**
4426 Louisburg Rd. Suite 100
Raleigh, NC 27616
919-431-0995
*www.nccasa.org*

**National Safety Council**
1121 Spring Lake Dr.
Itasca, IL 60143-3201
630-285-1121
*www.nsc.org*

## AIDS Information and Hotlines

| | |
|---|---|
| American Foundation for AIDS Research | 212-806-1600 |
| | *www.amfar.org* |
| American Red Cross AIDS Education Office | 202-303-4498 |
| Centers for Disease Control—Statistics: | *www.cdc.gov* |
| Hearing Impaired AIDS Hotline | 800-243-7889 |
| National AIDS Hotline | 800-342-AIDS |
| National AIDS Information Clearing House | 800-458-5231 |
| National AIDS Network | 202-293-2437 |
| National Gay/Lesbian Crisis Line | 800-777-2437 |
| National Sexually Transmitted Diseases Hotline | 800-227-8922 |
| Pediatric and Pregnancy AIDS Hotline | 212-430-3333 |
| Project Inform (Drug Information) | 800-822-7422 |
| Spanish AIDS Hotline | 800-344-7432 |

# Professional Organizations/Associations

**American Academy of Nurse Practitioners**
1111 19th St. NW Suite 404
Washington, DC 20036
202-659-2190
*www.nurse.org/acnpl*

**The American Assembly for Men in Nursing**
11 Cornell RD
Latham, NY 12110
518-782-9400 ext. 346

**American College of Nurse Midwives**
8403 Colesville Rd Suite 1550
Silver Spring, MD 20910
240-485-1800
*www.midwife.org*

**American Holistic Nurses' Association**
P.O. Box 2130
Flagstaff, AZ 86003-2130
*www.ahna.org*

**American Nurses Association**
Head office
600 Maryland Ave., SW Suite 100
West Washington, DC 20024
*www.nursingworld.org*

**Association of Nurses in AIDS Care**
3538 Ridgewood Rd.
Akron, Ohio 44333
800-260-6780
*www.anacnet.org*

**Association of Rehabilitation Nurses**
4700 W. Lake Ave
Glenview, IL 60025
*www.rehabnurse.org*

**The Association of Women's Health, Obstetric, and Neonatal Nurses (AWHONN—formerly NAACOG)**
2000 L Street NW Suite 740
Washington, DC 20036
800-673-8499
*www.awhonn.rog*

**Canadian Nurses Association**
50 The Driveway
Ottawa, Ont., Canada K2P 1E2
800-361-8404
*www.can-nurse.ca*

**Midwives Alliance of North America**
4805 Lawrenceville Hwy Suite 116-279
Lilburn, GA 30047
888-923-6262
*www.mana.org*

**National Association of Hispanic Nurses**
1501 16th Street NW
Washington, DC 20036
*www.thehipanicnurses.org*

**National Association of Neonatal Nurses**
4700 W. Lake Ave.
Glenview, IL 60025-1485
*www.nann.org*

**National Association of Nurse Practitioners in Reproductive Health (NANPRH)**
325 Pennsylvania Ave. SE
Washington, DC 20002

**National Black Nurses Association, Inc.**
8630 Fenton St. Suite 330
Silver Spring, MD 20910-3803
800-575-6298
*www.nbna.org*

**National League for Nursing (NLN)**
61 Broadway
New York, NY 10006
800-669-1656
*www.nln.org*

**Transcultural Nursing Society**
Department of Nursing
Madonna College
36600 Schoolcroft Rd.
Livonia, MI 48150-1173
888-432-5470
*www.tcns.org*

# Patient Education Materials

### Abbott Laboratories
Professional Services—D383
100 Abbott Park Rd.
Abbott Park, IL 60064-3500
847-937-6100
*www.abbott.com*

### Childbirth Graphics
PO Box 21207
Waco, TX 76702
800-229-3366
*www.childbirthgraphics.com*

### Eli Lilly and Company
Educational Resources Program
PO Box 100B
Indianapolis, IN 46206
*www.lilly.com*

### Healthy Mothers, Healthy Babies Coalition
121 North Washington St. Suite 300
Alexandria, VA 22314
703-836-6110
*www.hmhbb.org*

### National Woman's Health Network
514 10th Street NW Suite 400
Washington, DC 20004
202-347-1140
*www.nwhn.org*

### Nutrition Education Association
PO Box 20301
Houston, TX 77225
*www.eatright.org*

### Planned Parenthood Federation of America, Inc.
434 West 33rd St.
New York, NY 10001
212-541-7800
*www.plannedparenthood.org*

### Ross Laboratories
Creative Services and Information Department
625 Cleveland Ave.
Columbus, OH 43216
*www.rosslearningcenter.com*

### Schering Corporation
Professional Film Library
200 Galloping Hill Rd.
Kenilworth, NJ 07033
908-298-4000
*www.sch-plough.com*

# Nursing Journals

### "Bereavement" Magazine
4765 North Carefree Cir.
Colorado Springs, CO 80917
888-60-4HOPE
*www.bereavementmag.com*

### Birth: Issues in Perinatal Care
Blackwell Synergy
*www.blackwellpublishing.com*

### Canadian Nurse
The Canadian Nurses Association
50 The Driveway
Ottawa, Ont., Canada K2P 1E2
800-361-8404

### The Female Patient
Quadrant Health Com Inc
Chatham, NJ 07950

### Journal of Nurse-Midwifery
Elsevier Science BV
Amsterdam

### Journal of Obstetric, Gynecologic and Neonatal Nursing (JOGNN)
Sage Science Press/Publication
2455 Teller Rd.
Thousand Oaks, CA 91320

### Journal of Perinatal and Neonatal Nursing
Lippincott, Williams and Wilkins
*www.lww.com*

MCN The American Journal of Maternal Child Nursing

Lippincott, Williams and Wilkins

www.lww.com

Nursing Network on Violence Against Women Newsletter

www.nnvawi.org

# Websites of Interest to Maternal–Newborn Nurses

### Alliance for Transforming the Lives of Children

Website of ATLC providing guidance about consciously conceiving, birthing, and nurturing children.

http://www.atlc.org

### American Academy of Family Physicians

Website of AAFP

http://www.aafp.org

### American Academy of Husband-Coached Childbirth

Website for information on the Bradley Method of childbirth

http://www.bradleybirth.com

### American Academy of Pediatrics

Home page for the AAP

http://www.aap.org

### American Association for Therapeutic Humor

A resource for frazzled health professionals to help maintain a sense of humor about the world around them.

http://ideanurse.com/aath

### American College of Nurse-Midwives

Website of ACNM

http://www.acnm.org

### American College of Obstetricians & Gynecologists

Website of ACOG

http://www.acog.org

### American Medical Women's Association

The main women physicians' organization in the United States. The group focuses on women's health issues.

http://www.amwa-doc.org

### American Nurses Association

Website of the ANA

http://www.ana.org

### American Public Health Association

Website of the APHA

http://www.apha.org

### Association for Pre- & Perinatal Psychology and Health

Explores the many mental and emotional dimensions of pregnancy and birth in everything from scholarly articles to personal stories and late-breaking headlines.

http://www.birthpsychology.com/

### Association of Labor Assistants and Childbirth Educators

Home page for ALACE

http://www.alace.org

### The Baby Zone: Childbirth Choices

Links to sites and articles on childbirth options, part of a larger site addressing pregnancy and parenting issues.

http://babyzone.com/childbirthchoices.htm

### Cascade HealthCare Products, Inc.

Childbirth professionals find equipment and supplies, teaching aids, handouts and books at Cascade. Serving childbirth professionals for more than 20 years.

http://www.1cascade.com

### Centers for Disease Control and Prevention

Website of the CDC

http://www.cdc.gov

### Childbirth.org

Extensive list of links for educators, providers, and consumers alike.

http://www.childbirth.org

### Coalition for Improving Maternity Services

CIMS has created the Mother-Friendly Childbirth Initiative, an evidence-based document which provides guidelines for identifying and designating mother-friendly birth sites.

http://www.motherfriendly.org

**Doulas of North America**

Website of DONA

*http://www.dona.com*

**Global Maternal Child Health Association**

Comprehensive resource on waterbirth

*http://www.waterbirth.org*

**Health A to Z**

A comprehensive search engine for medical and health related sites. Health A to Z provides format and search capabilities for both medical professionals and consumers.

*http://www.healthatoz.com*

**Healthy People 2010**

Website of the Healthy People Initiative -

*http://web.health.gov/healthypeople/*

**International Childbirth Education Association**

Website of ICEA

*http://www.icea.org*

**International Lactation Consultant Association**

Website for ILCA

*http://www.ilca.com/*

**La Leche League International**

Website for La Leche League

*http://www.lalecheleague.org*

**Lamaze International**

Website of Lamaze International (*formerly* ASPO/Lamaze)

*http://www.lamaze-childbirth.com*

**Maternity Center Association**

For nearly 80 years as a national voluntary health agency, Maternity Center Association has worked to improve the maternity care system through family-centered maternity care and parenting education which supports and empowers women and their families.

*http://www.maternitywise.org*

**MedExplorer**

MedExplorer is a free medical/health related search engine with no membership or registration requirements. Utilized primarily by healthcare professionals and consumers.

*http://www.medexplorer.com*

**MIDIRS Midwifery Digest**

Home page for MIDIRS Midwifery Digest.

*http://www.midirs.org*

**MidwifeInfo.com**

A site dedicated to midwifery, it provides information and resources for midwives, aspiring midwives and consumers.

*http://www.midwifeinfo.com*

**Midwifery Today**

Midwifery Today: for midwives, nurses, doulas, childbirth educators, doctors, and parents

*http://www/midwiferytoday.com*

**Motherstuff's Midwifery Page**

Midwifery links of all sorts

*http://www.motherstuff.com/html/2midwifery.html*

**National Center for Education in Maternal and Child Health**

Comprehensive information on maternal and child health

*http://www.ncemch.org*

**National Coalition on Health Care**

Website for the National Coalition on Health Care–the nation's largest and most broadly representative alliance working to improve America's health care

*http://www.nchc.org*

**National Fire Protection Association**

Website of the NFPA — the standard-setting organization for Life Safety Codes

*http://www.nfpa.org*

**National Institutes of Health (NIH)**

Website of the NIH. A good resource for all health professionals

*http://www.nih.gov*

**Online Birth Center**

Many articles and abstracts on midwifery, pregnancy and birth.

*http://www.moonlily.com/obc/*

**UNICEF**

UNICEF information on the Baby Friendly Hospital Initiative

*http://www.unicef.org/newsline/bfhi.htm*

# Cervical Dilatation and Gestation Wheel

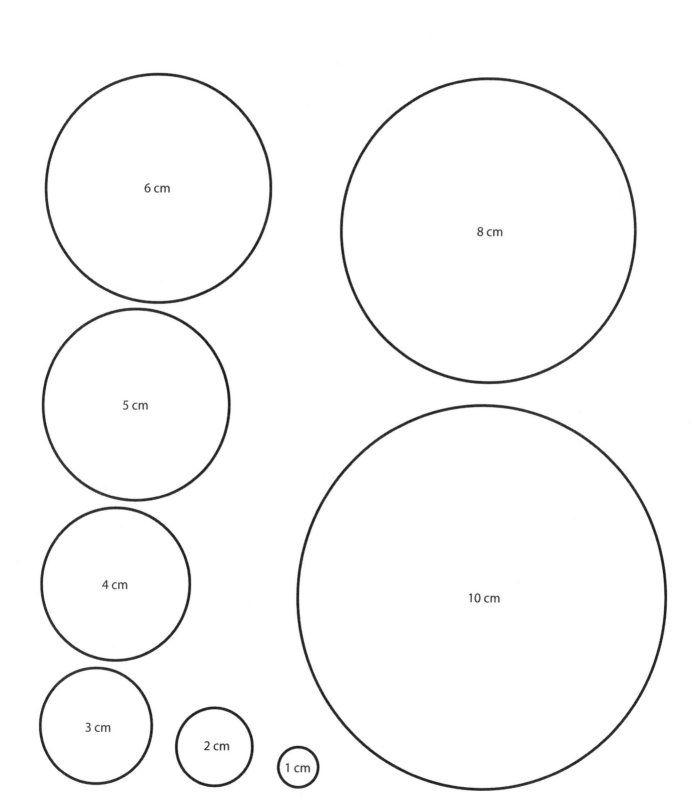

6 cm

8 cm

5 cm

4 cm

10 cm

3 cm

2 cm

1 cm

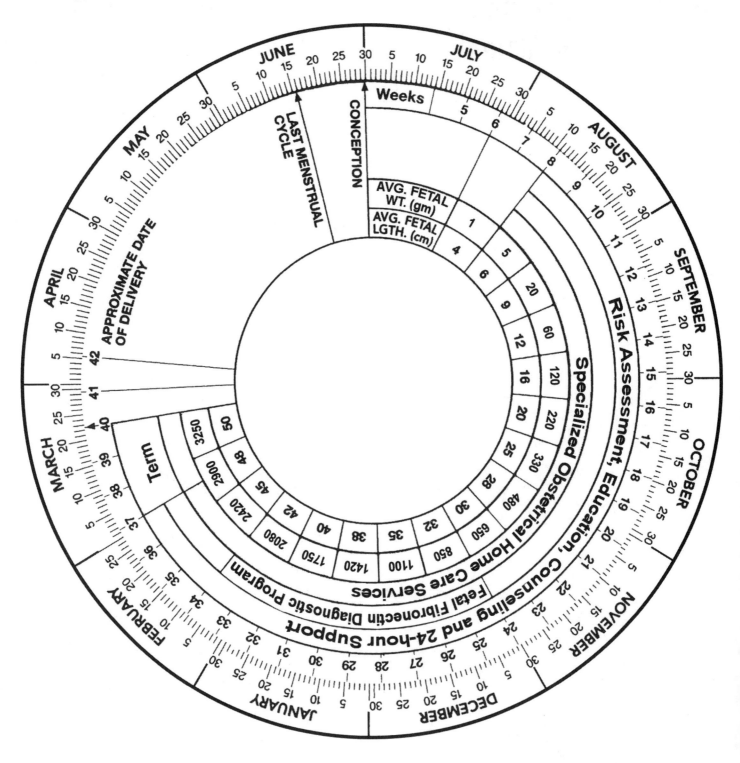

# BIBLIOGRAPHY

## Texts

Coad, J. *Anatomy and Physiology for Midwives*. St. Louis, Mosby

Craig, C., Stitzel, R.C., Stitzel, R.E., Stitzel, R. (Editor) *Modern Pharmacology with Clinical Applications* (6th ed). Philadelphia, Lippincott Williams & Wilkins

Cunningham, F.G., Gant, N.F., Leveno, K.J., Gilstrap, L.C., Hauth, J.C., Wenstrom, K.D. *Williams Obstetrics* (21st ed). New York, McGraw-Hill Professional

D'Avanzo, C.E., Geissler, E.M. *Cultural Health Assessment* (Mosby's Pocket Guide Series, 3rd ed). St. Louis, Mosby

Dildy, G.A., Belfort, M.A., Saade, G.R., Phelan, J.F., Hankins, G.D., Clark, S.L. *Critical Care Obstetrics* (4th ed). Ames, IA: Blackwell Science

Disaia, P., Creasman, W.T., Van Dinh, T. *Clinical Gynecology Oncology* (6th ed). New York, Elsevier Science

Guyton, A.C., Hall, J.E. *Textbook of Medical Physiology* (10th ed.) Philadelphia: W.B. Saunders

Kee, J.L., Hayes, E.R. *Pharmacology: A Nursing Process Approach* (4th ed). Philadelphia: W.B. Saunders Company

Ling, F.W., Duff, P. *Pocket Guide to Obstetrics and Gynecology: Principles for Practice*. New York, McGraw-Hill

Lowdermilk, D.L., Perry, S.E. *Maternity & Women's Health Care* (8th ed). St. Louis, Mosby

Meek, J. (ed) *The American Academy of Pediatrics: New Mother's Guide to Breastfeeding*. New York: Bantam

Olds, S.B., London, M.L., Ladewig, P.A., Davidson, M.R. *Clinical Handbook for Maternal Newborn Nursing & Women's Health Care* (7th ed). Upper Saddle River, NJ, Prentice Hall

Scott, J., Scott, J.R. (Editor), Gibbs, R.S. (Editor) *Danforth's Obstetrics and Gynecology* (9th edition). Philadelphia, Lippincott Williams & Wilkins

Varney, H., Kriebs, J.M., Gegor, C.L. *Varney's Midwifery* (4th ed). Sudbury MA , Jones & Bartlett Publishers, Inc.

Wong, D.L., Hockenberry, M.J., Wilson, D., Winkelstein, M.L., Kline, N.E. & Hockberry-Eaton, M. *Whaley & Wong's Nursing Care of Infants and Children* (7th ed). St. Louis, Mosby

## Journals

Bigelow, J.L., Dunson, D.B., Stanford, J.B., Ecochard, R., Gnoth, C., Colombo, B. Mucus observations in the fertile window: a better predictor of conception than timing of intercourse. *Hum Reprod*. 19(4):889-92, April 2004

Clemmens, D., Driscoll, J.W., Beck, C.T. Postpartum depression as profiled through the depression screening scale. *MCN Am J Matern Child Nurs*. 29(3):180-5, May-June 2004

Cluett ,E.R., Nikodem, V.C., McCandlish, R.E., Burns, E.E. Immersion in water in pregnancy, labour and birth. *Cochrane Database Syst Rev*. (2):CD000111, 2004

Fawole, B., Hofmeyr, G.J. Maternal oxygen administration for fetal distress. *Cochrane Database Syst Rev*. (4): CD000236, 2003

Gupta J.K., Hofmeyr, G.J. Position for women during second stage of labour. *Cochrane Database Syst Rev*. (1): CD002006, 2004

Hutti, M.H. New & emerging contraceptive methods: nurses can help women make wise choices. *AWHONN Lifelines*; 7(1):34-9, 2003

Kenyon, S., Boulvain, M., Neilson, J. Antibiotics for preterm rupture of membranes. *Cochrane Database Syst Rev*. (2): CD001058, 2003

Kremer, C.J., Duff, P. Glyburide for the treatment of gestational diabetes. *Am J Obstet Gynecol*. 190(5):1438-9, May 2004

Lee, B.B., Ngan-Kee, W.D., Ng, F.F., Lau, T.K., Wong, E.L. Epidural infusions of ropivacaine and bupivacaine for labor analgesia: a randomized, double-blind study of obstetric outcome. *Anesth Analg*. 98(4):1145-52, April 2004

Lund, C.H., Osborne, J.W. Validity and reliability of the neonatal skin condition score. *J Obstet Gynecol Neonatal Nurs*. 33(3):320-7, May-June 2004

Morse, C., Durkin, S., Buist, A., Milgrom, J. Improving the postnatal outcomes of new mothers. *J Adv Nurs*. 45(5):465-74, March 2004

Ofir, K., Sheiner, E., Levy, A., Katz, M., Mazor, M. Uterine rupture: risk factors and pregnancy outcome. *Am J Obstet Gynecol*. 189(4):1042-6, October 2003

Raines, D.A., Morgan, Z. Culturally sensitive care during childbirth. *Appl Nurs Res*. 13(4):167-72, November 2000

Roberts, J.E. A new understanding of the second stage of labor: implications for nursing care. *J Obstet Gynecol Neonatal Nurs*. 32(6):794-801, November-December 2003

Sheiner, E., Levy, A., Ofir, K., Hadar, A., Shoham-Vardi, I., Hallak, M., Katz, M., Mazor, M. Changes in fetal heart rate and uterine patterns associated with uterine rupture. *J Reprod Med*. 49(5):373-8, May 2004

Simpson, K.R., Knox, G.E. Obstetrical accidents involving intravenous magnesium sulfate: recommendations to promote patient safety. *MCN Am J Matern Child Nurs*. 29(3):161-9, May-June 2004

Stan, C., Boulvain, M., Hirsbrunner-Amagbaly, P., Pfister, R. Hydration for treatment of preterm labour. *Cochrane Database Syst Rev*. (2): CD003096, 2002

Thomas, K.A., Renaud, M.T., Depaul, D. Use of the parenting stress index in mothers of preterm infants. *Adv Neonatal Care*. 4(1):33-41, February 2004

# Classic Articles

Baines, C.J. Reflections on Breast Self-examination. *J Natl Cancer Org.* 89:339-340, 1997

Balcazar, H., Peterson, G.W., Krull, J.L. Acculturation and family cohesiveness in Mexican American pregnant women: social and health implications. *Family & Community Health*, 20(3): 16-31, 1997

Beck, C.T., Reynolds, M.A., Rutowski, P. Maternity blues and postpartum depression. *JOGNN* 21:287, 1992

Davis, M.S. Natural family planning. *NAACOG Clin Issues Perinat Women Health Nurs.* 3:280, 1992

Denehy, J.A. Interventions related to parent-infant attachment. *Nurs Clin North Am.* 27:425, 1992

Horn, B. Cultural concepts and postpartal care. *J Transcultural Nurs.* 2:48, 1990

Horner, N.E., & Lampe, J.W. Potential mechanisms of diet therapy for fibrocystic breast conditions show inadequate evidence of effectiveness. *Journal of the American Dietetic Association*, 2000

Jackson, K.B. Men and midwifery. Paternal presence at delivery. *British Journal of Midwifery* 5(11): 682-4, 1997

Luegenbiehl, D.L., et al. Standardized assessment of blood loss. *MCN*, 15:241, 1990

McKay, S., Roberts, J. Obstetrics by ear. Maternal and caregiver perceptions of the meaning of maternal sounds during second stage labor. *J Nurse Midwife*, 35:266, 1990

Rizvi, F., Mackey, R., Barrett, T., McKenna, P., Geary, M. Successful reduction of massive postpartum hemorrhage by use of guidelines and staff education. *BJOG.*111(5):495-8, May 2004

Ruchala, P.L., James, D.C. Social support, knowledge of infant development, and maternal confidence among adolescent and adult mothers. *J Obstet Gynecol Neonatal Nurs.* 26(6):685-9, November-December 1997

Thomas, D.B., Gao, D.L., Self, S. et al. Randomized Trial of Breast Self Examination in Shanghai: Methodology and Preliminary Results. *J Natl Cancer Inst.* 89:355-65, 1997

# INDEX